Tracing the Path of Yoga

Tracing the Path of Yoga

The History and Philosophy of Indian Mind-Body Discipline

STUART RAY SARBACKER

SUNY
PRESS

Cover: Vajrasattva Buddha (anonymous devotional art; author's collection)

Published by State University of New York Press, Albany

For information, contact State University of New York Press, Albany, NY
www.sunypress.edu

Library of Congress Cataloging-in-Publication Data

Name: Sarbacker, Stuart Ray, author.
Title: Tracing the path of yoga : the history and philosophy of Indian mind-body discipline / Stuart Ray Sarbacker, author.
Description: Albany : State University of New York Press, [2021] | Includes bibliographical references and index.
Identifiers: ISBN 9781438481210 (hardcover : alk. paper) | ISBN 9781438481234 (ebook) | ISBN 9781438481227 (pbk. : alk. paper)
Further information is available at the Library of Congress.

10 9 8 7 6 5 4 3 2 1

To My Parents, John and Margaret Sarbacker

pitrośca pūjanaṃ kṛtvā prakrāntiṃ ca karoti yaḥ /
tasya vai pṛthivījanyaṃ phalaṃ bhavati niścitam //

And one who, having revered the parents, performs circumambulation [of them];
That one, indeed, obtains merit equal to that arising from [circumambulating] the earth.

—*Śiva Purāṇa* 2.4.19.39

Contents

Acknowledgments

The work that follows was inspired by a number of scholars of Indian philosophy and religion whose work has deeply informed my research on the history and philosophy of yoga traditions. Perhaps foremost among them is Mircea Eliade, whose work *Yoga: Immortality and Freedom* (1954) continues to produce insight into yoga traditions for me after numerous readings, to the point that I wonder if I will ever fully get to the bottom of it. Another important figure in the field of yoga studies whose work has provided a context for the development of my own has been Georg Feuerstein, whose books, including *Yoga: The Technology of Ecstasy* (1989) and *The Yoga Tradition* (1998), have been some of the most well-known, scholarly informed popular narratives of yoga's history. I was touched when Georg wrote an appreciative review of my first book, *Samādhi: The Numinous and Cessative in Indo-Tibetan Yoga* (2005), encouraging me to pursue my research further. Another major source of inspiration and influence has been the work of David Gordon White, whose monographs, such as *The Alchemical Body* (1996), *Kiss of the Yogini* (2003), and *Sinister Yogis* (2009), and edited volumes, such as *Tantra in Practice* (2000) and *Yoga in Practice* (2012), have brought a critical eye and historical consciousness to the academic study of yoga traditions. White's determined attention on the pursuit of spiritual accomplishment or perfection (*siddhi*) in yoga as a counterpart to the larger emphasis in the field on liberation (*mokṣa*) was a key catalyst for my thinking on the topic, and I am grateful for his formative influence on my work. Geoffrey Samuel's work on the history of yoga and tantra has deeply informed my understanding of the social and political contexts that frame the practice of yoga, a topic he investigates at length in his book *The Origins of Yoga and Tantra: Indic Religions to the*

Thirteenth Century (2008). I have similarly benefitted from my engagement with Ronald Davidson's *Indian Esoteric Buddhism: A Social History of the Tantric Movement* (2005) with respect to the social and political context of Buddhist tantra. Gavin Flood's coherent model of the larger Hindu tradition in his *An Introduction to Hinduism* (1996) was also formative in my conceptualization of the larger historical context of yoga, and he offered valuable advice and encouragement to me at an early stage of the project. David Gitomer, similarly, provided critical perspective and support to me with respect to research and teaching on yoga during the formative early phase of the project, and his influence pervades the text in many ways. The work of a range of scholars of yoga philosophy, including Johannes Bronkhorst, Chris Chapple, Knut Jacobsen, Gerald Larson, Philipp Maas, Andrew Nicholson, LLoyd Pflueger, T. S. Rukmani, and Ian Whicher, had a significant impact on the way I conceived of this project, and their collective influence is apparent throughout the text. I have drawn extensively in this project upon the groundbreaking work being done under the aegis of the Haṭha Yoga Project at the School of Oriental and African Studies in London, including that of Jim Mallinson, Jason Birch, Mark Singleton, and their many talented colleagues and students. With respect to scholarship on yoga and Hindu tantra, I have also significantly benefitted from the publications of, and conversations with, Somadeva Vasudeva and Gudrun Bühnemann, the latter of which was my original Sanskrit teacher. Likewise, the pioneering publications of Norman Sjoman, Joseph Alter, and Elliott Goldberg on modern yoga have informed and inspired my research in numerous ways. Last, I am grateful for the support and advice I have received over the years from my many teachers, including Sriram Agashe, John Dunne, Indira Junghare, David Knipe, and Robert Tapp, among others.

A number of scholars provided helpful feedback on the manuscript, including the two anonymous reviewers for SUNY Press who helped provide a roadmap for revision that improved the work as a whole in significant ways. Colleagues who provided helpful feedback and comments on the manuscript included George Bond, Jason Birch, Chris Chapple, Anya Foxen, Elliott Goldberg, Patrick McCartney, Andrew Nicholson, and Mark Singleton. A special note of thanks to Seth Powell and Adam Miller, who provided extensive comments on the style and substance of the manuscript as it neared completion, helping me bring closure and coherence to the work. Tracy Pintchman similarly helped me with technical issues related to the final stages of the preparation of the manuscript, in addition to providing input and advice on my research. I am deeply grateful to all of those who have provided assistance along the way, and I take full responsibility for all errors and omissions in the work as a product of my own lack of understanding and/or misunderstanding (*avidyā*).

I received critical support for the project in its various stages from my home institution, Oregon State University. This included two fellowship periods at the Center for the Humanities at Oregon State, which were overseen by David Robinson and Chris Nichols, respectively. I particularly appreciated Chris Nichols's enthusiastic support and encouragement during the final stages of writing and revision of the manuscript. The Oregon State University College of Liberal Arts, led by Dean Larry Rodgers, along with the Center for the Humanities, provided funding for my research at the Krishnamacharya Yoga Mandiram in Chennai, and the School of History, Philosophy, and Religion and the Horning Foundation helped support my research at various locations in Rishikesh. In Chennai, the faculty of the Krishnamacharya Yoga Mandiram, especially Jayaraman Mahadevan, T. Swaminathan, V. Srinivasan, and Nrithya Jagganathan were gracious and informative hosts, as were Swami Veda Bharati and his staff at the Swami Rama Sadhaka Grama in Rishikesh. I received release time from the University Research Office at Oregon State as well. I am particularly grateful for the support I received from the Hundere Chair in Religion and Culture at Oregon State, Courtney Campbell, who provided both material and logistical resources for my research and writing at several critical phases in the development of this project. I want to thank Courtney and all of my excellent colleagues in the School of History, Philosophy, and Religion, including our former director, Ben Mutschler, and current director, Nicole von Germeten, for helping create an outstanding academic environment for the pursuit of substantive and transformative research and teaching.

I want to express my gratitude for the work of Nancy Ellegate, the former South Asia editor at SUNY, with whom I had originally developed the project, and to Chris Ahn and James Peltz, who took up the project upon Nancy's untimely passing. I also want to express my appreciation for the work of my production editor, Diane Ganeles, my copyeditor, John Wentworth, and my marketing manager, Michael Campochiaro. I am also very grateful for the work of Rachel Nishan at Twin Oaks Indexing, who diligently and patiently built the index for the book.

I want to thank Jacob Darwin Hamblin and Richard Miller for their friendship and intellectual and moral support as I worked my way through this project. I particularly appreciated Jake's willingness to patiently listen to me work through ideas on long runs through the McDonald-Dunn Forest near Corvallis. As a result, he probably knows more about yoga than any other historian of science in the United States. The many insights that Rich, a professor of English composition, has shared with me about the writing and revision process have been and continue to be part of the bedrock of my approach to writing. Both Jake and Rich have kept me engaged with musical endeavors, providing an excellent counterpart to, and reprieve from, my academic work, and I hope to return the favor many times over. I also want to express gratitude to my friend, kindred spirit, and collaborator Freedom (Kevin) Kimple, whose depth and gravitas in the study and practice of yoga is uniquely matched by his capacity for laughter.

My family has shared in the intellectual journey of this project in both direct and indirect ways. My wife Sara and my daughters Stella and Tara continue to push me to reflect on the relationship, or lack thereof, between my study and practice of yoga and the concrete realities of life in the world. And I should not forget to mention our Australian Shepherd, Kiki, who every day teaches me another lesson about the virtue of spontaneous (*sahaja*) joy.

I have dedicated this book to my parents, John and Margaret Sarbacker. I hope this acknowledgment communicates at least a small part of the gratitude I feel for the care and support they have offered me over the years.

Pronunciation Guide for Sanskrit Terms

The terminology used in this study is primarily drawn from Sanskrit (*saṃskṛta*) and related languages, including Pāli, Buddhist Hybrid Sanskrit, and various vernacular languages. When Sanskrit terms are transliterated into the Roman script ("Romanized"), special symbols (diacritic marks) are used to capture their distinct sounds. The following guide, adapted from Winthrop Sargeant and Christopher Key Chapple, *The Bhagavadgītā* (SUNY Press, 2009), provides examples of Sanskrit letters in the Indic Devanāgarī script and Roman script and instructions for pronunciation in (U.S.) English.

a (अ) as in h*u*t
ā (आ) as in f*a*ther
i (इ) as in *i*t
ī (ई) as in pol*i*ce
u (उ) as in p*u*sh
ū (ऊ) as in cr*u*de
ṛ (ऋ) as in b*ir*th
ṝ (ॠ) lengthened *ṛ*
ḷ (ऌ) as in simp*le*
e (ए) as in tempo
ai (ऐ) as in *ai*sle
o (ओ) as in st*o*ne
au (औ) as in m*ou*se
ṃ (ं) nasal ending of previous vowel
ḥ (ः) echo of previous vowel
k (क) as in *k*ill
kh (ख) as in bun*kh*ouse
ṭ (ट) as in *t*rue
ṭh (ठ) as in an*th*ill
ḍ (ड) as in *d*rum
ḍh (ढ) as in re*dh*ead
ṇ (ण) as in no*n*e
t (त) as in *t*one
th (थ) as in nu*th*atch
d (द) as in *d*ot
dh (ध) as in a*dh*ere
n (न) as in *n*ut
p (प) as in *p*ot
ph (फ) as in u*ph*ill
b (ब) as in *b*eer
bh (भ) as in a*bh*or
m (म) as in *m*an
y (य) as in *y*oung
r (र) as in *r*ed

g (ग)	as in *g*o
gh (घ)	as in lo*gh*ouse
ṅ (ङ)	as in si*n*g
c (च)	as in ri*ch*
ch (छ)	as in bir*ch h*ill
j (ज)	as in *j*ump
jh (झ)	as in hed*geh*og
ñ (ञ)	as in hi*n*ge
l (ल)	as in *l*aw
v (व)	as in *w*ind
ś (श)	as in *s*ure
ṣ (ष)	as in *sh*ut
s (स)	as in *s*ay
h (ह)	as in *h*ero
oṃ (ॐ)	as in h*om*e

Introduction

The History and Philosophy of Yoga

The history of the physical and mental disciplines referred to collectively as "yoga" extends into the distant past of India's religious and cultural heritage, perhaps as far back as 2,500 years or more. Yoga has played a crucial role in the development of the doctrine and practice of a range of Indian religious traditions, including Hinduism, Buddhism, and Jainism, and its influence has extended out of India to touch nearly all parts of the world, especially in the past two centuries. Its manifestation as a popular mode of physical and athletic culture in Europe and the Americas in the twentieth and twenty-first centuries represents one chapter in a fascinating history that has seen both great change and remarkable continuity. The goal of this work is to examine a wide range of meanings and permutations of theory and practice that are associated with the term "yoga," and thereby bring coherence and nuance to our understanding of its historical formulations and contemporary manifestations.

In the contemporary context, the range of ideas and practices commonly referred to as "yoga" is represented, in large part, by a constellation of transnational traditions emphasizing the physical practice of yogic posture (*āsana*), often without apparent connection to sectarian religious commitment or identity. The term "yoga" may bring to mind images of a room of practitioners bent into various shapes, such as the "lotus posture" (*padmāsana*), the "warrior pose" (*vīrabhadrāsana*), and the "head[stand]" posture (*śīrṣāsana*). In this context, yoga exists as a form of nonsectarian, if not secular, body discipline or as a vaguely Indian- or Hindu-inflected spirituality, in contrast to the more tangible sectarian doctrines and practices of mainstream institutional religion. Upon closer examination, however, it becomes evident that even the most athletic or calisthenic forms of yoga have their roots in Indian traditions that have complex philosophical and religious histories behind them. Modern yoga is the product of a process that bridged the worlds of Indian spirituality and European physical culture, laying a foundation for its extraordinary international and cross-cultural appeal. Modern yoga has been sculpted to suit modern aspirations and inclinations that are the common heritage of a cosmopolitan culture that crosses the boundaries of modern nation-states and traditional societies. The success of yoga in the modern era is, in part, a function of the entrepreneurial spirit of its formulators who consciously sought to bridge cultural worlds in the late nineteenth to the mid–twentieth century. Such innovation remains unabated into the twenty-first century and is likely to stretch well into the future.

The term "yoga" is derived from the Sanskrit verbal root *√yuj*, which is cognate with, and roughly equivalent to, the English infinitive verb form "to yoke." This meaning provides one of the most basic and universal definitions of yoga, as a "yoking" or disciplining of the body and mind. In explicitly theistic or monistic contexts, this yoking may also refer to the "union" of one's innermost self or soul (*ātman*) with a personal deity (*devatā, īśvara*), a supreme self (*paramātman*), or an impersonal absolute reality (*brahman*) through devotional or contemplative practice. These two senses of the term, as "discipline" and as "union," which are among a number that will be explored in this work, give a sense of the spectrum of interpretive possibilities available with respect to understanding what the Sanskrit term "yoga" means. Yoga, as such, might be conceived of as referring generically to a method of disciplining mind and body, a mode of practice not unique to any particular religious or philosophical tradition—thus making sense, for example, of the expressions "Christian Yoga" or "Jewish Yoga." It might alternately be framed as a particular vision of achieving spiritual liberation through insight into or identity with an ultimate being or reality, such as that expressed in the Hindu Vedānta formula equating the individual self (*ātman*) with absolute reality (*brahman*). Though a number of central concepts link together the range of definitions of yoga, it nevertheless varies dramatically in meaning, scope, and purpose within the various contexts in which it is found. Examining the theory and practice of yoga in its various historical situations brings to light the ways in which yoga has unique and distinctive manifestations, while at the same time illustrating how the practices of even the most thoroughly modernized forms of yoga can be, and often are, understood within conceptual frameworks established in their premodern ancestors.

Although references to yoga are pervasive in the history of Indian religion and philosophy, considerable disagreement persists among different Indian religious traditions over the degree of centrality of yoga within the spiritual path. Yoga ranges from being viewed as essential to spiritual realization, to being an aid to it, or, conversely, to being an impediment to or distraction from the goals of the religious life. Its practices have also often been viewed as a means to gain power or mastery over the world as much as a way to obtain spiritual knowledge or liberation. The image of the yoga practitioner (the *yogī*, *yogin*, or *yoginī*) is, in many cases, deeply informed by the great powers they are said to obtain through their disciplining of body and mind. Such powers may be alternately viewed as an impediment to spiritual liberation, as indicators of spiritual progress, or as facilitating the compassionate activity of an enlightened or liberated being. In some cases, yoga has been critiqued as overly ascetic in its orientation, as a form of self-mortification that causes undue pain to the practitioner and thereby impedes their progress toward spiritual liberation. The great range of understandings, interpretations, and applications of yoga in the Indian tradition are, in part, a function of these varied viewpoints on its purpose and efficacy.

This study is focused on the origin and development of yoga in its Indian contexts, primarily within the Indian religious traditions of Hinduism, Buddhism, and Jainism, with an eye to its impact on other traditions in India and beyond.[1] Yoga has been explored and explained at greatest length and in most detail by scholars and practitioners within Hindu, Buddhist, and Jain traditions, who frequently sought to define and defend yoga in connection with their core religious and philosophical principles. It is within these traditions that yoga has found its broadest range of formulations in terms of theoretical understanding and practical application. The role and function of yoga varies significantly within these sectarian divisions of the Indian tradition as well as among them. Formulations of yoga are also affected, over time, by major shifts in Indian philosophy, literature, and ritual practice, such as the advent of pan-Indian traditions of scholastics (*śāstra*), personal devotion (*bhakti*), and ritual extension (*tantra*) over the course of the first millennium of the Common Era. Likewise, encounters with Islam and Christianity, and with European cultures during the colonial and modern eras in India, shaped Indian religion, philosophy, and physical culture, and thereby the formulation of yoga, in important ways. These shifts culminated in the transformation of yoga into a popular transnational phenomenon in the nineteenth and twentieth centuries and the elevation of yoga within India to a status as iconic of Indian, and especially Hindu, spirituality and even of the Indian nation itself in the twenty-first century.

The scope of this work is broken down into historical eras with topically focused sections, augmented by discussions of academic issues in the contemporary study of the theory and practice of yoga, such as questions regarding the origins of yogic concepts and practices, the role of founding figures in yoga traditions, the relationships between Hindu, Buddhist, Jain, and other traditional formulations of yoga, the content of major texts, and the social and cultural contexts in which yoga developed. Emphasis is placed on the ways in which yoga is seen as a means of obtaining power and mastery over the world, termed the *numinous* dimension of yoga, as well as a means to achieve deep insight and freedom from worldly pain and misery, referred to as the *cessative* dimension of yoga. This numinous-cessative dynamic is connected to broader issues regarding the relationship between renouncer and householder traditions in Indian religion, in which other-worldly and this-worldly orientations are represented. It is also related to important philosophical and theological questions regarding the goals of the practice of yoga and the nature of liberation as it is represented in relative states of embodiment and disembodiment and of worldly perfection and transcendence. These issues extend in various ways into the formulation of modern yoga traditions, where the mundane goals of material success, personal health, and communal well-being exist in tension with more soteriologically oriented inclinations and aspirations. Overall, this study aims to provide a nuanced philosophical (phenomenological) examination of the conceptual and pragmatic frameworks utilized in the theory and practice of yoga in its different eras, framed within the historical (sociocultural) contexts in which they were developed and utilized. As such, it aims to finds a middle ground between scholarly works on the topic that have, respectively, principally focused on the description of yoga philosophy and practice, such as Mircea Eliade's *Yoga: Immortality and Freedom* (1954) and Georg Feuerstein's *The Yoga Tradition* (1998), or on the social, political, and economic forces in yoga's history, such as Geoffrey Samuel's *The Origins of Yoga and Tantra: Indic Religions to the Thirteenth Century* (2008).

For those primarily interested in the origin and structures of modern yoga traditions, chapters 1 and 8 together provide an overview of various definitions of yoga and the principal structural elements and formulators of modern yoga traditions. Chapter 1 introduces a number of concepts used throughout the text and a broad chronological framework for understanding the development of yoga traditions over time. Particular focus is placed on the issues at stake in defining yoga, given its wide semantic range, with an emphasis on an approach that validates both generic and contextual meanings. Chapter 2 focuses on the prehistory of yoga as represented in the earliest theorized strata of yoga or "proto-yoga" practices in the Indus Valley Civilization and the Vedic tradition. This includes a discussion of theories regarding evidence for the origin of yoga in the Indus Valley Civilization and a discussion of the models of ascetic practice and agency found in the *brāhmaṇa* (priestly) literature of the Vedic tradition, the earliest documented form of Hinduism. Building on this foundation, chapter 3 examines the emergence of the yogic-ascetic paradigm in the mainstream of the emergent orthodox traditions of *brāhmaṇa* asceticism and the respectively heterodox *śramaṇa* renouncer traditions of Jainism and Buddhism.

Chapter 4 examines the classical Hindu model of yoga, the "yoga view" (*yoga darśana*), referred to as Pātañjala Yoga, Sāṃkhya-Yoga, Yoga Philosophy, or simply as Yoga, drawing upon Patañjali's *Yogasūtra* and the larger *Yogaśāstra*, the primary discourse (*sūtra*) and treatise (*śāstra*) texts of the *yoga darśana*. The first part of the chapter focuses on the conceptual framework of the Yoga philosophy in relationship to the ontology and metaphysics of the Sāṃkhya system of Indian philosophy, introducing the shared vision of reality in these two systems. The second part of the chapter focuses on the *aṣṭāṅgayoga* or "eight-limbed yoga" system of practice as developed in the *Yogasūtra*, with an emphasis on how the practice of yoga is presented as a discipline for realizing supernormal accomplishments and powers (*siddhi*, *vibhūti*) of perception and action, leading ultimately to the attainment of spiritual liberation (*kaivalya*). Chapter 5 focuses on the emergence of yoga as a recurrent topic within the Hindu epic and narrative literature (*itihāsa-purāṇa*) and in priestly scholastic and legal treatises (*dharmaśāstra*). Emphasis is placed on the elevated status of yoga and its human and divine practitioners within the *Bhagavadgītā* and Hindu

Purāṇa literature and the mainstreaming of yoga into householder culture as represented by the integration of yoga into the Hindu legal (*dharma*) and philosophical (*darśana*) literature.

Chapter 6 explores the role of yoga within sectarian and scholastic treatises of the classical *śramaṇa* traditions of Buddhism and Jainism within the context of the flowering of Indian philosophy in the early to mid-centuries of the first millennium of the Common Era. Particular attention is paid to the development of Buddhist and Jain path literature that situates yoga within systematic presentations of doctrine and practice that delineate the stages on the path to spiritual liberation. Chapter 7 examines transformations of yoga with respect to emerging paradigms of personal devotion (*bhakti*) and ritual extension (*tantra*) in medieval Indian traditions of Hinduism, Buddhism, and Jainism. It also provides an overview of the principles of the formative Siddha, Mahāsiddha, and *haṭhayoga* traditions of this era, with significant attention to their relationship to Hindu and Buddhist tantric traditions and the development of modern modes of yoga practice that draw upon their methodologies. Chapter 8 focuses on modern yoga traditions and contemporary practice, demonstrating how modern yoga traditions represent a fusion of Indic and modern cosmopolitan, especially European, forms of bodily discipline, philosophy, and spirituality. It also provides an overview of a range of prominent gurus and institutions in modern and contemporary forms of yoga, emphasizing the role of entrepreneurial teachers in their formulation and documenting the ways in which modern yoga is connected to and disconnected from its premodern counterparts, in some cases in unexpected and counterintuitive ways.

The study of yoga in its various manifestations sheds light on a number of aspects of Indian religious traditions, including their philosophies, theologies, rituals, and soteriologies. Yoga embodies and reflects conceptions of the nature of the religious life as framed in Hindu, Buddhist, Jain, Sikh, and other traditions. In the modern era, yoga has become iconic of India itself, taking the form of a global and universalizing Indian physical culture and spirituality that has transcended its sectarian origins. As a popular transnational phenomenon, it has thrived at the boundaries between the religious and the secular and among a multitude of cultural and religious identities and commitments, from Hindu, Buddhist, and Jain to Sikh, Christian, and Jewish. The examination of these roots and branches of yoga provides insight into the history of Indian religion and spirituality and into our contemporary globalized and cosmopolitan world culture. The impact of modern yoga extends from the realm of personal physical, spiritual, and religious practices and commitments to the larger spheres of economics, politics, and public health on a national and global level.

Though this study is intended primarily for students and researchers at the collegiate or university level in Religion, Philosophy, and Contemplative Studies, it also is addressed more broadly to nonspecialists and students of yoga who seek a foundational understanding of yoga in theory and practice in the Indian traditions and a sense of the continuities and discontinuities between modern traditions of yoga and their precursors. With that in mind, it is hoped that the following will be of interest and useful for a range of readers, from scholars of Indian religion and philosophy to practitioners of modern yoga systems and all of the various permutations in between.

Chapter 1

Defining Yoga

The term "yoga" has a wide range of meanings, due to its use in a variety of religious and secular contexts over the course of its over two-thousand-year history and its wide geographical representation across the globe. In the context of Indian religion and philosophy, especially within the traditions of Hinduism, Buddhism, and Jainism, the term "yoga" is used to signify both universal concepts and unique, contextual ones. Definitions of the term also vary within the range of modern nonsectarian and secular traditions of yoga that are distant from the cultural and religious moorings of the Indian traditions in which they originated. It might be suggested that beyond the simple fact that the term "yoga" is employed frequently by its various adherents, it is difficult to find a unitary thread that links the diversity of practices and ideas referred to as "yoga" together. In some cases, the religious roots of the traditions that gave rise to yogic practices have been left behind in a break from sectarian identity or have faded into the background in the process of modernization. In other cases, yoga is seen as a primarily, if not purely, spiritual or religious exercise that has been obscured, or even desacralized, by its adoption in modern secular contexts for the pursuit of physical fitness and beautification. Some scholars of religion have argued that yoga is the heart of the religions of India, while others have argued that yoga had been a relatively obscure, if not largely insignificant, facet of Indian religious life previous to the modern era.[1]

In order to negotiate such various interpretations and evaluations, this chapter will begin with a brief examination of various contextual uses of the term "yoga" derived from different phases of its historical development.

Having done this, a tentative definition for the term will be provided, focusing on its primary and secondary usages. The goal is to provide a heuristic, or constructive and pragmatic, definition of yoga applicable to its various contexts, thereby facilitating greater understanding, even if such a definition is incomplete or lacking in some respects. Much like in other fields of inquiry, it is helpful to think of defining yoga in terms of "family resemblance," or common features or elements, rather than in essentialist terms. This is sometimes referred to as a "polythetic" or "prototype" approach, one that recognizes common features while acknowledging the dynamic and variable nature of the object of study. Even within traditional sources, such as Patañjali's *Yogasūtra*, yoga has been defined or framed in multiple ways. In addition, practitioners and scholars of yoga often apply chronologically later, and more systematic, conceptions of yoga retroactively—for example, applying systematic or "classical" definitions of yoga developed in the early centuries of the Common Era to practices found in earlier *brāhmaṇa* asceticism and *śramaṇa* traditions.[2] The primary and generic sense of yoga that will be examined here, yoga as a "discipline," points to a common semantic and conceptual thread in how yoga is understood and practiced across various traditional boundaries.[3] The broader focus, however, will be on examining the various historical and philosophical themes that demonstrate both continuity and discontinuity in yoga's theory and practice in its various contexts over time.

Yoga as "Discipline"

Archeological evidence from the Indus Valley Civilization (2500–1500 BCE), an ancient Indian civilization contemporaneous with Near Eastern civilization in Egypt and Mesopotamia, shows numerous figures in seated positions that appear similar to what would later be known as a form of seated yoga posture (*āsana*). This has suggested to some scholars that the origins of yoga might be tied to the rise of this ancient urban Indian civilization in the Indus valley.[4] Though such archeological relics are intriguing, they are nonetheless of questionable authority in establishing the history of yoga in comparison to later and more clearly verifiable textual representations.[5] At this point in time, the writing system of the Indus Valley Civilization has not been deciphered to such an extent as to provide clarity on these issues, so it is difficult to evaluate these claims satisfactorily.[6] However, the Sanskrit term *yoga* does appear in Hindu Vedic (*vaidika*) literature (1500–500 BCE) frequently, providing a basis for understanding the semantic development of this concept in the early Vedic Sanskrit literature and later in the Classical Sanskrit literature. It also appears in Pāli Buddhist (Skt. *bauddha*) literature (500 BCE–100 CE) and in later Buddhist Hybrid Sanskrit literature in ways that anticipate, parallel, and expand upon its meaning and usage in the Hindu Vedic ritual compilation (*saṃhitā*) texts and philosophical correspondence (*upaniṣad*) literature. Likewise, early Jain (Skt. *jaina*) literature (500–300 BCE), such as the *Ācārāṅgasūtra*, references ascetic principles and practices that parallel, if not anticipate, cognate developments in Hinduism and Buddhism.

In its early literary contexts, such as in the Hindu Upaniṣads, including the *Kaṭha Upaniṣad* and *Śvetāśvatara Upaniṣad*, and in the Buddhist Nikāya literature, notably in the *Dhammapada*, yoga is represented as a means of developing restraint of the body and senses and concentration of mind.[7] Yoga is, in this respect, an aspect of asceticism, a discipline or method of cultivating self-control and enhancing the application of mind. The conception of yoga as an instrument of self-mastery expresses the literal meaning of yoga as a "yoking" or "harnessing," in this case of physical and mental faculties. This notion of yoga as a means of obtaining control over one's embodiment through self-discipline is tied into conceptions of the physical and mental structure of the human organism as much as it is tied into a unique sectarian tradition, philosophical position, theology, or metaphysics. This conception of yoga as a mode of mind-body discipline is arguably at the root of yoga's adaptability to different Indian sectarian contexts and its success as a cosmopolitan practice in the modern era. As a set of techniques of physical and mental discipline, it is, in principle, not subservient to a particular philosophy or religious view beyond the understanding that mind and body can be fruitfully disciplined and brought under control. Where different traditions diverge, in part, is in their understanding of the fruits or benefits of such practice—whether they are understood in terms of worldly or otherworldly goals, for example. Traditions of yoga, from the most esoteric to the most mundane and secularized, place it within the domain of practice. Even traditions that view yoga as ultimately facilitating spiritual "union" with an inner self (*ātman*) or with a deity (*devatā*), for example, frame such union within the context of a spiritual discipline that prepares one for or precipitates the state. Though many modern traditions of yoga eschew formal sectarian religious identity, they implicitly, if not explicitly, value the disciplining of mind and body and contain an ethos regarding the benefits of performing yoga practice, even if they are simply mundane achievements such as relaxation, physical health, or beautification.

Though developing mastery of mind and body through practical discipline links the spectrum of yoga practices together, yoga traditions differ significantly with respect to relative emphasis on the mental and physical aspects of embodiment. This is particularly evident in the contrast between modern types of yoga that focus on meditation (*dhyāna*) and those that focus on physical posture (*āsana*). In the context of meditation-oriented conceptions of religious practice, such as the eight-limbed yoga (*aṣṭāṅgayoga*) of the Hindu Yoga Philosophy (*yoga darśana*), the practice of yoga is viewed as a means of establishing mastery of mind, especially the development of deep concentration. In these contexts, yoga is equated with meditation (*dhyāna*) or mental cultivation (*bhāvanā*) and the practice of contemplation (*samādhi*). In the *Yogasūtra*, for example, Patañjali refers to yoga as *cittavṛttinirodha*, "the cessation of fluctuations of mind," a process of meditative isolation from the datum of ordinary experience through the achievement of mental stillness.[8] The primary commentary on Patañjali's work, the *Yogabhāṣya*, emphasizes this focus on mind by stating that yoga is, in essence, contemplation (*samādhi*).[9] This is consistent with a technical and etymological definition of *yoga* as "concentration," one that is advocated in the larger commentarial literature to the *Yogasūtra*.[10] Another well-known definition of yoga found in the *Bhagavadgītā* refers to yoga as *samatva*, referring to the cultivation of mental equilibrium or "even-mindedness." The Buddhist conception of the eightfold path (*aṣṭāṅgamārga*), common to the major sectarian divisions of Buddhism (Theravāda and Mahāyāna) culminates in the development of contemplation (*samādhi*), which is understood as the basis for developing spiritual insight or wisdom (*prajñā*) and supernormal powers of manifestation and perception (*nirmāṇa, abhijñā*). In late medieval *haṭhayoga* and modern yoga traditions, on the other hand, the body is a principal locus for yogic mastery, and an embodied state of perfection—immortality and power, or simply health and beauty—either takes precedence over, or is seen as facilitating, mastery of mind, in some cases without the need for a formal meditative praxis.

However, even in meditation-focused types of yoga, a progression from physical to mental practice occurs, from outer life to inner life. In the Upaniṣads, for example, spiritual practice is associated with the successive mastery over various levels of embodiment, referred to as "sheaths" (*kośa*), that range from the concrete physical body to the subtle spiritual self. Patañjali's *aṣṭāṅgayoga* system focuses successively on the mastery of social relationships, the body, and the breath as preliminaries to meditative praxis, and Buddhist mindfulness practices (Skt. *smṛti*, Pāli *sati*) utilize the contemplation of the body and breath to cultivate serenity, concentration, and insight. Traditions of *layayoga*, *kuṇḍalinīyoga*, and *haṭhayoga* develop sophisticated conceptions of an inner spiritual architecture, in which the physical body is informed by a "subtle body" (*sūkṣma-śarīra*) comprised of channels (*nāḍī*) and energetic centers or wheels (*cakra*) through which vital energy (*prāṇa*) flows. The subtle body may be viewed as the locus for latent spiritual forces of intense energy and heat (*kuṇḍalinī, caṇḍālī*), and the manipulation of *prāṇa* and of vital fluids (*bindu*, *bīja*, *rajas*) through its channels seen to facilitate rapid spiritual as well as physical transformation. Nonetheless, in the contemporary context, a distinction between body-centered and mind-centered types of practice is readily apparent, in that most popular and cosmopolitan modern yoga traditions are typically oriented toward either a meditative or postural model of yoga practice.[11]

"Limbs" (*aṅga*) of Yoga

One of the paradigmatic presentations of yoga that serves as an introduction to a core set of practices is the *aṣṭāṅgayoga* or "eight-limbed yoga." The use of the Sanskrit term *aṅga*, much like the metaphorical use of the English term "arm," is typically interpreted by scholars of yoga as technically referring to an "instrument," "accessory," or "auxiliary" of yoga rather than as a "limb" per se.[12] The *locus classicus* for *aṣṭāṅgayoga* is the *Yogasūtra* of Patañjali and the *Pātañjalayogaśāstra*, a Hindu priestly text and commentary tradition that dates from the early first millennium CE. The *aṣṭāṅgayoga* system is referenced extensively in Hindu narrative and philosophical literature and informs Jain perspectives as well, providing one of the principal paradigms for authoritative yoga in the Indian context. Patañjali's *aṣṭāṅgayoga* is often represented as an orthodox expression of yoga practice in the Hindu tradition, though it appears to be a synthesis of Hindu, Buddhist, and Jain conceptions of yoga developed in the early centuries before the Common Era. Later Buddhist and Jain traditions were in turn influenced by Patañjali's presentation of yoga, as were later Hindu sectarian yoga traditions, demonstrating an important reflexivity and counter-influence among traditions of yoga in India.[13]

Patañjali's presentation of *aṣṭāṅgayoga* assumes a progression of development from outer (*bahir*) to inner (*antar*) limbs. The individual limbs of Patañjali's *aṣṭāṅgayoga* are restraint (*yama*), observance (*niyama*), posture (*āsana*), breath control (*prāṇāyāma*), sense withdrawal (*pratyāhāra*), fixation (*dhāraṇā*), meditation (*dhyāna*), and contemplation (*samādhi*). The first two limbs situate yoga practice within an ethical framework of social, bodily, and spiritual concerns, invoking the need for a nonviolent attitude (*ahiṃsā*), physical and mental purity (*śauca*), ascetic discipline (*tapas*), and self-recitation (*svādhyāya*), among other requirements. The withdrawal of the senses (*pratyāhāra*), which appears as the fifth limb of yoga, links the *aṣṭāṅgayoga* system to some of the earliest documented techniques of yoga found within the Hindu Upaniṣads. Of particular importance with respect to modern traditions of yoga are the third and fourth components of posture (*āsana*) and breath control (*prāṇāyāma*), techniques emphasized within modern postural yoga traditions, in part due to their proximity to medieval *haṭhayoga* traditions that expanded on the classical *āsana-prāṇāyāma* repertoire.[14] Likewise, meditative components such as *dhāraṇā*, *dhyāna*, and *samādhi* serve as the focus of contemporary meditation-oriented traditions of yoga such as Transcendental Meditation (TM).

A number of medieval *haṭhayoga* and Hindu and Buddhist tantric texts forward a six-limbed yoga (*ṣaḍaṅgayoga*) model quite similar to, and perhaps derivative of, the eight-limbed yoga (*aṣṭāṅgayoga*).[15] These systems put significant emphasis on the relationship between posture, breath control, and meditation. Within traditions that focus distinctly on meditation (*dhyāna, bhāvanā*), such as Pātañjala Yoga and Theravāda Buddhism, the practices of fixing the mind (*dhāraṇā*) and creating continuous meditation (*dhyāna*) leading to deep contemplation (*samādhi*) are viewed as a gateway to supernatural agency or accomplishment (*siddhi*) and liberating knowledge or wisdom (*jñāna, prajñā*). The inner (*antar*) or cognitive dimension of yoga is fostered through the use of objects of meditation such as mantras, breath and bodily sensations, and images of divine and liberated beings, among others. In some tantric traditions, mastery over the limbs of yoga is presented as a basis for entering into sophisticated forms of ritual practice (*sādhana*) that aim to accelerate the process of spiritual development.

Paths (*mārga*) of Yoga

A common framework for defining yoga within contemporary Hinduism is that of the "three yogas" of the "yoga of action" (*karmayoga*), the "yoga of knowledge" (*jñānayoga*), and the "yoga of devotion" (*bhaktiyoga*). This threefold framework, often said to have its origin in the popular Hindu epic (*itihāsa*) narrative of the *Bhagavadgītā*, offers different religious methods, framed as forms of yoga, that suit the distinct inclinations of practitioners. A clear articulation of this view is found in another Vaiṣṇava Hindu text, the *Bhāgavata Purāṇa*, in which *karmayoga* is prescribed to those attached to material life, *jñānayoga* to those averse to it, and *bhaktiyoga* to those who are neither attached nor averse to material life.[16] In the modern context, the category of *rājayoga* or "royal yoga" is sometimes added as a fourth mode of practice. This is due in part to the work of the influential modern Hindu teacher Swami Vivekananda, who emphasized the uniqueness of meditative yoga (*dhyānayoga*) in relation to the other forms of yoga in his lectures and writings.[17] The threefold *karma-*, *jñāna-*, and *bhaktiyoga* distinction frames yoga as an adaptable means, method, or path (*mārga*) for obtaining religious goals, especially spiritual liberation (*mokṣa*). The division also illuminates the fact that action, knowledge, and devotion have all been legitimate components of the practice of Hindu-based forms of yoga. With respect to action (*karma*), the fact that moral principles such as duty (*dharma*) and nonviolence (*ahiṃsā*) are seen as the foundation of the practice of yoga indicates the significance of the social context of yoga practice.[18] *Karmayoga*, in its popular formulations in the *Bhagavadgītā* and elsewhere, expresses the notion that one's personal career or duty (*dharma*) can be a religious path and that world renunciation is unnecessary. *Jñānayoga*, on the other hand, suggests that spiritual liberation is a product of a special type of knowledge (*jñāna*) or wisdom (*prajñā*) regarding the true nature of the self and the world obtained through renunciation and contemplation. Lastly, *bhaktiyoga* methodologies present devotion as a means to liberation, principally through worship of and surrender to a supreme being. *Bhaktiyoga* is arguably the foremost path in popular Hindu Vaiṣṇava texts such as the *Bhagavadgītā*, and a critically important aspect of many Hindu sectarian traditions of yoga. In the larger Hindu, Buddhist, and Jain context, devotion (*bhakti*) to divine beings and to human exemplars, often through formal rituals of worship (*pūjā*), is a central aspect of ritual and communal life.

Formal worship is often complemented by the practice of mantra recitation (*japa*) and the singing of hymns (*bhajana*, *kīrtana*). Even in contexts in which action (*karma*) or knowledge (*jñāna*) is in a preeminent position, the development of faith or confidence (*śraddhā*) is considered essential to success on the spiritual path (*mārga*).[19] Though modern nonsectarian and postural forms of yoga often downplay the devotional aspect of yoga, the genealogy of many modern yoga lineages is linked to Hindu teachers who saw faith and devotion as essential components of yoga practice.[20]

In Hindu sectarian forms of *bhakti*, the goal of yoga may be viewed as unification or intimate relationship with a personal deity, such as Śiva, Devī, Viṣṇu, or Kṛṣṇa, or as absorption into an impersonal ultimate self or ultimate reality (*paramātman*, *brahman*). The Hindu gods Śiva and Viṣṇu are themselves referred to by devotees as the "Lord of Yoga" (*yogeśvara*) and other titles that indicate their mastery of the practice and powers of yoga. Śiva is commonly portrayed in Hindu art with the iconographic features of a *yogin*, seated in the forest in lotus posture (*padmāsana*) with his hands in meditation gesture (*dhyānamudrā*) and his eyes half-closed in deep contemplation (*samādhi*). In Sikhism, devotion (*bhakti*) to an all-powerful creator deity through the chanting of his name (Hindi *nām*) is presented by a tradition of teachers (*guru*) as a means of obtaining liberation from *saṃsāra*. Where unification with a deity is not emphasized, such as in the Hindu *yoga darśana*, Theravāda Buddhism, and in Jainism, spiritual archetypes and religious leaders become the object of veneration and identification. The practices of dedication to Īśvara (*īśvarapraṇidhāna*), or the "Lord [of Yoga]," in Pātañjala Yoga and the recollection of the Buddha (*buddhānusmṛti*) in Theravāda Buddhism exemplify the notion that contemplation of the qualities of perfected beings is spiritually efficacious. In tantric traditions, a similar dynamic is represented by deity yoga (*devatāyoga*), wherein a practitioner seeks to meditatively cultivate (*bhāvanā*) and merge with an image of a powerful enlightened being, thereby assimilating their wisdom and power.

As with *karmayoga*, *bhaktiyoga*, and *jñānayoga*, different paths of yoga can be indicated by the compounding of the term "yoga" with a concept encapsulating a methodology of practice. Unlike the generic term *tapas*, which refers to the "heat" or "friction" of ascetic self-discipline, yoga is generally associated with the development of systems of practice that subsume other techniques like *tapas* into a larger framework. Yoga is, in this respect, associated with sects or schools of practice that have distinct methods and goals. Indian literature provides various typologies of yoga, the threefold analysis (of *karmayoga*, *jñānayoga*, and *bhaktiyoga*) being one of the major instantiations. Others include a distinct rubric of a fourfold yoga of the "yoga of incantation" (*mantrayoga*), "the yoga of dissolution" (*layayoga*), the "yoga of force" (*haṭhayoga*), and the "yoga of kings" or "royal yoga" (*rājayoga*), drawing upon tantric paradigms and other emergent post-classical systems.[21] The various "limbed" yoga systems such as the eight-limbed and six-limbed yogas (*aṣṭāṅgayoga*, *ṣaḍaṅgayoga*) likewise indicate methods of practice adapted to fit into various philosophical and religious frameworks in Hinduism, Buddhism, and Jainism.

Yoga as "Union"

A common definition of yoga found in the modern Indian religious context is that of yoga as "union," specifically as derived from the verbal root √*yuj* as meaning "to join" or "to unite." This etymology can be connected to some earliest appearances of the term in Hindu Vedic literature, where it refers to the linkage of a horse and chariot or an ox and cart. The horse-and-chariot metaphor for yoga is extended in the Indian epic *Mahābhārata*, where yoga appears as a discipline for chariot-mounted warriors to reach immortality through death in battle, who are represented as being "yoked to yoga" or "joined in yoga" (*yogayukta*).[22] A more pervasive modern conception of yoga as union is that of the unification of the individual soul, or *ātman*, with the ultimate self (*paramātman*) or ground of being (*brahman* or *parabrahman*), a view rooted in Neo-Vedāntic interpretations of the Hindu Upaniṣads and Vedānta philosophy. A variant of this formulation with significant historical precedent is the notion of yoga as a union of the individual self with a personal deity, such as Viṣṇu or Śiva, who represents an ultimate person or cosmological principle. Formulations of yoga as union with a deity typically situate yoga within a distinctly theistic and sectarian context, most commonly one associated with the god Śiva.[23] As such, yoga relates to both the method and the goal of spiritual practice; spiritual practice aims at, or ultimately expresses, a foundational relationship between the human and the divine.[24] These notions of yoga as union are prominent in contemporary yoga traditions with Hindu sectarian leanings and those that utilize scholastic reconstructions of Hindu philosophical, especially tantric, frameworks for practice. However, secularized traditions of modern yoga—such as those with a strong athletic, calisthenic, or gymnastic emphasis—may, in contrast, frame yoga as a "union" of the more mundane factors of body and breath, or of body, senses, and mind in a manner distinct from the language of devotion, theism, or transcendence.[25]

Lastly, the term "yoga" may also be associated with the goal of disjunction (*viyoga*), or "disunity," rather than with unity or unification, indicating what is to be avoided rather than what is to be pursued in the spiritual life. In in the Yoga Philosophy (*yoga darśana*) of Patañjali, yoga refers to the stoppage of mental fluctuations (*cittavṛtti*) that leads to liberation (*kaivalya*), where the soul or person (*puruṣa*), the seer (*draṣṭṛ*) of reality, achieves a state of freedom from the turmoil of material existence (*prakṛti*), or that which is seen (*dṛśya*). This conception of spiritual liberation is referred to as a form of disunion (*viyoga*) that effectively ends the conjunction (*saṃyoga*) of *puruṣa* and *prakṛti*.[26] Similarly, in Buddhism and Jainism, the term "yoga" can refer to a form of clinging or attachment to the world that is to be eliminated, in addition to serving as a term for a mode of self-discipline viewed as spiritually productive.[27]

The Numinous and Cessative in Yoga

It its Hindu, Buddhist, and Jain contexts, yoga has often appeared within a framework of ideas regarding an endless cycle (*saṃsāra*) of birth and rebirth that is driven by the force of action (*karma*) and characterized by suffering or unsatisfactoriness (*duḥkha*). As such, practitioners sought liberation (*mokṣa*) through special knowledge (*jñāna*) or wisdom (*prajñā*) facilitated through spiritual discipline (*yoga*). Liberating knowledge was framed positively in terms of an understanding of the nature of the spiritual self or soul (*ātman, jīva*) and negatively in the form of the discernment of the non-self or non-soul (*anātman, ajīva*) in the mind, body, and world.[28] As such, yoga served the soteriological goal of liberation from death and rebirth (*punarjanma*) or re-death (*punarmṛtyu*) through facilitating liberating knowledge and experience. Restraint of the senses, for example, served as a means of weakening attachment and thus bondage to the phenomenal world and ultimately to *saṃsāra*. In this aspect, the goal of yoga can be said to be a *cessative* one, exemplified by the Sanskrit term for cessation (*nirodha*), which signifies bringing the process of *saṃsāra* and its attendant misery to an end. In Theravāda Buddhism, the attainment of *nirodha*, epitomized by the attainment of the state of extinction (*nirvāṇa*), is viewed as a disjunction from the phenomenal world and conditioned existence. In this context, yoga facilitates extricating oneself from the process of birth and rebirth, the goal of the religious path being the transcendence of worldly affliction (*duḥkha*) through the cessation (*nirodha*) of conditioned existence. In the *Yogasūtra*, this state of liberation (*mokṣa*) is referred to as separation (*kaivalya*) and in Jainism by the related term of isolation (*kevala*), and represents a transcendence of nature (*prakṛti*) and its elements (*bhūta*) and principles (*tattva*). Spiritual transformation in the cessative model is tied to ethical transformation, in that virtue, as expressed in moral principles such as non-harm (*ahiṃsā*), is seen as both supporting the path of renunciation and as being supported by it.

Though liberation (*mokṣa*) is often represented as the principal goal, yoga is also understood throughout the Indian tradition to be a means of obtaining extraordinary powers. Through the development of mastery of body, mind, and nature, yoga practitioners are said to obtain various forms of accomplishment (*siddhi*) or power (*vibhūti*) that provide extraordinary capacities of knowledge and agency. This accomplishment of divine-like power can be referred to as the *numinous* dimension of yoga, in that these powers transform the practitioner in such a way that they become "other," effectively like a deity or spirit (*numen*), thereby transcending the limits of human agency. In contrast to the cessation (*nirodha*) of the process of birth and rebirth (*saṃsāra*), the numinous dimension of yoga represents mastery (*aiśvarya*) over the world of experience and its constituents.[29] It is a transfiguration or apotheosis of the yoga practitioner into a quasi-divine being, who possesses preternatural capacities of knowledge and action such as the ability to read others' minds and to see and hear distant things. The minds of adept practitioners are also correlated cosmologically with beings, especially deities, at higher levels in the spiritual hierarchy of the universe.[30] In Hindu religious literature, a common expression of yogic powers is as a set of eight accomplishments (*aṣṭasiddhi*): smallness (*aṇimā*), lightness (*laghimā*), obtaining (*prāpti*), irresistible will (*prākāmya*), greatness (*mahimā*), lordship (*vaśitva*), mastery (*īśitva*), and suppression of desire (*kāmāvasāyitva*).[31] Others include the ability to become invisible (*antardhāna*), to know the past and future (*atītānāgata*), to transcend or "fly up" (*utkrānti*) at death, and to enter or possess (*āveśa*) the bodies of others. In Buddhist literature, a list of powers, referred to as forms of higher knowledge (*abhijñā*), includes six attainments: magical accomplishment (*ṛddhi*), mind reading (*paracittajñāna*), divine ear (*divyaśrotra*), divine eye (*divyacakṣus*), memory of former lives (*pūrvanivāsānusmṛti*), and the knowledge of the cessation of mental pollutants (*āsravakṣayajñāna*).[32]

Narratives in Jain and Buddhist traditions recount how their historical founders—Mahāvīra Vardhamāna and Siddhārtha Gautama, respectively—defeated opposing ascetics and drew followers through the display of such accomplishments.[33] *Siddhi* or *vibhūti* are alternately represented as temptations that can lead a practitioner astray and as sources of confidence in the power and success of yogic practice. In some contexts, such powers function as a means to instill faith in and serve the needs of others, a notion exemplified by the compassionate activities of Buddhas and Bodhisattvas in Mahāyāna Buddhism. The numinous dimension of yoga is particularly apparent in traditions that focus on the idea of liberation-in-life (*jīvanmukti*), or embodied liberation, most notably in Hindu tantric traditions and the systems of *haṭhayoga*.[34] Given the fluidity of the boundary between the human and divine, it is not surprising that Hindu deities such as Śiva are represented as practitioners of yoga and that human masters such as the Buddha and Mahāvīra come to be objects of veneration as embodiments of liberating insight and ascetic power.[35] In some cases, practitioners of yoga are associated with powerful elemental beings such as serpents (*nāga*) and nature spirits (*yakṣa*), linking the forces of nature and yogic accomplishment.[36] It has also been argued that the image of the yogi in Indian narrative literature is as often that of a terror-inspiring sorcerer as it is of an enlightened saint, and yogis are said to inspire both awe and fear, the latter being a point that evokes classical theories of numinous religious experiences.[37] Displays of yogic mastery through mental feats and the manipulation of the body make the inner dimensions of yoga explicit and tangible, evoking emotions of awe, wonder, and joy in observers.[38] Given this, the demonstration of, or reputation for, virtuosity by yoga practitioners supports the establishment of their charismatic authority, especially in environments without a clear institutional structure.[39]

The pervasive enumeration of yoga powers found in the philosophical and narrative literatures of Hinduism, Buddhism, and Jainism testify to the appeal that obtaining occult powers has had over the course of the development of yoga. Nearly one quarter of the verses in Patañjali's *Yogasūtra* are dedicated to explicating the means whereby one can obtain powers such as strength, flight, invisibility, bodily perfection, and supersensory perception.[40] Likewise, the *Haṭhapradīpikā*, one of the late encyclopedic texts of *haṭhayoga*, describes yoga as a means of obtaining physical strength and freedom from a range of diseases as well as a means of cultivating the liberating experience of *rājayoga*.[41] In some cases, it is not a great distance between the claims of medieval *haṭhayoga* texts and the claims of modern yoga proponents with respect to the mundane health benefits of yoga. Though it is commonly argued that modern yoga practices focused on worldly goals such as professional success, health, or beautification are "inauthentic," it is clear that yoga has historically served a variety of motivations, both this-worldly and other-worldly, rather than simply the goal of spiritual liberation.

Householder and Renouncer Traditions

Though it is often assumed that yoga is first and foremost a renouncer methodology, it exists within a range of permutations between the poles of worldly householder life and otherworldly asceticism. In some cases, the distinction between the householder and renouncer is framed as the distinction between world-affirming (*pravṛtti*, lit. "turning toward") and world-negating (*nivṛtti*, lit. "turning away") modes of life. Indian conceptions of householdership (*gṛhastha*) are rooted deeply in Hindu priestly (*brāhmaṇa*) traditions of sacrificial ritual and worship (*yajña*, *pūjā*), social duty (*dharma*), and stratification of class and caste (*varṇa*, *jāti*). This priestly ethos, which emerged in the Vedic period of Hinduism (1500–500 BCE), can be contrasted with the principles of the "striver" (*śramaṇa*) traditions of Buddhism and Jainism (c. 500 BCE), which idealized the rejection of householder responsibilities for the sake of pursuing spiritual liberation (*mokṣa*). Priestly forms of renunciation, or Brāhmaṇical asceticism, arose parallel to, and perhaps in conversation with, *śramaṇa* traditions and offered Hindu practitioners the option of pursuing a comparable ascetic mode of living within a Vedic framework.[42] The *śramaṇa* traditions and Brāhmaṇical asceticism diverged in important ways from the mainstream of Vedic *brāhmaṇa* householder traditions, leading some scholars to speculate that they represent the reemergence of pre-Vedic traditions, such as the Indus Valley

Civilization, or the influence of non-Vedic communities from the region of Magadha in eastern India.[43] However, the Vedic tradition contained a number of practices that anticipate the development of yoga, among them the notion of the power of ascetic heat (*tapas*) developed through self-denial and self-mortification. Much like yoga, *tapas* is represented in Vedic texts and later Hindu tradition as producing a morally ambiguous spiritual power through the force of self-discipline. This ambiguity is illustrated in Indian narrative literature, such as the Indian epics, where despotic villains obtain dangerous, world-threatening powers through *tapas,* particularly by means of intense self-mortification.[44]

In the Hindu priestly ideology of the duties of stage and class (*varṇāśramadharma*), performing one's duty (*dharma*) in life through proper action (*karma*) is perceived as a means to happiness in this life and peace after death. In the renouncer paradigm, liberation (*mokṣa*) becomes the primary goal, and so abandoning householder aims such as wealth (*artha*) and pleasure (*kāma*) serve as a means of clearing the path to the pursuit of a superior goal. In Jainism and in early Buddhism, the ideal or noble (*ārya*) life was exemplified by the homeless monk or nun who had given up all worldly attachments in order to pursue liberation. Likewise, in the renouncer (*saṃnyāsa*) traditions of Hinduism, as with the *śramaṇa* traditions, the forest became the locus for the cutting off of worldly attachment and the realization of spiritual knowledge (*jñāna*). Though renunciation may have been, at one time, a vocational option within the Vedic priestly tradition, perhaps in response to the *śramaṇa* traditions, eventually liberation (*mokṣa*) was established as the final goal of Hindu life, to be pursued in old age after discharging one's worldly responsibilities.[45] Buddhist, Jain, and Hindu renouncer traditions all differentiate between higher and lower levels of practice and observance, especially those of monastic and lay. This is represented in Jainism and Yoga Philosophy by the distinction between the great vow (*mahāvrata*) and lesser vow (*aṇuvrata*), the former characteristic of monastic practitioners and the latter of laypeople. Among other terms, those who abandon the world are referred to with titles such as striver (*śramaṇa/śramaṇerī*), renouncer (*saṃnyāsin/saṃnyāsinī*), virtuous one (*sādhu/sādhvī*), and mendicant (*bhikṣu/bhikṣuṇī*). In addition to their own spiritual and ethical commitments, laypeople provide material support to monastic practitioners, gaining spiritual merit (*puṇya*).

The notion of ascetic heat (*tapas*) demonstrates a logic that is broadly characteristic of asceticism, namely that acts of personal sacrifice, especially in the form of enduring bodily pain or discomfort, are spiritually profitable. Disciplining the body, in this paradigm, creates an inner heat (*tapas*) that purifies body and mind and serves as the basis for a continuum of worldly and otherworldly powers.[46] *Tapas* includes practices such as fasting, standing on one leg, holding one arm up in the air, undergoing piercing penances, hanging upside down, sitting in the sun or near blazing fires, and taking an oath of silence, among other possibilities. In the literature of *haṭhayoga* and tantric traditions, correspondences are drawn between the heat of self-discipline and the mastery of the subtle body (*sūkṣma-śarīra*), with both householders and renouncers being admonished to practice the discipline of yoga for the sake of purity, power, and liberation. The focus on the purifying power of heating the body and of sweating in modern yoga traditions connects modern postural yoga and *tapas*-based asceticism, although the former typically appeal to physiological and therapeutic conceptions of practice rather than spiritual or soteriological ones.[47] Much of postural practice in modern yoga may be fruitfully understood as an expression of *tapas*, particularly in the form of the endurance of pain and discomfort of physical exertion and a resultant emotional catharsis.[48] In its classical contexts, *tapas* is subsumed under a broader rubric of yoga discipline, serving as part of the corpus of yogic techniques as an aid to liberation (*mokṣa*) and source of spiritual perfection (*siddhi*).[49]

Tapas is also integrally connected to a language of purification found within the larger Indic ideological framework that informs *brāhmaṇa* and *śramaṇa* thinking. In the priestly (*brāhmaṇa*) context, bodily cleanliness (*śauca*) and, by extension, purity (*śuddhi*), can be contrasted with uncleanliness (*aśauca*) and impurity (*aśuddhi*). These conceptions frame individual and social identity, which is conceived of as informed by a hierarchy of purity extending downward from the highest of the gods to the lowest of humans. In *śramaṇa* thought, establishing purity of body and mind is seen as a means of freeing oneself from the bonds of action (*karma*) and for facilitating liberating insight (*jñāna*, *prajñā*). In Theravāda Buddhism, this is reflected in scriptural passages in which the Buddha states the religious path of all of the Buddhas as being one of "avoidance of all sin, performance of the right, [and] purifying one's thoughts."[50] In the context of the eight-limbed yoga (*aṣṭāṅgayoga*) in Patañjali's system, *śauca* is one of five observances (*niyama*), and *brahmacarya* or sexual restraint is one among five elements of restraint (*yama*). *Haṭhayoga* traditions often place great emphasis on purificatory practices, referred to as *kriyā*, which are a range of external and internal physical cleansings of the body. *Haṭhayoga* also includes teachings regarding the preservation of the *bindu*, or essence of bodily vitality, which is believed to be lost in the process of sexual activity through the emission of sexual fluids. Hindu and Buddhist tantric traditions, on the other hand, are known for their deliberate inversion of conventional conceptions of purity, including, in rare cases, the utilization of sexual intercourse and its physical products within yogic and tantric ritual practice.

The *Guru-Śiṣya* Relationship

Another point of intersection between *brāhmaṇa* and *śramaṇa* traditions is an emphasis on authoritative succession (*guru-paramparā*), in which teachings are formally passed directly from teacher (*guru*), literally "the [one] heavy [with experience]," to disciple (*śiṣya*). The *guru* is often popularly referred to as a "dispeller of darkness" for the *śiṣya*.[51] Variants on the term *guru* include those of preceptor (*ācārya*) and master (*svāmin*) or "swami." The *guru-śiṣya* relationship often presupposes a preliminary process of investiture (*upanayana*), initiation (*dīkṣā*), or both. For *brāhmaṇa* traditions, the investiture (*upanayana*) of the sacred thread has been the means of establishing entry into Vedic discipleship and learning the oral tradition of the Vedas since its earliest period. Discipleship in the priestly context has traditionally been tied to heredity, particularly to one's class (*varṇa*) and, more specifically, one's birth or caste identity (*jāti*). To authoritatively receive the teachings of the Vedas, the revealed (*śruti*) scriptures of early Hinduism, a person has traditionally had to be located within the three upper classes, and ideally within that of the priestly *brāhmaṇa* class. This is illustrated by genetic lineages of *brāhmaṇa* identity, where the *guru-śiṣya* relationship is principally that of father and son, with the patrilineal passage of teaching and authority dominating the transmission of the Vedas. Within *śramaṇa* traditions, such as Buddhism, and in *brāhmaṇa* ascetic traditions, ordination (*upasaṃpadā*) and various forms of initiation (*abhiṣeka*) take the place of such familial ties, creating a "spiritual family" among the initiated.

The *guru-śiṣya* relationship hinges on the conception that true teachings can be properly received only from someone who embodies the mastery of them. The concept of the true teacher (*sadguru*) encapsulates the idea of the *guru* as embodying the truth and as capable of passing it on to others. Practices such as *guruyoga* emphasize the transformative potential of viewing one's guru as a fully liberated or realized being who embodies the truth of the tradition in a complete way.[52] As such, the *guru* becomes a model or archetype of mastery for practitioners, and the body of the *guru* symbolically represents the body of the community of disciples as a whole.[53] To the degree that yoga is understood to be mastered through personal practice, instruction by a teacher who knows the terrain of the path and its landmarks is particularly highly valued. In Buddhism, the doctrine of *upāya-kauśalya* or "skillful means" suggests that a skilled teacher can discern a student's propensities and capabilities and thereby provide teaching suitable to allow the student to progress most effectively on the path.[54] The related Buddhist concept of the "beneficial friend" (*kalyāṇamitra*) encapsulates the idea that spiritual progress is, in part, a function of the people one associates with.[55] Access to the *guru* is highly valued and, as a result, leads to a politics of access to the *guru*, whose presence becomes charged with value and therefore is often rationed carefully, especially with respect to those outside an inner circle of disciples. A *guru* might transmit teachings in a range of ways, through didactic or discursive means such as verbal teachings, through performance and initiatory ritual, and through physical contact that facilitates a direct transmission or contagion of spiritual activation, such as the practice of the "descent of power" (*śaktipāta*).

Because of the inherent power imbalance, the *guru-śiṣya* relationship is open to a significant danger of abuse. In contemporary usage, the term *guru* is often associated with the dangers of blind submission to spiritual authority, social parasitism, psychological manipulation, and sexual abuse.[56] *Guru* figures may emphasize an exclusivism in which practitioners are not allowed to study with other teachers, ostensibly to prevent a dilution of their practice, creating territorialism and, in some cases, conflict between yoga communities. The common model of male preceptor and female student within modern yoga also reflects an unbalanced distribution of power and authority in the *guru-śiṣya* relationship. The *guru-śiṣya* relationship is rooted in Indian priestly and ascetic traditions that historically have been administered by males, with women typically excluded from leadership, if not from participation entirely. In orthodox Hinduism, women's ascetic practice has often been primarily performed as a vehicle for domestic prosperity, especially the physical welfare of the husband, as opposed to individual spiritual progress.[57] However, some of the most influential modern yoga systems, such as that of the Krishnamacharya tradition, have been adapted to accommodate changing gender roles, allowing expanded access to practice for Indian women and, in some cases, organizational leadership roles. It is notable that the daughters of a number of prominent modern yoga teachers, including Geeta Iyengar, the daughter of B.K.S. Iyengar, have served in important leadership positions in yoga organizations in India and internationally.

In modern transnational yoga traditions, authority is often more diffuse and formal initiatory ritual less common than in traditional Indian contexts. However, official modes of entry into authoritative modern practice in nonsectarian traditions do exist. This includes a range of formalized teacher training sequences and authorizations that serve to determine the authority of various strata of practitioners. Placing higher expectations on the certification of teachers, such as the requirement for personal authorization, may help leadership establish control over a tradition's dissemination and the economic and cultural capital involved.[58] Practitioners within the global community enhance their authority through establishing relationships with teachers and lineages in India or through traveling to practice in highly reputed locations for the study of yoga such as Mysore (Mysuru) or Rishikesh. Formal practice sequences connect transnational communities of practitioners and, in some cases, form a basis for legal and economic disputes.[59] Initiatory structures such as formal teacher training sequences and workshops also establish authority within and among yoga traditions, providing clear pathways for professional development.

Yogī, Yogin/Yoginī, Sādhaka, and Siddha

In Sanskrit, the term *yogī* is a nominative masculine noun formed from the stem *yogin*, the latter having the female equivalent form of *yoginī*. The term *yogī* is, however, often used in anglophone, or English-language-mediated, modern yoga traditions in a gender-neutral manner.[60] Prototypes of the *yogin* from the early Indian Vedic tradition include the Keśin, or "long-haired one," an ecstatic figure who is portrayed as drinking a poison or psychoactive agent (*viṣa*) and flying through the air with the gods; ascetic figures, such as the Yati, Muni, and Brahmacārin, who restrain action, speech, and sexuality; fraternal brotherhoods of the Vrātya or "avowed ones;" and, perhaps most notably, the Vedic Ṛṣi or "seer," a class of ancient sages at the roots of the *brāhmaṇa* tradition. In the Upaniṣads, the final strata of the Vedic literature, the word *guru* appears as a referent for various sages, such as Yājñavalkya, who are represented as embodying the living wisdom of the tradition.[61] In the epic and Purāṇa literature, images of the *yogin* and *yoginī* range from that of warriors and ascetics to powerful human sorcerers and sorceresses, with Śiva, Viṣṇu, and other gods and saints, such as Kapila, being represented at practitioners of yoga.[62] Narratives of the Buddha and Mahāvīra describe their extraordinary virtue, knowledge, and power, and they are represented visually in postures of ascetic austerity and meditation. Notions of *yoga* of the *yogin* appear with increasing frequency in Buddhist literature over time, and are further referenced in terms of practice such as meditator (Skt. *dhyānin*, Pāli *jhāyin*), applying the teaching (Skt. *dharmayogī*, Pāli *dhammayogī*), engaged in yoga (*yogāvacara*), practitioner of yoga (*yogācāra*), and yoga-practicing monk (*yogācāra-bhikṣu*).[63] By the medieval period in India, the terms *yogin* and *yoginī* have a wide semantic range, referring to tantric practitioners and "heroes" (*sādhaka*, *vīra*), such as the Hindu Nāths, Mahāsiddhas, and warrior-ascetics, as well to practitioners of mainstream ascetic discipline (*tapasvin*, *tapasvinī*).[64] The transfiguration of practitioners of yoga into a higher order of being is indicated by the notions of becoming a "lord of yoga" or "lord of the practitioners of yoga" (*yogeśvara*, *yogīśvara*) or a "perfected one" or "great perfected one" (*siddha*, *mahāsiddha*). In Buddhist and Jain contexts, the terminology of accomplishment includes those of "awakened one" (*buddha*), "thus-gone one" (*tathāgata*), "lord" (*bhagavat*), "crossing-maker" (*tīrthaṃkara*), "great hero" (*mahāvīra*), and "victor" (*jina*), among others. Other terms that relate ascetic and yogic mastery in the Indian context include those of "great soul" (*mahātma*), "great king" (*mahārāja*), "king of yoga" (Skt. *yogarāja*, Hin. *yogirāj*), "(grand)father" (*bābā*), "mother" (*mātā*, *mā*), and "honored one" (*śrī*).

Yoga literature often contains admonitions of the need for men to restrain their sexual impulses in response to temptation by immodest or seductive women, as part of a larger trope regarding gender in Indian asceticism.[65] However, ascetic and yogic principles are, in some contexts, presented as equally relevant to both men and women, and numerous examples in Indic literature have women exemplifying ascetic and yogic virtues.[66] Early Hindu literature provides many examples of prototypes for the *yoginī*. Female ascetics who gain insight through contemplation and power through austerities appear in the Upaniṣads and in the Hindu Epic and Purāṇa literature. These examples include female sages such as Gārgī and Sulabhā and various female celibates (*brahmacāriṇī*), forest-dwellers (*vānaprasthinī*), renouncers (*bhikṣuṇī, saṃnyāsinī*), and accomplished ones (*siddhā*) who possess considerable realization and power.[67] Other female ascetics also are represented as pursuing worldly goals through acts of asceticism (*tapas*), demonstrating the numinous power available to women through self-discipline.[68] Hindu devotional (*bhakti*) literature highlights the power and impact of female saint-poet (*sant*) figures such as Mīrābāī.[69] Buddhist literature celebrates the accomplishments of Buddhist nuns (*bhikṣuṇī*), and one of the earliest Buddhist references to the term *yogī* as indicating an enlightened sage appears in the Therīgāthā, a compilation of the wisdom of female Buddhist elders.[70] The notion of the *yoginī* as a female counterpart to the *yogin* has a broad application in Indic context.[71]

The term *yoginī* is also prominent in medieval Hindu and Buddhist tantric literature in reference to human and divine tantric adepts that serve as objects of worship and as facilitators of tantric ritual, especially initiation.[72] Yoginīs may have played an important role in the formulation and dissemination of medieval yoga and tantra practices, some of which had transgressive sexual components.[73] The tantric *yoginī* may have also been connected to traditions of possession ritual that existed as a counterpart to *brāhmaṇa* culture, conferring power and authority on female ritualists, paralleling a mode of religious practice that continues in many parts of India today.[74] This mode of practice can be referred to as a form of *positive possession*, brought about through rituals of evocation, or adorcism, as opposed to *negative possession*, which is addressed through rituals of elimination, or exorcism.[75] Yoginī figures appear in tantric texts as initiatory deities and consorts that facilitate the rapid attainment of power and knowledge. The integration of women's ritual traditions into the patriarchal priestly and monastic traditions may have led to the elevation of women and female deities within tantric practice.[76] The fluidity of human and divine *yoginī* categories also demonstrates the potential of yoga to transfigure human practitioners, as the divine *yoginī* can be conceived of, in some circumstances, as an apotheosis of the human *yoginī*.

Class, Gender, and Sexuality

In Indian literature, yoga has often been associated with higher-class (*varṇa*) and higher-caste (*jāti*) male members of Indian society. As a result, the historical role of women and marginalized social groups in the formulation of yoga traditions is, in many cases, relatively obscure when compared to male and higher-class practitioners. The founders of Jainism and Buddhism, Mahāvīra Vardhamāna and Siddhārtha Gautama, are represented as having been born into the warrior (*kṣatriya*) or ruling (*rājanya*) class of Indian society, and although the Jain and Buddhist traditions accepted members from all classes, it appears that higher classes were disproportionally represented in their communities.[77] Early Hindu narratives highlight the status of important figures as members of the priest (*brāhmaṇa*) or warrior (*kṣatriya/ rājanya*) class of Vedic society. One theory suggests that the warrior class may have had a critical role in the development of renouncer traditions, highlighted by the import of the *kṣatriya*-renouncer figure in Jainism and Buddhism and in the Hindu Upaniṣads.[78] In the Hindu epic literature, ascetic techniques and yoga are utilized by forest sages of the *brāhmaṇa* class and by members of the ruling class (*rājanya*), notably the five Pāṇḍava brothers, who are the heroes of the *Mahābhārata* and exemplify the virtues of the warrior (*kṣatriya*) in Indian society, such as truth, social order, and duty (*dharma*). Some medieval traditions of yoga, such as *haṭhayoga*, and *bhakti*-influenced traditions, especially Siddha traditions in southern India, contain threads of both nonsectarian and anti-caste thinking that anticipate the universalist views found in many modern yoga traditions.

Much of the literature of yoga has been preserved in elite scholastic languages, including Vedic Sanskrit, Pāli, Classical Sanskrit, and Buddhist Hybrid Sanskrit, though a number of oral and literary traditions exist in regional or vernacular languages, such as the south Indian languages of Tamil, Telegu, and Kannada and northern Indian dialects related to Sanskrit and Hindi, such as Brajbhasha. The *aṣṭāṅgayoga* system of Patañjali's *Yogasūtra* contains elements, such as the terminology of *brahmacarya, tapas*, and *svādhyāya*, that would be principally familiar to members of the Vedic *brāhmaṇa* class, and the commentarial tradition of the *Yogasūtra*, beginning in the *Pātañjalayogaśāstra*, offers explicit instructions for *brāhmaṇa* practitioners.[79] Hindu renunciation has often had caste restrictions, and many important figures within Hindu traditions of asceticism are represented as having been from the *brāhmaṇa* class, such as the renowned philosophers Śaṅkara and Rāmānuja.[80] The development of the major schools of the Kashmir Śaiva tradition, in which various forms of tantric yoga were developed and codified, were championed by *brāhmaṇa* linguists and philosophers such as Utpaladeva and Abhinavagupta. The texts of *haṭhayoga* appear to appeal to a literate *brāhmaṇa* audience, but occasional references to female practitioners and to nonsectarian practice traditions appear in some *haṭhayoga* texts, suggesting a range of degrees of elite orthodoxy.[81] Tantric narratives, such as those of the medieval Mahāsiddha traditions, represent working- and lower-class occupations as being a locus for spiritual mastery, playing on the purity concerns of high-class and -caste society.[82] However, many of the key figures in such stories come from the *brāhmaṇa* and *kṣatriya* classes, and it is clear that tantra was an integral part of religious and political life at the highest echelons of Indic society during the medieval era.[83] Many influential modern yoga teachers who have played a role in its visibility in India and its transmission on a global scale, such as B.K.S. Iyengar and Swami Sivananda, have been from the *brāhmaṇa* class, even if publicly emphasizing yoga's universal applicability.[84]

The literature of yoga is more limited in its representation of lower-class and marginalized members of Indian society, or subalterns, as well as in its representation of women, though there are significant exceptions. Traditions of *bhaktiyoga* often highlight subaltern concerns, framing devotion (*bhakti*) as transcending class (*varṇa*), caste (*jāti*), and, in some cases, identity as Hindu or non-Hindu. Likewise, as noted above, female ascetics and *yoginī* figures do appear in Indian literature, such as the Purāṇas, embodying the principles of yoga in concrete ways. Women's renunciation is validated to varying degrees within Hindu, Buddhist, and Jain traditions, though the asymmetry between male and female practitioners is evident in the working principles of Indian asceticism, which often place emphasis on the retention of male sexual fluids as a physical representation of spiritual power and control. This is evident in narrative tropes in which a *yogin* is "tempted" by a seductive nymph (*apsaras*), often sent by the gods to impede the practitioner's success, which would otherwise threaten the given order of the world. This motif is found in narratives of the Buddha's awakening, in the *Kaṭha Upaniṣad*, and in the principal commentary to *Yogasūtra*, among other places. Additionally, women may use ascetic or yogic mastery to coerce or seduce gods, a theme found in the great poem (*mahākāvya*) of the *Kumārasambhava*, in the Vedic literature, and in the *Mahābhārata*.[85] Women's asceticism within Hinduism is also often associated with the domestic *pativrata*, or "husband-vow," in which a woman's spiritual self-discipline, akin to *tapas*, is a vehicle for domestic prosperity. Tantric traditions validate the power and capability of the *yoginī* in some contexts, while representing them as mere instruments for the achievement of power and liberation by a male agent in others.[86] Women have played an extraordinarily important role in modern anglophone traditions of yoga as one of the principal audiences for instruction by Indian teachers, and, in some cases, as the inheritors of those teachers' authority or as the progenitors of new transmission lineages.[87]

The Origins of Yoga

As mentioned above, historical and archeological evidence provides an unclear picture as to when yoga first appeared in India.[88] Some scholars suggest that yoga originated in the Indus Valley Civilization (2500–1500 BCE), though evidence of the term *yoga* in Indian literature appears significantly later, during the Vedic period (1500–500 BCE). In the case of the Indus Valley Civilization, steatite, or soapstone, seals portray a figure seated in what some later interpreters have suggested is a yogic posture, though no known textual tradition supports this assertion. The word "yoga" appears in an early stage of the literature of the Vedas, in reference to the yoking of oxen and horses to carts and to chariots, and as a systematic spiritual discipline only significantly later. The Vedic literature prior to the Upaniṣads, however, does offer descriptions of religious specialists concerned with visionary and ecstatic experience, facilitated through ascetic practice (*tapas*), ritual, and the use of psychoactive substances. These iconic figures, which range from the ancient seers (*ṛṣi*) to the priestly (*brāhmaṇa*) performers of ritual sacrifice (*yajña*), possess many characteristics attributed to later yoga practitioners. The Vedas, the foundational texts of the Hindu tradition, are self-represented by the tradition as the product of the poetic, if not meditative, vision (*dhī*) of the ancient Vedic seers. The description of the consumption of psychoactive substances, including a poison or agent (*viṣa*) and juice or extract (*soma*), indicates the importance of extraordinary states of action and vision among certain Vedic practitioners. The use of ascetic self-discipline (*tapas*) in the Vedic tradition as a preparation for ritual and, later, as a source of extraordinary capacities demonstrates an important link between Vedic ritual traditions and *brāhmaṇa* and *śramaṇa* renouncer traditions. The use of ritual and psychoactive agents to induce visionary experiences and the use of ascetic techniques to facilitate the attainment of spiritual experience and knowledge also have larger connections to shamanic traditions, including the use of psychoactive substances and possession ritualism in its positive and negative manifestations.[89] The roots of yoga are to be found, in part, in early Indian quests for obtaining numinous experiences of power and transcendence through ritual, the sacramental use of psychoactive substances, and ascetic self-discipline.[90]

With the rise of Indian renouncer traditions (c. 500 BCE) and the development of yoga as a systematic discipline of restraint and self-mastery, an emphasis on cessative concerns became particularly prominent within Hindu, Buddhist, and Jain contexts. The emergence of the problem of suffering (*duḥkha*) represented a critical development in the post-Vedic yoga traditions. In Brāhmaṇical asceticism and in the *śramaṇa* traditions, especially Buddhism and Jainism, yoga is framed as a method of service in the pursuit of a cure for the problem of suffering (*duḥkha*), which is the defining characteristic of the endless cycle (*saṃsāra*) of birth and rebirth. Early Indian medical paradigms, which culminated in the medical system of *āyurveda*, viewed physical illness and metaphysical suffering as continuous with one another, and likely helped spurn the development of the soteriological models of yoga practice.[91] The transformation of Vedic civilization from a village-based tribal and pastoral mode of life to a centralized urban civilization was likely another major factor in the emergence of *brāhmaṇa* asceticism and *śramaṇa* traditions. Such socioeconomic changes in Indian civilization allowed for networks of support and patronage for renouncer traditions to develop.[92] *Śramaṇa* leaders, such as the Buddha and Mahāvīra, saw themselves in competition with each other for the support and patronage of local rulers and merchants, and commanded considerable political power with respect to their access to and advising of the ruling elite of their time. The worldview and practices of the *brāhmaṇa* elite of the Vedic tradition, in which priests served as intermediaries to the gods and goddesses (*deva*, *devī*), may have become less relevant to people's lives in an increasingly urban society, with renunciation opening the door for broader participation in the religious life. Renouncer traditions may have also served as a counterpart to the world-affirming Vedic tradition, acting as a sort of "release valve" for the tensions of its hierarchical society.[93] Nonetheless, *śramaṇa* teachings, such as those in Buddhism, placed emphasis on establishing skillful modes of living for both lay and monastic practitioners, suggesting that ascetic principles are of value to both the individual and to society.

Living Yoga Traditions

Within the contemporary traditions of Hinduism, Buddhism, and Jainism, yoga continues to be an important area of religious discourse and sectarian identity as a set of textual and performative traditions. Yoga has also become part of mainstream Indian, especially Hindu, society, as an extension of *brāhmaṇa* priestly traditions and as part of a householder ideology that connects self-discipline and this-worldly health and success on the individual and communal level.[94] This is exemplified by the rise of Indian celebrity yoga gurus, such as Swami Ramdev and Sadhguru Jaggi Vasudev, who have brought yoga in India to a level of visibility and political influence beyond any point in its history, melding physical fitness discourse with a Hindu-rooted universalizing spirituality. Interest among European and American audiences has also encouraged the revival and reconstruction of traditional methods of yoga in India to appeal to modern cosmopolitan audiences, especially those within anglophone transnational yoga traditions.[95] The globalization of yoga has been facilitated by its reinterpretation within modern, especially scientific, discourses that deemphasize its metaphysical superstructures and focus on its therapeutic applications.[96] Yoga has been integrated into secular culture on a large scale, but continues to inform the practice of a diverse range of religious traditions, from Hinduism and Buddhism to Jainism, Sikhism, Judaism, Christianity, and Islam. Its adaptability to suit various cultural and religious contexts parallels the development of modern physical disciplines such as Pilates and the modern Chinese, Japanese, and Korean martial arts.[97]

The most visible and globally representative type of yoga in the twenty-first century is what has come to be referred to as "modern postural yoga."[98] The practices and ideologies associated with this form of yoga are rooted in the integration of late medieval and early modern yoga practices of *haṭhayoga* and a range of nineteenth- and twentieth-century physical disciplines, such as Indian and European traditions of gymnastics, dance, martial arts, and wrestling. Modern traditions of postural yoga are also situated in an ideological framework informed by Hindu spirituality and European physical culturist thought, metaphysical religion, and occultism.[99] What stands out most prominently in the modern postural adaptations of *haṭhayoga* is an emphasis on a narrow set of physical practices, particularly posture (*āsana*) and breath control (*prāṇāyāma*), and a widely variable emphasis on the metaphysical concerns of premodern yoga and Euro-American spirituality and occultism.[100] A counterpoint to postural traditions of yoga are those of "modern meditative yoga," which draw on Hindu, Buddhist, and Jain practices of meditation or cultivation (*dhyāna*, *bhāvanā*) and contemplation (*samādhi*).[101] In Hindu-derived traditions such as Transcendental Meditation, meditation is performed on a mantra, such as the syllable *oṃ*, though Hindu or Hindu-inspired meditative traditions may utilize a variety of objects, from the breath and body to the image of deities such as Śiva or Viṣṇu. Buddhist traditions of meditation involve the cultivation of concentration on particular objects, such as the breath and body, and techniques for developing insight into the nature of body and mind. The Theravāda Buddhist tradition, or "Southern Buddhism," places emphasis on "insight meditation" (Pāli *vipassanā*, Skt. *vipaśyanā*), in which a seated meditator observes the arising and falling of mental and physical experiences. In Mahāyāna, or "Northern Buddhism," meditative techniques include the contemplation of principles such as emptiness (*śūnyatā*) and visualization and contemplation of the qualities of spiritually awakened beings such as the Buddha. As with postural practices, meditation has become a topic of considerable interest with respect to its therapeutic applications, especially in the psychological and neurobiological sciences.[102] In its secularized forms, it has become an integral part of discourses of psychological therapy and self-help, stress reduction, and athletic and professional performance, especially with reference to the concept of mindfulness (*smṛti*).[103]

Defining "Yoga" and "Tantra"

Having established some of the key parameters of the theory and practice of yoga, a heuristic definition can be provided as a conceptual foundation for the broader study that follows. In its primary sense, yoga is a set or a system of techniques of mind-body discipline, rooted in Indian religion and philosophy, that aims to transform a practitioner into a more perfect being so as to (1) make them more powerful and/or to (2) facilitate liberation from worldly affliction. In its secondary sense, yoga refers to specific modes and goals of practice, and thus may be qualified by compounding the term with particular categorical designations of technique, such as *rājayoga*, *haṭhayoga*, *aṣṭāṅgayoga*, *ṣaḍaṅgayoga*, *mantrayoga*, *layayoga*, *bhaktiyoga*, and so forth.[104] In the modern context, such categorical designations may be supplanted by references to the progenitors of systems of yoga or schools of yoga, such as Iyengar Yoga, Sivananda Yoga, Integral Yoga, Siddha Yoga, Yantra Yoga, and others, each of which implies particular modes and goals of practice. This relatively simple heuristic approach to defining yoga is useful in capturing the universality of Indian notions of a goal-oriented spiritual discipline found throughout the range of traditions of yoga, while respecting the fact that the nature of the discipline and the goals of practice in yoga may differ significantly depending on the philosophical, sectarian, or nonsectarian contexts in which they have been developed and practiced. Different degrees of systematization are found among the various premodern and modern forms of yoga, with some traditions largely equating yoga with asceticism (*tapas*), and others incorporating *tapas* into a larger framework of yoga practice, such as *aṣṭāṅgayoga*. Some schools of yoga incorporate different modes of practice (*haṭhayoga*, *bhaktiyoga*, etc.) together, whether as stages of practice or as alternative or complementary modes of practice. Similarly, some sectarian traditions and schools of yoga are strongly tied to renouncer ideologies, others to householder traditions, and some mediate or integrate these models.

The closely related Sanskrit term *tantra* refers to a network of concepts that connect to and overlap with yoga in important ways, and it is useful to offer a working definition of *tantra* at this point as well. The term is derived from the Sanskrit verbal root √*tan*, which means "to stretch" or "to extend," and thus can be defined as "[ritual] extension." *Tantra*, in this context, refers to a mode of practice, drawn from Indian religion and philosophy, that aims to accelerate spiritual development, in the form of obtaining power and liberation, through the invocation of and identification with deities, often fierce in character, and the utilization of the forces of nature and embodiment, including the use of transgressive actions and substances.[105] The term can also refer to a class of texts, which are alternately termed as *tantra*, *āgama*, or *saṃhitā*, in which such practices are outlined, with *yoga* being the subject of one of the four principal divisions of these texts.[106] As such, *tantra* may refer to a particular approach to the practice of yoga, or as an umbrella under which yoga is incorporated as an element. The notion of *tantra* as a supplementary mode of practice is demonstrated in the threefold distinction in Hinduism between *vaidika* (Vedic, or early Hindu, ritual methodologies and ideologies), *paurāṇika* (classical Hindu ritual methodologies and ideologies, based in the *sūtra* and *itihāsa-purāṇa* literature), and *tāntrika* (medieval Hindu ritual methodologies and ideologies, based in the *tantra* and *āgama* literature) modes of priestly (*brāhmaṇa*) practice. In Jain and Buddhist traditions, this progression is paralleled by the division of early *śramaṇa* practice and ideology, classical scholastic practice and ideology (*sūtra* and scholastic commentarial literature), and tantric practice and ideology. Tantra became a pervasive part of Indic religion in the medieval era (500–1500 CE) and has been highly influential with respect to broader religious and cultural life in India to the present.[107]

Much of what is referred to as "tantra" in the contemporary global context only distantly resembles tantric practices in Hinduism, Buddhism, and Jainism. Instead, such "neo-Tantric" traditions are often uniquely focused on sexual practices and integrate a range of modern, including Theosophical, New Age, and popular psychological, ideas and practices into its expression.[108] In contemporary India, tantric practitioners are often viewed as providing ritual assistance for patrons seeking health and romantic and material success, as opposed to being concerned with spiritual liberation.[109] In some contexts, tantric practitioners are seen to be particularly adept at managing spirit-based illness, especially possession by malevolent spirits and other occult-inspired mental and physical disorders.

The Chronology of Yoga Traditions

The primary academic model of the formation of Indian society posits two streams of language and culture that merged over time, those of the Dravidians and Indo-Aryans. In this model, the Dravidians, who entered India in an early migration around 3000 BCE or earlier, developed the earliest large-scale indigenous civilization in India, referred to as the Indus Civilization. Known for its cities on the Indus River, Harappa and Mohenjodaro, the Indus Civilization was a thriving and cosmopolitan society, establishing trade widely, most notably with the civilizations of Mesopotamia and Egypt. Conservative estimates place the height of the Indus Civilization at approximately 2500 BCE, though some scholars, primarily in India, place this date significantly earlier. The second source of Indian society in the "two culture" model is the Vedic, or Indo-Aryan, Civilization, the product of the consolidation of nomadic tribes from Central Asia that entered northwestern India around 1500 BCE, displacing but also mixing with the indigenous Dravidian population and culture of India. Archeological and linguistic evidence clearly indicates that early Indian culture demonstrated a plurality of cultural and ethnic influences, thus supporting such a "two cultures" model.[110] However, scholarly disagreement, principally between European and Indian scholars, has led to a range of different views on the nature and antiquity of ancient Indian civilization.[111] This has, by extension, resulted in a broad range of dates being associated with the earliest developments of the practice of yoga.

The chapters that follow examine the transformation of yoga over time, following its chronological development through the changing cultural and religious environment of India, culminating in its emergence as a global, transnational phenomenon. We will begin with an examination of the prehistory of yoga as represented in the archeological records of the Indus Civilization (2800–1500 BCE) and in the Vedic tradition (1500–500 BCE). This will be followed by a discussion of concepts and practices related to yoga and renunciation within Vedic Brāhmaṇical asceticism and in the *śramaṇa* traditions of Jainism and Buddhism (500 BCE). We will subsequently examine the classical Hindu model of yoga as found in the *yoga darśana* as articulated in Patañjali's *Yogasūtra* and its principal commentarial literature (200–400 CE), focusing on the paradigmatic framework of the eight-limbed yoga (*aṣṭāṅgayoga*) system. We will then explore the development of representations of yoga in Hindu epic (*itihāsa*) and narrative (*purāṇa*) literature and in Hindu scholastic, theological, and legal literature (500 BCE–500 CE). This will be complemented by an examination of classical and scholastic *śramaṇa* models of yoga as represented in contemporaneous Jain and Buddhist literature. The larger discussion of the classical era will be expanded through an exploration of the transformation of yoga during the medieval period (500–1500 CE) in light of the impact of devotional (*bhakti*) movements and the development of tantric methodologies and formal classification systems such as the fourfold set of *mantrayoga, haṭhayoga, layayoga*, and *rājayoga*. Lastly, we will examine the development of modern yoga systems (1500 CE–present), with an emphasis on the dynamic transformation of yoga in the past two centuries into a global phenomenon of extraordinary impact and scope.

While it is recognized that no academic study of a religious practice that has a complexity such as that of yoga can be fully comprehensive, the goal of this work is to establish a narrative arc of the history and philosophy of yoga that brings an informed scholarly perspective to its many facets. It will become clear that while the practice of yoga often embodies the aspiration to realize an unchanging truth, it has been adapted time and again to suit novel historical and cultural situations. This is perhaps most dramatically demonstrated in the contemporary context, in which the processes of globalization have radically changed the cultural landscape of the world and with it the discipline of yoga in its manifold variations and permutations.

Chapter 2

The Prehistory of Yoga

The Indus Civilization and the Vedic Tradition

The roots of yoga are found deep within the earliest strata of Indian civilization, theorized to be a composite of two principal cultural and linguistic groups, the Dravidians and Indo-Aryans, who came in separate migrations to India in the millennia before the Common Era, beginning in the vicinity of 3000 BCE or earlier.[1] Dravidian linguistic traditions are principally associated with modern populations in southern India and the languages of Tamil, Telegu, Kannada, and Malayalam. Indo-Aryan linguistic traditions are principally associated with the languages of populations in northern India that have a genealogical relationship to Sanskrit (Skt. *saṃskṛta*), such as modern Hindi, Marathi, Gujarati, and Bengali, which are extensions of the medieval Sanskrit dialects of the Prakrits (Skt. *prākṛta*). Given the wide historical influence of the Sanskrit language, the admixture of the two linguistic families over time, the influence of Persian and Arabic on Indic language during the Delhi Sultanate and Mughal imperial periods, and the establishment of English in education and commerce in the British colonial era, India is linguistically quite complex. Distinct Indo-Aryan and Dravidian language heritages cannot be geographically circumscribed in simple ways, given the diffusion that has taken place. However, contemporary political tensions between northern and southern India, such as controversies over attempts to establish Hindi as India's national language, point to differences in cultural self-perception between north and south India that are rooted in the distinction between the two larger cultural and linguistic heritages.

Scholarly knowledge about the Indus Valley Civilization (2800–1500 BCE) is limited to archeological evidence. Although what appears to be an Indus script is found on objects, understanding of the language of the Indus Civilization remains conjectural due to a lack of consensus on accepted decipherment, with some scholars arguing that the so-called script is not, in fact, writing at all.[2] With respect to the later Indo-Aryan or Vedic Civilization (1500–500 BCE), the opposite is the case. The Indo-Aryans were nomads who built temporary structures, leaving behind little archeological evidence of their civilization. However, the Indo-Aryans created an expansive body of texts, the Vedas (*veda*), which was preserved in oral and, eventually, written form, and provides much information about their language, culture, and self-perception. The principal theory of cultural dissemination in India is that of the Aryan Migration Thesis (AMT), which identifies the Indus civilization as culturally and linguistically Dravidian, distinct from that of the Indo-Aryans who arrived in India later. This thesis is based on evidence for disjunctions between the archeological records of the Indus civilization and the self-representation of Aryans in the Vedas. There are, however, some scholars who have suggested that the Indus Civilization may have, in fact, been the homeland of the Aryans, a hypothesis referred to as the Cultural Transformation Thesis (CTT) or the Out of India Thesis (OIT).[3] For practical purposes, it makes sense to examine the Indus and Vedic Civilizations separately, given the distinct nature of the archeological and textual evidence that each provides. The material and textual sources the Indus Civilization and the Vedic tradition provide likely represent the elite viewpoints and culture of their societies disproportionately. However, they provide a useful set of data points for theorizing on the development of yoga in early Indian civilization.

Indus Valley Civilization and the "Yogi" Seal (2800–1500 BCE)

The Indus Civilization may be the source of the earliest known physical representations of yoga practice, and it is common for narratives of the history of yoga to proceed with the Indus archeological evidence as the logical starting point for the topic. The issue has particularly strong import with respect to larger issues of yoga's identity as being indigenous to India. To the degree to which the Indus Civilization is considered the place where yoga began, it can be argued that yoga has been an integral part of Indian culture from the dawn of documented civilization. It is also significant with respect to the larger tradition of Hinduism, where links to the Indus Civilization are often seen to signify its uniquely indigenous nature, in contrast to narratives of Indo-Aryan migration.

The argument for the origins of yoga in the Indus Civilization is based on two principal types of archeological evidence: first, small steatite (soapstone) seals with figures seated in a yoga *āsana*-like position; and second, terracotta figurines that appear to show individuals in a range of different postures, perhaps suggestive of various types of yoga *āsana*. The first case, represented by Mohenjodaro seal number 420 and others, portrays a central figure wearing a headdress and sitting with bent knees and feet together, with hands resting on both knees.[4] The figure is surrounded by animals and seated upon a dais. Though the figure is sometimes referred to as sitting in the lotus posture (*padmāsana*), the posture illustrated in the seal perhaps more closely resembles perfected posture (*siddhāsana*) or, alternately, root-lock posture (*mūlabandhāsana*).[5] The figure has, in some cases, been identified with the later Hindu deity Śiva in his form as "animal-lord" (*paśupati*), who is associated with the divine bull Nandi and represented as a seated, meditating ascetic practitioner or *yogin*.[6] The Indus figure is also represented in seal 420 as ithyphallic, perhaps suggesting a connection between the figure and the later worship of Śiva in the form of the *liṅga*, or phallic icon. Some of the seated figures also have multiple faces, suggestive of later representations of Śiva and other Hindu deities as having multiple faces and multiple limbs. The second case, focusing on small terracotta figurines that appear in a range of *āsana*-like poses, presents a generic association between the culture of the Indus and an interest in disciplines of the body, suggesting the possibility of yoga along with dance as part of the Indus repertoire. Female figurines have also been the subject of speculation as possible precursors of later Hindu Śākta (goddess) traditions associated with Hindu yoga and tantra.

Indus seal figures have been alternately identified by some scholars with later Jain representations of their liberated masters (*jina*, *tīrthaṃkara*), suggesting that the connections to animals and plants portrayed in the seals illustrate care and concern for the natural world and the principle of *ahiṃsā*.[7] Connections have also been made between later representations of the Buddha and of other Buddhist religious figures, who are represented as being flanked by two disciples who have their hands held together in a gesture (*mudrā*) of obeisance (*namaskāra*) or offering (*añjali*).[8] The inclusion of two deer or antelope below the seated Mohenjodaro figure similarly elicits potential connections to later representations of the figure of the Buddha, as does the iconography of the *pippala* or fig tree found in a number of seals, a tree that has important associations with Indian religion in general and specifically with Buddhism.[9] Lastly, the representation of human figures covered by a hood of a serpent (*nāga*) that appears in the context of at least one of the Indus seals may suggest a connection to later representations of Hindu, Buddhist, and Jain figures who are portrayed iconographically as being shielded by the hood of a *nāga*.[10]

Despite the intriguing nature of such claims, there is reason for considerable skepticism regarding the conceptual leaps necessary to connect such archeological evidence to significantly later, and more clearly documentable, representations of yoga.[11] Among other issues, seated figures similar to those of the Indus figures appear independently in a range of cultural contexts in the ancient world.[12] It is, perhaps, all too easy to connect later manifestations of yoga and Indian religion to the material archeological record without substantive knowledge of what such objects meant for the Indus people in their original contexts.

The Indo-Aryans and the Vedic Brāhmaṇical Tradition

Archeological and linguistic evidence indicates that around 1500 BCE nomads from Central Asia began to enter into northwestern India via a passageway into India that would be later used by the Greeks and Persians, among others. They likely encountered the remnants of a dwindling Indus Civilization as they pressed south and east. These nomads, the Indo-Aryans, spoke an ancient language called Vedic Sanskrit, or simply Vedic, which was part of a larger family of languages that are collectively referred to by linguists as Proto-Indo-European (PIE). Vedic Sanskrit was related to the Indo-Iranian language of Avestan, which was spoken in ancient Persia. The Indo-Aryans and Indo-Iranians developed a body of texts, referred to as the *veda* and *avesta*, respectively, that prescribed ritual procedures, notably for fire sacrifice, and codified the ideology of their societies. In the case of the Indo-Iranians, the vestiges of this legacy can be found within the Zoroastrian religion, practiced by one of India's religious minorities, the Parsis. With respect to the Indo-Aryan tradition, the Vedic tradition became the foundation for the development of virtually all branches of the Hindu tradition. Even traditions that formally reject the authority of the Vedas, such as Buddhism and Jainism, are deeply informed by Vedic language, principles, and practices. The central textual collection of the Vedas was a resource for the establishment of Vedic ritual and ideology, and the focus of the career of a class (*varṇa*) of priests (*brāhmaṇa*, often anglicized as "Brahmin"). Hinduism eventually shifted away from the strict observance of Vedic ritual, but elements of this ancient strata of religious practice can still be found in contemporary India in small pockets of Vedic (*vaidika*) priestly (*brāhmaṇa*) traditions that seek to keep the ancient mode of practice, including fire sacrifice, alive. The *vaidika* mode of practice can be contrasted with the later strata of *brāhmaṇa* practice, namely the "remembered" or "traditional" (*smārta*, *paurāṇika*) and tantric (*tāntrika*) modes of priestly life.

Composed over a number of centuries, the religious literature of the Vedic period provides insight into the nature and development of the early Hindu tradition. Modern traditions of *vaidika* practice also provide a window to the world of early Hindu practice, though *vaidika* traditions, as conservative as they might be, have demonstrated significant adaptability over time.[13] At the heart of the Vedic tradition is the textual corpus of the *veda*, its name being derived from the Sanskrit root √*vid*, meaning "to know," which is qualified as being a "heard" (*śruti*) or revealed set of texts, as opposed to those that are "remembered" (*smṛti*) or of human composition. The Veda is the textual locus for ritual and ideological authority for the *vaidika brāhmaṇa* tradition. The Vedic tradition establishes many concepts and practices that are building blocks of yoga and provides an important part of the larger ideological and metaphysical context out of which yoga traditions ultimately emerge.

Structure of the Vedic Tradition

The Vedas portray life in Vedic society as intimately tied up with the nomadic-pastoralist mode of living in Indo-Aryan culture. As nomads, the Indo-Aryans migrated with various livestock, which represented a key part of their wealth and livelihood. It is not surprising, then, that pastoral animals, in particular the cow, were highly valued to such an extent that they came to be viewed as quasi-sacred beings in the Vedic and later Hindu traditions. The language describing gods (*deva*) and goddesses (*devī*) often refers to the deities as being like cows in their supreme generosity.[14] The products of the cow, particularly the so-called "five essences" (*pañcagavya*), milk, yogurt, butter, urine, and dung, were utilized in various ways in Vedic ritual, particularly for sacrifice (*yajña*) and purification. Whether the Indo-Aryans were originally vegetarian is a subject of scholarly dispute, though considerable evidence exists that an emphasis on vegetarianism, especially within higher-class society, was a later development within *smārta brāhmaṇa* traditions.[15] The Indo-Aryans appear to have driven light horse-drawn chariots and, as a result, were quite accomplished in warfare.[16] The chariot, over time, became an iconic element of Indian narrative literature, and military battles in the Indian epic literature feature chariot-borne heroes prominently. This is famously illustrated in the *Bhagavadgītā*, in which a key discourse on yoga unfolds between the warrior Arjuna and his charioteer Kṛṣṇa in the moments before battle. The language of yoga as a spiritual discipline is drawn, in part, from the language of the yoking (*yoga*) of a horse and a chariot, and the chariot becomes an important metaphoric device in elucidating philosophical principles in both Hindu and Buddhist traditions.[17]

The *brāhmaṇa* class had two overarching roles in Vedic society, the performance of domestic (*gṛhya*) and public or ordained (*śrauta*) sacrifice (*yajña*) and the interpretation and articulation of justice (*ṛta*) and law (*dharma*). These obligations continue to inform orthodox *brāhmaṇa* culture in contemporary Hindu practice and observance. During the Vedic era, priestly life was rooted in the mastery of the Vedas, which articulated the structure of priestly ritual and ideology. The Vedas are counted as four in number by contemporary Hindu traditions, though they developed sequentially over time, with the fourth Veda being composed relatively late compared to the others. It is common in early Hindu literature to see the expressions "the Three Vedas" (*vedatrayī*) and "the Threefold Knowledge" (*trayīvidyā*), which indicate that the fourth was not yet considered canonical. The Vedic corpus was ultimately compiled as the set of the Four Vedas, the *Ṛg-*, *Yajur-*, *Sāma-*, and *Atharvaveda*, which dealt with verse (*ṛc*), formula (*yajus*), song (*sāma*), and fire [ritual] (*atharva*), respectively. The *Ṛgveda Saṃhitā* is the earliest of the Vedas and the root source of the Vedic literature, as the others are largely derivative of it. Each Veda was ultimately divided into four parts, a compilation (*saṃhitā*) of verse, a priestly (*brāhmaṇa*) commentary, a forest-treatise (*āraṇyaka*), and a correspondence (*upaniṣad*) text, yielding a set of sixteen textual categories among the Four Vedas. The additional sections expanded and transformed the root text of the *saṃhitā*, providing variants upon which various priestly schools (*śākhā*) formed. In some cases, there exist more than one recension of a particular *veda*, such as the White (*śukla*) and Black (*kṛṣṇa*) variations of the *Yajurveda*. *Brāhmaṇa* traditions were characterized by the memorization of one or more of the Vedas, which were passed down orally from teacher to student, often from father to son, for hundreds of years. Students of the *veda* strove to "become" a *veda* through internalizing its text, a tradition that continues in present-day *vaidika* traditions.[18] Elaborate rules for the pronunciation and recitation of the Vedas and the performance of connected rituals helped ensure faithful transmission of these texts from generation to generation. In some *vaidika* rituals, priests are differentiated by their mastery of a particular *veda* collection and its rituals, notably the *hotṛ* with the *Ṛgveda*, the *udgātṛ* with the *Sāmaveda*, the *adhvaryu* with the *Yajurveda*, and the *brahman* with the *Atharvaveda*.[19]

Ṛṣi, Deva, Devī, Asura, Asurī

The composition of the *veda* is traditionally credited to the work of ancient seers (*ṛṣi*), who heard (*śruta*) the *veda* in a state of poetic inspiration through the power of their meditative vision (*dhī*).[20] Through this power, the *ṛṣi* came to know the forces that govern human existence in a direct way, and on that basis composed verses (*ṛc*), referred to as the "well-said" (*sūkta*), containing incantations (*mantra*) and ritual formulae (*yajus*) for aligning human life with those powers. These powers were conceived of as gods (*deva*) and goddesses (*devī*), literally "shining [ones]," and also referred to as *asura* and *asurī*, literally "incorporeal [ones]." These Vedic deities represented the forces that govern nature and human society, from fire, water, wind, earth, sun, and moon to justice, law, and sovereignty. At the head of the pantheon of the Vedic gods, sometimes enumerated as a set of thirty-three principal deities, were Agni (the embodiment of fire),

Indra (the embodiment of sovereignty), and Soma (the embodiment of the sacred extract).

The gods were viewed in the Vedic period as dwelling within a threefold structure of earth (*bhūr*), atmosphere (*bhuvas*), and heaven (*svar*), though various divisions of the three appear in Vedic texts and separate systems, including a sevenfold division, appear over time.[21] In some traditional sources, the deities of the *veda* are classified with respect to the threefold division as terrestrial (*pṛthivīsthāna*), aerial or intermediate (*antarikṣasthāna*, *madhyamasthāna*), and celestial (*dyusthāna*).[22] The terrestrial deities include Agni (fire), Pṛthivī (earth), Bṛhaspati (prayer), and Soma; the atmospheric deities include Indra, Vāyu (wind), Rudra (tempest), the Maruts (lightning), and Āpas (water); and the celestial deities include Dyaus (sky), Varuṇa (order), Mitra (sustenance), Sūrya, Savitṛ, Viṣṇu, Puṣan (sun), and Aryaman (stars).[23] Other important Vedic figures include the major deities Aditi (infinity), Prajāpati (creation), and Yama (death), and the twin Aśvin (light) gods, in addition to a range of minor deities and human sages (such as the *ṛṣi*) and heroes. The boundaries between Vedic deities are remarkably fluid, as the Vedic texts often identify them with one another and attribute similar cosmological functions and powers to various gods and goddesses. This is a precursor to classical Hindu theological conceptions in which deities are worshipped independently as representing different cosmological functions and as having particular qualities (*saguṇa*) as aspects of the ultimate nature of the divine, which is unlimited by such qualities (*nirguṇa*). Similarly, the categories of *deva-devī* and *asura-asurī* become two prototypical categories of divine typology in later philosophical and narrative contexts, in which they are portrayed as competitors for divine sovereignty and possessing distinct divine attributes.[24]

Sacrifice (*yajña*) and Worship (*pūjā*)

The ritual life of the *brāhmaṇa* in the Vedic period was centered on sacrifice (*yajña*), specifically fire sacrifice (*homa*) involving oblations (fire-offerings) to the Vedic deities, with the incantation (*mantra*) of the Vedic hymns serving as the foundation of their liturgy. Vedic priests made offerings, especially clarified butter (*ghṛta*), animals, grains, and fruit and vegetable products, into the sacrificial fire while reciting mantras invoking the various deities being worshipped and propitiated. Over time, highly structured ritual processes emerged, including a standardized ritual enclosure and sacrificial fire system, the principal permutation being the three-fire system utilized in contemporary *vaidika* practice.[25] Agni played a critical role in these sacrifices as the messenger of the gods, consuming the offerings as the "mouth" of the gods and carrying it to other deities in the form of smoke. A sacred extract (*soma*) was prepared and consumed by the sacrificers that might have originally contained a psychoactive substance derived from a plant. *Soma* has been theorized alternately to have been derived from the herb Ephedra, the mushroom *amanita muscaria*, the mountain rue *peganum harmala*, opium poppy, or *cannabis*, among other substances.[26]

Yajña had two principal forms in the Vedic context, ordained rites (*śrauta*) that were performed in public, such as the praise of Agni (*agniṣṭoma*), the coronation of a king (*rājasuya*), and the horse sacrifice (*aśvamedha*), and domestic rites (*gṛhya*), such as the investiture of the sacred thread for boys (*upanayana*) and rites of marriage (*vivāha*). The latter are examples of what are referred to as occasional (*naimittika*) and life-cycle (*saṃskāra*) rituals. These are in addition to the numerous daily (*nitya*) rites and rituals for fulfilling desires (*kāmya*) performed by the observant *brāhmaṇa*. The goals of *yajña* are represented in the Vedic literature as health, wealth, sons, and immortality, obtained through an economy of the sacred in which deities rewarded the priests and the patrons of the sacrifice as an exchange for their gifts. *Yajña* was considered a vehicle for the attainment of both worldly and otherworldly goods, the latter being a successful transition to the realms of the heavens (*svarga*) or ancestors (*pitṛloka*). The valuation of sons was tied to the patriarchal nature of Vedic society, in which sons remained in the household and inherited the family name and wealth, while women left the natal household at marriage, as is the case in much of Hinduism today. Likewise, having a son to light the father's funeral pyre at death was considered particularly auspicious, and life was conceptualized as a linear process from birth to the finality of death, in contrast to later conceptions of rebirth in *saṃsāra*.[27] Though women appear to have been principally responsible for domestic matters in the Vedic tradition, there is some indication that the wife of the sacrificer might have played an important role in the performance of *yajña*.[28]

Over time, the performance of *yajña*, especially public ordained rites (*śrauta*), faded from its central role in priestly practice, except within the isolated pockets of *vaidika brāhmaṇa* tradition, giving way to the classical *smārta* or *paurāṇika* mode of practice, in which formal rituals of worship (*pūjā*) of individual deities such as Śiva, Viṣṇu, and Devī largely took the place of Vedic *yajña*. However, the performance of *pūjā* builds on the Vedic heritage, incorporating a number of aspects of *vaidika* practice, such as the use of sacred fire and *mantra* to invoke and honor deities that are the object of worship. Adapted forms of the Vedic *yajña* ritual form continue to be performed by Vedic (*vaidika*), classical (*smārta, paurāṇika*), and tantric (*tāntrika*) priestly traditions in India, especially for life-cycle rituals and other special occasions such as the end of festivals and ceremonies.

The performance of mantra is a pervasive part of Indic religion and spirituality, and its practice is deeply rooted within the Vedic tradition. This is evident in the longevity of popular Vedic mantras such as the *gāyatrī*, which invokes the three cosmic regions and the power of the sun's effulgence to impel the mind. Similarly, popular peace (*śānti*) mantras derived from the late Vedic texts of the Upaniṣads are used to calm the mind and remove spiritual obstacles through the invocation of Vedic deities such as Indra and Varuṇa and through encouraging peaceful relations between *guru* and *śiṣya*. The performance of mantra can be understood as a contemplative as well as a ritual process, one that cultivates mental agility and intensity of concentration and aligns the human being with the cosmic forces that govern nature.[29] This is coextensive with yogic ideals of mastering the forces of embodiment and of nature such as the elements (*bhūta*) and vital air (*prāṇa*), and of union (*yoga, saṃyoga*) with divine beings that link the microcosm of the body to the macrocosm of the world. Sacrifice (*yajña*), fueled by *mantra*, allowed the Vedic priests to reconstitute and renew the world periodically, serving as a template for the development of ascetic practices that sought to reach perfection and wholeness through practices of internal or interior sacrifice.[30]

Vedic Justice (*ṛta*), Law (*dharma*), and Social Order

As a sacerdotal elite, the *brāhmaṇa* class in the Vedic tradition was central to the development and articulation of the ideological foundations of society as revealed in the *veda*. Particularly important were the notions of cosmic law and order, represented by the concepts of *ṛta* and *dharma*. The concept of *ṛta*, the earlier of the two concepts, was associated with the Vedic god Varuṇa, a sky god said to observe all of the actions of humanity from the celestial regions. Over time, the focus on the concept of *ṛta* gave way to the more expansive notion of *dharma*, which was fleshed out in later Vedic literature and in classical Hindu sources. *Dharma*, which is derived from the root √*dhṛ*, meaning "to hold," is a term comparable in some respects to the English term "religion," which, according to one prominent etymology is drawn from the Latin root √*leig*, meaning "to bind," plus the prefix *re-*.[31] *Dharma* refers to the given law, order, and structure that govern the universe and are reflected in human society. Human society was represented as having four classes (*varṇa*): priest (*brāhmaṇa*), warrior (*kṣatriya*) or ruler (*rājanya*), merchant (*vaiśya*), and servant (*śūdra*). The top three classes were eligible for initiation (*upanayana*) as twice-born (*dvija*) and thus full participation in Vedic society. The ruling (*rājanya*) or warrior (*kṣatriya*) class played a particularly important role in patronizing the ritual activities of the priestly class and served as the executive force behind the propagation of priestly ideology. In the *Ṛgveda*, the *varṇa* structure is established as part of the cosmic order in a narrative in which the world is created out of the sacrifice of a primordial person (*puruṣa*), whose body parts correlate with the structures of human society.[32] Human society is represented as being formed from the mouth (*brāhmaṇa*), torso (*kṣatriya*, *rājanya*), legs (*vaiśya*), and feet (*śūdra*) of the *puruṣa*, respectively. A separate category appears later for those who are considered outside of or non-class (*avarṇa*) members, as well as a term for foreigners (*mleccha*).

Sanātanadharma, *Varṇāśramadharma*, and *Puruṣārtha*

The priestly commentaries of the *veda* and later *dharma* literature outline class-related responsibilities, connecting the notion of *dharma* as the law or order of the universe to *dharma* in the form of human duties. The goal of *dharma*, in this respect, is the harmonious operation of society in a manner analogous to the harmonious operation of the parts of the human body. As these concepts crystallized during the classical period, they were codified in terms of the eternality of the *dharma* (*sanātanadharma*), as *dharma* for class and station of life (*varṇāśramadharma*), and in terms of goals of human life (*puruṣārtha*) known as the four divisions (*caturvarga*). These include independent notions of "men's own duty" (*svadharma*) and "women's own duty" (*strīsvadharma*), which hinge on the differentiation of men's and women's responsibilities in Vedic society. Over time, the category of class (*varṇa*) was expanded into a much more sophisticated classification system, known by the term "birth" (*jāti*), often translated as "caste." The term *jāti* communicates the conception that social identity is a function of birth, and became associated with notions of physical cleanliness (*śuci*) and purity (*śuddhi*), with *jāti* ranked in a human hierarchy capped by the supremely clean and pure deities (*deva, devī*). Classical Hindu tradition later came to associate *jāti* with conceptions of birth and rebirth, linking a person's current *jāti* with the legacy of their actions (*karma*) from previous births, a concept foreign to the earlier Vedic worldview. Priestly traditions have, at times, viewed social groups at low or non-*varṇa* and *jāti* levels as "untouchable" due to their occupation-related uncleanliness (*aśuci*) and thus impurity (*aśuddhi*). This has led members of these groups to refer to themselves as "oppressed" (Hin. *dalit*, from Skt. *dal*, "to break, to expel"), and the social reformer Mohandas K. Gandhi referred to them collectively as the "people of God" (Skt. *harijana*, Hin. *harijan*), though the latter rubric has been criticized as patronizing by *dalit* scholars and activists.[33]

Proto-Yogic Concepts and Practices in the Vedic Literature

The Vedic literature of the *brāhmaṇa* traditions represents many examples of proto-yogic concepts and practices, especially with respect to principles of ascetic self-mastery and the attainment of spiritual knowledge through visionary experiences. Among them are those that relate to facilitation of ecstatic or visionary states, including incantation (*mantra*), asceticism (*tapas*), breath control (*prāṇāyāma*), celibacy (*brahmacarya*), vow (*vrata*), station (*āśrama*), extract (*soma*), agent (*viṣa*), and herb (*auṣadhi*).[34]

Mantra

The use of incantation (*mantra*) forms a thread of practice that runs from the Vedic tradition through the history of yoga to the present. The depiction of *mantra* as the product of the visionary experiences of the Vedic sages (*ṛṣi*) demonstrates the Vedic idealization of religious specialists who gain spiritual knowledge through contemplative processes. *Vaidika brāhmaṇa* traditions utilize ritual processes as a way to engage with divine forces for the sake of worldly happiness and salvation. Similarly, the mastery of *mantra* is a means to connection, if not identification, with deities, and thereby assimilation of their powers in later yoga systems. In Pātañjala Yoga, for example, self-recitation (*svādhyāya*), a Vedic term for mantra performance, is portrayed as leading to union with one's chosen deity (*iṣṭadevatā*). In traditions of tantric yoga, *mantra* formulas, sometimes referred to in terms of support (*dhāraṇī*) or knowledge (*vidyā*), facilitate worship of and identification with divine beings and are linked to the activation of the subtle energetic centers (*cakra*) in the body. In Theravāda Buddhism, often portrayed as especially antagonistic to the Vedic heritage, particularly with respect to sacrifice, the use of formulaic chanting to preserve religious discourse (Pāli *sutta*, from Skt. *sūtra* or possibly *sūkta*) and the performance of protective chants (*paritta*) are core elements of liturgical life. The use of *paritta* in Buddhism bears significant resemblance to the use of mantras in the late Vedic text of the *Atharvaveda*, among other sources.[35]

Perhaps the most well-known example of a Vedic mantra that pervades the history and philosophy of yoga is that of the seed (*bīja*) syllable *oṃ* (*oṃkāra*, *ekākṣara*) which appears as early as the Veda Saṃhitā literature and becomes prominent in the late Vedic literature of the Upaniṣads.[36] In the Upaniṣads, *oṃ* is represented as the sonic embodiment of the ultimate nature of things, a sound that contains all sounds and represents the ultimate reality (*brahman*) that encompasses and contains all other realities. In later Hindu traditions, it is sometimes identified as the ultimate reality in the form of the "word" (*śabdabrahman*). The mantra *oṃ*, or *praṇava*, is represented in the *Muṇḍaka Upaniṣad* 2.2.4 as a bow that fires the arrow of the self (*ātman*) to the target of the ultimate reality (*brahman*). In the Pātañjala Yoga tradition, *oṃ* is represented as the word or signifier (*vācaka*) of Īśvara, the "Lord [of Yoga]," the recitation of which removes spiritual obstacles (*antarāya*) and facilitates *samādhi*. Mantra is represented in the *Yogasūtra* as being one of five principal sources for obtaining extraordinary accomplishments (*siddhi*), along with birth (*janma*), herbs (*auṣadhi*), asceticism (*tapas*), and contemplation (*samādhi*).

Tapas, *Prāṇāyāma*, and *Brahmacarya*

The term *tapas* refers to ascetic "heat," derived from the Sanskrit root √*tap*, meaning "to burn." *Tapas* is the heat or friction of self-denial and self-mortification, illustrated in its literal sense in bearing the heat of the elements through subjecting oneself to exposure to the sun or to burning fires. *Tapas* can also be linked to the Vedic notion of the purity of the sacrificial fire, signifying the force of the heat of asceticism generated within the body, with the term *tapas* possibly having an etymological link to the pain and burning of hunger endured while fasting.[37] In the early Vedic context, *tapas* operated as a method for a *brāhmaṇa* to obtain purification as a preparation for sacrifice, but was also understood to confer extraordinary power and knowledge.[38] Indian tradition contains a wide range of practices of *tapas*, including fasting, celibacy (*brahmacarya*), physical ordeals such as standing in the sun, standing on one leg, or holding one or both arms up in the air, and control or extension of the breath (*prāṇāyāma*). The empowering nature of restraint represented in *tapas* is a theme found throughout the world's religious traditions. Asceticism is rooted in a logic or economy of embodiment, in which self-discipline and self-denial strengthen spiritual faculties and remove physical and mental impurity. It also parallels the give-and-take of sacrificial ritual, in which the physical destruction of offerings yields reciprocal rewards for the individual or community performing the sacrifice.

These inner and outer modes of sacrifice come together in the conception of ritual interiorization that appears in the Upaniṣads, in which the Vedic sacrifice is seen as a template for an inner contemplative process.[39] This interiorization process is also evident with respect to the Vedic practice of *prāṇāyāma*, the control or extension of the breathing process and its vital air or energy (*prāṇa*). *Prāṇāyāma* operates first in the Vedic context as a preliminary to ritual performance, especially as a ritual means of expelling the impurity associated with unvirtuous actions. It takes on a more sophisticated role, however, in its articulation as an inner representation of Vedic ritual as the "breath-fire-sacrifice" (*prāṇāgnihotra*), providing a template for continuity between Vedic priestly practice and traditions of renunciation.[40]

The control of sexual impulses, in particular the practice of celibacy, is represented by the Vedic principle of *brahmacarya*, a term closely associated with the life of the Vedic apprentice. The logic of asceticism with respect to *brahmacarya* is that the restraint of sexual impulses leads to spiritual power, purity, and physical vitality, as well as providing the time and energy necessary to focus on religious matters. As with *prāṇāyāma*, *brahmacarya* is often represented in the Vedic tradition as a preparatory practice for ritual performance, paralleling the later prescription of *brahmacarya* as a foundation for the practice of yoga as a form of restraint (*yama*).[41]

Vrata and *Āśrama*

The Vedic concepts of vows (*vrata*) and stations (*āśrama*) similarly provided additional semantic fields for the emergence of ideas and practices of renunciation and yoga. The Vedic tradition linked moral observance, spiritual development, and social relationships together as expressions of divine order.[42] Conceptions regarding the taking of vows (*vrata*) were of significance with respect to the development of not only *brāhmaṇa*-based ascetic traditions, but also likely laid the groundwork for non-Vedic *śramaṇa* traditions, such as Buddhism and Jainism.[43] The use of *vrata* may have originally indicated an individual or communal commitment to worship of a particular deity for the sake of particular boons, a practice evident in contemporary women's practices such as the *pativrata*, that eventually evolved into renunciatory, and especially communal, vows. The related term *āśrama* is derived from the Sanskrit root √*śram*, "to strive," and refers to a place of exertion, whether that be a phase, stage, or station in life, or a physical location. The classical Hindu tradition of later centuries set various *āśrama* states, like those of the student (*brahmacārin*) and householder (*gṛhastha*), in a serial sequence, whereas in the Vedic context they were viewed as alternatives. The Vedic tradition recognized a plurality of stations (*āśrama*) of the priestly life, characterized by particular vows (*vrata*), some of which involved turning away from conventional urban life, such as the forest-dwelling *vānaprastha*. These were codified in the classical era into the stages of student (*brahmacārin*), householder (*gṛhastha*), forest-dweller (*vānaprastha*), and renouncer (*saṃnyāsin*). This plurality of roles in the late Vedic to early classical Hindu period anticipates the range of careers associated with the practice of yoga, which was adapted to suite a range of modes of religious life, including those of householder and renouncer.

Soma, *Viṣa*, *Auṣadhi*

The use of psychoactive substances in the Vedic tradition in order to inspire visionary and transformative experiences stands out as a precursor to the ecstatic dimension of yoga traditions, especially the use of herbs (*auṣadhi*) to secure spiritual accomplishments (*siddhi*) and immortality (*nirjara*). The ritual pressing and consumption of the extract of *soma* is represented in Vedic texts as stimulating vigor and ecstasy among the sacrificers, and ultimately as conferring immortality upon them in addition to producing worldly goods. Indra, one of the principal deities of the Vedic pantheon, is portrayed in Vedic texts as a drinker of *soma*, and the extract itself is referred to as a deity, called Soma. A widely known theory regarding *soma* is that it was a juice extracted from pressing the *amanita muscaria* mushroom, which contains a highly potent psychoactive compound and needs to be prepared carefully to avoid toxicity.[44] Such an association would provide a link between Vedic ritual and traditions of shamanism that utilize the *amanita muscaria* or other psychoactive mushrooms in ritual performance. However, other scholars have argued that *soma* was far more likely a product of the Ephedra plant, especially given the evidence of the relationship of the Vedic *soma* with Iranian *haoma*, the latter of which has clear associations with Ephedra.[45] Other theories, as mentioned above, have suggested a range of other psychoactive substances, including *cannabis*, *peganum harmala*, opium poppy, and *ayahuasca*-analogs. Regardless of its pedigree, the Vedic *brāhmaṇa* tradition used this extract to augment the performance of ritual, whether for the sake of inducing visionary experience or to provide extraordinary stamina during protracted ritual performances.

The use of substances to generate ecstatic states may also be indicated by the term "poison" or "agent" (*viṣa*), which appears in *Ṛgveda* 10.136, in which a "long-haired [one]" (*keśin*) consumes a presumably psychoactive-substance-infused beverage in communion with Rudra, the "howler," a fierce, and perhaps dreaded, Vedic deity. In 10.136, the *viṣa* is ritually prepared and consumed by the Keśin, who is referred to as a "silent [one]" (*muni*). The use of *soma* and *viṣa* in the Vedic context suggests that such ritually prepared beverages were represented as inducing powerful and profitable mental and physical transformations and producing extraordinary capacities of knowledge and action that anticipate those of later yogic traditions. The Vedic use of such substances can also be tied to the larger tradition of "the way of essences" (*rasāyana*), especially as associated with later alchemical and *haṭhayoga* traditions, as well as the extensive popular use of *cannabis* within Hindu renouncer traditions.[46] Though some scholars have viewed the use of psychoactive substances as an accretion, it makes more sense to view them as an integral element of yoga traditions, as they appear consistently within the sphere of yoga over time.[47] Likewise, the connections between the Vedic god Rudra and ecstatic and visionary experience carries into the classical era of Hinduism, particularly in the elevation of the deity Śiva, who is identified with the Vedic Rudra and represented as the root-guru (*ādiguru*) of tantric Hindu traditions and the systems of *layayoga* and *haṭhayoga.*

Virtuosos and Proto-Yogis in the Vedic Literature

With respect to practitioners of yoga, though the early Vedic literature does not use the explicit terminology of *yogin* or *yoginī*, a number of religious specialists in the *veda* appear as religious virtuosos and "proto-yogis." Conceptions regarding the obtaining of supernatural power and vision through ascetic and ecstatic practices are amply demonstrated in the case of these various Vedic figures. These include the Vedic "seer" (*ṛṣi*), "long-haired one" (*keśin*), "silent [one]" (*muni*), "celibate [one]" (*brahmacārin*), "restrained [one]" (*yati*), ascetic (*tapasvin*), and "avowed [one]" (*vrātya*).

Ṛṣi

The *ṛṣi* are referred to as poets (*kavi*) and serve as the paradigmatic agents of revelation in the Vedic tradition. They are credited with composing the Vedic hymns on the basis of their poetic or meditative vision (*dhī*) of the principles that govern human existence. The mantras themselves are considered nonhuman (*apauruṣeya*) in origin, in that the *ṛṣi* are capable of perceiving the Veda, but are not the creators of it.[48] The Seven Ṛṣi (*saptarṣi*) are commonly viewed as the root source of the Vedic, if not the Hindu, tradition, being the formulators of the revealed or heard (*śruti*) tradition of the Vedas, which was, in turn, passed down orally through the generations of twice-born (*dvija*) Vedic, especially priestly, families. In some cases, the name of the principal *ṛṣi* associated with a *maṇḍala* or cycle of Vedic hymns is later identified with a particular family of priests and the namesake of sages identified with the yoga tradition, such as is the case with the *ṛṣi* named Vasiṣṭha.[49] Over time, multiple categories of *ṛṣi* developed, stretching from the human to the divine, paralleling the fluidity of the boundary between the human and divine in yoga traditions. The Vedic power of poetic or meditative vision (*dhī*) anticipates the development of the renouncer soteriology of visionary experience, where the truth of things is revealed through a special form of knowledge referred to as yogic direct perception (*yoga-pratyakṣa*). It also anticipates the conception in later yoga and tantric traditions of transfiguration of a practitioner through mastery of *mantra*, leading to extraordinary accomplishments (*siddhi*) and the attainment of the status of "perfected one" (*siddha/siddhā*).

Keśin and *Muni*

The *Ṛgveda* hymn that portrays ascetic and ecstatic figures referred to as "the long-haired [one]" (*keśin*) anticipates later figurations of the yogi in a number of ways. The intentional growth of one's hair (*keśa*), often leading to matted locks, became a mark of ascetic commitment in a number of Indian traditions, being widely practiced among contemporary Hindu renouncers. It is also an iconographic element in the narrative and visual portrayal of the Hindu god Śiva, who is cast in the image of a renouncer and viewed as the patron deity of yogis. In *Ṛgveda* hymn 10.136, the *keśin* is portrayed as wearing red or yellow (*piśaṅga*) clothing, suggestive of later common forms of ascetic garb. The *keśin* is also described as being possessed by the gods, who enter his body, as riding on the wind, and as scanning the cosmos while traveling with celestial companions, *apsaras* and *gandharva*, whose minds and desires he knows.[50] The final verse of this passage describes the *keśin* consuming a poison or agent (*viṣa*) with Rudra.[51] The *keśin* is a prototype of the yogi in physical form and in terms of the range of extraordinary capacities he obtains through his asceticism and through consumption of an agent (*viṣa*). He is referred to as a sage (*muni*), literally one who practices silence (*mauna*), and an object of veneration.

Brahmacārin

The *brahmacārin* provides another Vedic model of the ascetic life that is a foundation for Indian traditions of asceticism and yoga. The *brahmacārin* is a practitioner of *brahmacarya*, a state of celibacy connected with Vedic apprenticeship. Its principal expression is the vow (*vrata*) of celibacy and self-restraint or ascetic discipline (*tapas*) of the Vedic student in training.

However, it may have also related to a particular mode of priestly practice in which a practitioner distanced themselves from conventional modes of living.[52] In the Atharvaveda, the *brahmacārin* is portrayed in cosmic terms, tapping into the generative power of the universe through *tapas* and *brahmacarya*.[53] The Atharvaveda also indicates that *brahmacarya* is a power utilized by women to attract an ideal mate, foreshadowing later classical Hindu narratives in which female ascetics attract the amorous attention of gods through the power of *tapas*.[54] *Brahmacarya* serves as a mode of preparation for the performance of Vedic ritual, anticipating the role of *brahmacarya* and *tapas* as preliminaries to the performance of yoga practice in the formal yoga systems, such as Pātañjala Yoga. Likewise, the relationship between a Vedic preceptor and the *brahmacārin* anticipates the formal teacher-student (*guru-śiṣya*) relationship that is the pedagogical basis for virtually all sectarian and many modern yoga traditions in the Indian context.

Yati, *Tapasvin*, *Vrātya*

Over the course of the development of the Vedic traditions, a number of titles came to signify ascetic practitioners and members of fraternal brotherhoods, such as the "restrained one" (*yati*), the "performer of *tapas*" (*tapasvin*), and the "vow-holder" (*vrātya*). The first two terms relate broadly to the notion of a religious path centered on self-control and self-discipline, and the third points to the notion of the observance of external vows (*vrata*) that regulate behavior within the norms of a communal identity. The Vedic traditions of the Vrātyas, or "avowed ones," have been of particular interest to scholars of Indian yoga and asceticism, as they are represented in Vedic literature as a fraternal brotherhood that existed outside of mainstream Vedic society. The brotherhood of the Vrātyas may be a precursor to communal striver (*śramaṇa*) traditions and the formation of monastic traditions.[55] The Vrātyas practiced many of the proto-yoga practices found in the Vedic tradition, notably *tapas* and *prāṇāyāma*, and demonstrated proto-tantric elements as well, such as the use of consorts in initiatory rituals.[56] The link between fraternal warrior brotherhoods and the structure of ascetic sects anticipates associations between warrior culture and yoga in the *Mahābhārata* and the development of medieval yoga traditions of warrior-asceticism in fraternal (Hin. *akhāṛā*, Skt. *akṣavāṭa)* organizations. It also anticipates the homologies of sovereignty and spiritual attainment in Jainism and Buddhism, such as the notion of Mahāvīra as a conqueror or victor (*jina*) and the symbolism of the Buddha as possessing the physical marks of a universal emperor (*cakravartin*).

The Vedic Roots of Yoga

Considerable debate persists as to whether the development of traditions of asceticism and renunciation in the Vedic tradition was the product of an organic, internal process or one that reflected the impact of external cultural and religious influences. It is clear, however, that the Vedic tradition as represented in the early Vedic literature and as practiced in living *vaidika brāhmaṇa* traditions demonstrates a range of concepts and practices that have a close relationship to systems of yoga in the late Vedic literature, the *śramaṇa* traditions, and in classical Hinduism. Among them are notions of cultivating visionary experience through psychoactive agents (*soma* and *viṣa*), the utilization of *mantra*, practices of *tapas*, *prāṇāyāma*, and *brahmacarya*, and the development of systems of vows (*vrata*) that govern social and religious life. The range of models of ascetic and virtuoso practice, including those of the *ṛṣi*, *keśin*, *muni*, *brahmacārin*, *yati*, *tapasvin*, and *vrātya*, anticipate many of the characteristics of later yogi figures, with whom these terms often become synonymous or interchangeable. Even in Buddhism, which explicitly rejects the ritualism of the Vedic heritage, there is explicit appeal to Vedic terminology with respect to notions of ascetics and yogis of old, perhaps the clearest case being that the Buddha himself is referred to as Śākyamuni, the "Sage of the Śākyas." The traditions of Brāhmaṇical asceticism and the *śramaṇa* sects of Jainism and Buddhism are built on a foundation of concepts and practices drawn from the Vedic tradition. Though they deviate in significant ways from their Vedic precursors, especially in turning away from the world-affirming views of the Vedic tradition, they nevertheless build on existing concepts and practices well documented in the early Vedic literature.

Chapter 3

Brāhmaṇical Asceticism and Śramaṇa Traditions

Early Indian renunciation can be divided into Brāhmaṇical, or *brāhmaṇa*, asceticism and *śramaṇa*, or "striver," traditions, such as Jainism and Buddhism.[1] This division represents the distinction between emergent traditions of renunciation that respectively accepted or rejected the authority of the texts, rituals, and social obligations of the Vedic tradition. Though the *śramaṇa* traditions reject many of the pillars of Vedic religion and society, they are nevertheless connected deeply to Vedic civilization and its culture and values. The historical founders of Jainism and Buddhism, Mahāvīra Vardhamāna and Siddhārtha Gautama, are represented as having been born into the ruling class (*kṣatriya, rājanya*) of Vedic society, and their respective traditions are framed by an adapted Vedic worldview. Vedic concepts such as *tapas*, *prāṇāyāma*, and *brahmacarya*, and the models of Vedic religious specialists such as the *ṛṣi*, *keśin*, and *muni* link Vedic and later Brāhmaṇical and *śramaṇa* ascetic and yogic traditions. However, the rapid emergence of renouncer movements at the end of the Vedic era raises the question of whether Indian asceticism and yoga were products of organic development within the Vedic tradition or the culmination of external influences on the mainstream of Indian religious life. One theory suggests that this emergence was the product of a late-Vedic era confluence of a northwestern Vedic civilization with distinct culture in northeastern India associated with the region of Magadha.[2] Other theories suggest a reemergence of Indus or other non-Aryan cultural influences that had been suppressed for centuries. It is very difficult to precisely date the late Vedic, Jain, and Buddhist literature and thereby determine the sequence of transmission of ideas of asceticism and renunciation among sectarian groups. However, it is clear that in the mid-first-millennium BCE the religious landscape of India was transformed by the rise of the *brāhmaṇa* and *śramaṇa* renouncer traditions that challenged the dominant *vaidika brāhmaṇa* models of religion and of society.

Within the scope of Brāhmaṇical asceticism, as discussed earlier, degrees of commitment to ascetic life varied widely, as priestly traditions provided an expanding range of lifestyle options as renunciation became increasingly validated as a legitimate approach to the religious life.[3] In the *śramaṇa* traditions, aside from some exceptional cases of world-affirmation such as that found in the "world-aimed" (*lokāyata*) school of Cārvāka, world-renunciation and asceticism were viewed as essential to liberating spiritual practice, giving rise to formal monastic orders. Brāhmaṇical ascetic and the early *śramaṇa* traditions of Jainism and Buddhism represented renunciation and yoga as facilitating liberation (*mokṣa*) from the cycle (*saṃsāra*) of birth and rebirth and as a means to achieving a range of worldly and otherworldly goods. In contrast, the *śramaṇa* Ājīvika tradition, an early competitor of Jainism and Buddhism, embraced a Stoic-like asceticism in the face of an impersonal fate (*niyati*) that would unravel to produce liberation (*mokṣa*), turning away from the emphasis on human agency in spiritual development characteristic of *brāhmaṇa* and Jain and Buddhist *śramaṇa* renouncer traditions.[4]

The Emergence of Asceticism and Renunciation in Indic Religion

One of the primary theories regarding the rapid emergence of world-renouncing ascetic traditions during the mid-first-millennium BCE is that the rapid urbanization of northern India, especially the region of the Gangetic plain, resulted in a profound cultural and religious shift away from the early Vedic worldview. According to this theory, as the Indo-Aryan people spread across northern India and settled into increasingly dense population centers, the nature of Vedic religion and culture began to change. The increasing challenges and problems of urban life may have tempered the world-affirming, and more pastoral, assumptions of Vedic life, and led to changing structures of power, wealth, and authority that upended the existing social and economic order. Brāhmaṇical asceticism and *śramaṇa* traditions represent the forest as the ideal locus for spiritual practice, suggesting the development of a city-forest dichotomy in which the latter was viewed with nostalgia and idealization. Early Buddhism appears to have utilized a monastic organizational structure closely aligned with the pre-urban tribal, as opposed to the urban and hierarchical monarchial, model of governance, suggesting a conservativism in Buddhist social thinking that may have appealed to the displaced and dispossessed.[5]

It is not difficult to imagine that the process of urbanization would have coincided with increasing concerns regarding the large-scale problem of human suffering and the emergence of a worldview in which life was viewed in cyclical terms, as an endless cycle (*saṃsāra*) of rebirth (*punarjanma*) or redeath (*punarmṛtyu*), rather than in linear terms. Knowledge of this worldview was presented in Brāhmaṇical asceticism and in the *śramaṇa* traditions as the product of an experiential knowledge obtained through contemplation. The *Bṛhadāraṇyaka Upaniṣad*, likely the oldest text in the corpus of the Upaniṣads, discusses various facets of the birth-rebirth process, indicating that by the late Vedic era, ideas of birth and rebirth were widespread and taking hold in the religious mainstream.[6] The early Vedic worldview had promised worldly happiness and a final peace at death as products of the efforts of the priestly class in the performance of ritual (*yajña*) and the discharge of social obligations or duty (*dharma*) by society as a whole. In the Vedic view, life culminated at death with entry into the realm of heaven (*svarga*) or of the ancestors (*pitṛ*). The introduction of the cyclical worldview of *saṃsāra* reconfigured the order of the universe such that the attainment of heaven was viewed an insufficient goal, a temporary state at best, with true spiritual freedom viewed as a radical rupture from or transcendence of the world. The *Muṇḍaka Upaniṣad* refers to the Vedic sacrifice as "floating unanchored," capable at best of yielding a temporary rebirth in heavenly realms that would inevitably lead to a fall from that elevated state, in contrast to the final liberation offered through knowledge of, and identity with, the highest truth. This critique may have been, in part, a reference to the state of ecstasy and immortality obtained through the performances of *soma*-ritual, suggesting that Vedic sacrifice leads to exalted but ultimately temporary achievements, which are inferior to the supreme and lasting achievements arising out of Brāhmaṇical asceticism.[7] Renouncer methodologies may have also appealed to those sated with the experience of wealth and luxury, dramatically illustrated in Siddhārtha Gautama's rejection of his palace life of pleasure for the life of renunciation.

Brāhmaṇical Asceticism in the Āraṇyakas and Upaniṣads

Brāhmaṇical asceticism builds on the principles and practices of the Vedic period, while likely borrowing elements from the non-Vedic *śramaṇa* traditions developing simultaneously. As discussed above, the four divisions of Vedic literature, or Four Vedas (*Ṛg-*, *Yajur-*, *Sāma-*, and *Atharvaveda*) were, over time, composed of four units, including a collection (*saṃhitā*), a priestly commentary (*brāhmaṇa*), a forest-treatise (*āraṇyaka*), and a correspondence-text (*upaniṣad*). These four units represent four strata of Vedic text, corresponding in sequence to the development of priestly ideas and practices over time. The earlier strata of Vedic texts, the *saṃhitā* and *brāhmaṇa*, conform most closely to the *vaidika* mode of religious practice, in which a priestly elite performs sacrifice (*yajña*) on behalf of themselves and others and establishes a social ethos centered on notions of justice (*ṛta*) and law (*dharma*). The Āraṇyaka and Upaniṣad texts represent a transition toward a new model of *brāhmaṇa* practice, one that moves incrementally toward rejecting the sacrificial model of *vaidika* tradition altogether. On this basis, in commentarial literature, the earlier sections of the Vedic texts are sometimes referred to as the branch of action (*karmakaṇḍa*) and the later sections as the branch of knowledge (*jñānakaṇḍa*).

The term *āraṇyaka* means "product of the forest," indicating an authorship outside the locus of urban civilization, intimating the movement toward the model of forest-asceticism found in the Upaniṣads. The close conceptual proximity of the Āraṇyaka and Upaniṣad literature is evident in the case of the *Bṛhadāraṇyaka Upaniṣad*, which is considered both an Āraṇyaka and an Upaniṣad.[8] The Upaniṣads, the final stratum of the Vedic literature, is referred to as the "end of the Vedas" (*vedānta*), a concept that encapsulates its philosophical principles as the furthest development of Vedic thought and practice, if not the essence of it. The term *upaniṣad* literally means "correspondence," though an alternate etymology suggests instead the expression "sit up near to," connecting the term to the transmission of teachings from student (*guru*) to disciple (*śiṣya*), a familiar trope in the Upaniṣads. The Upaniṣads successively turn away from the *vaidika* sacrificial model of the religious life toward a contemplative one in which a practitioner gains liberation (*mukti*) through a special knowledge (*jñāna*) of the ultimate reality (*brahman*). The early Upaniṣads, written between the seventh century BCE and the first century CE, articulate a range of conceptions of yoga that are increasingly organized and methodical, ultimately anticipating the development of the formal systems of yoga in the classical era. A separate set of late medieval, if not early modern, Upaniṣads, collectively referred to as the "Yoga Upaniṣads," present a variety of systems of yoga that had developed in the classical and post-classical period.[9] Many of the core concepts associated with yoga, including those of the laws of action (*karma*) and resultant cyclical existence (*saṃsāra*), the cultivation of knowledge (*jñāna*), and of the ultimate self (*ātman*) and ultimate self or reality (*paramātman, brahman*), develop in increasing sophistication over the literary arc of these Upaniṣads. Though freedom from rebirth through ascetic discipline and contemplation resulting in liberating spiritual knowledge (*jñāna*) is a primary focus of the Yoga Upaniṣads, numerous references are made to worldly attainments that can be achieved through spiritual discipline, indicating an ongoing dynamic between numinous and cessative applications of ascetic and yogic practice.

From Sacrifice (*yajña*) to Knowledge (*jñāna*)

The paradigmatic shift from a focus on *yajña* as the center of priestly and of religious life toward one in which obtaining spiritual knowledge (*jñāna*) and thereby liberation (*mukti*) is viewed as the *summum bonum* is documented in the literature of the early Upaniṣads. In the *Muṇḍaka Upaniṣad*, the sage Aṅgiras distinguishes between two types of knowledge, one higher (*para*) and one lower (*apara*), that are the foundational truths of the Vedic tradition.[10] The lower consists in the knowledge of the Vedic literature, ritual performance, and its ancillaries such as grammar and astronomy; the higher consists of the knowledge of the imperishable (*akṣara*) reality of *brahman*, the ultimate foundation of all things.[11] The Vedic rites are said to be represented by its proponents as a gateway to the heavens, in which the powers of the sun, mirroring the flames of the offering-fire, carry the ritualist up to the heaven of *brahman* as a reward for ceremonial action (*karma*). But Aṅgiras refers to these ritualists as fools, the "blind leading the blind," who do not realize that their heavenly ascent is temporary and in the end they will return again to this lower world.[12] Instead, those who live in the wilderness in a contemplative mode of existence, begging, practicing *tapas*, and cultivating peace, reach the true self (*puruṣa*) through the "door of the sun" (*sūryadvāra*).[13] The earnest student is implored to seek out a teacher rooted in the knowledge of *brahman*, and submit themselves as a disciple, establishing the *guru-śiṣya* relationship in which the teacher can impart the requisite knowledge of *brahman*.[14] This *brahman* is viewed as the source of all the structures of the universe, and the many phenomena of the world, animate and inanimate, are like sparks that fly out of a fire, only to return to their source in the end.[15] One's own self is represented as an arrow, shot from the bow of the mystical syllable *oṃ* toward the target of the imperishable *brahman*.[16] Liberation (*mukti*) is achieved through the discipline of renunciation (*saṃnyāsayoga*) in which the restrained one (*yati*) obtains immortality or "deathlessness" (*amṛta*) through the knowledge of Vedānta (*vedāntajñāna*).[17]

Methods of Yoga in the Upaniṣads

The term "yoga," used in a technical sense, appears as early as the *Taittirīya Upaniṣad*, and explicit references to practices of *pratyāhāra* and *prāṇāyāma* appear early in the *Chāndogya Upaniṣad* and *Bṛhadāraṇyaka Upaniṣad*, respectively.[18] The idea of multiple bodies or selves (*ātman*), later termed "sheaths" (*kośa*), made up or arising out of food (*annamaya*), breath (*prāṇamaya*), mind (*manomaya*), knowledge (*vijñānamaya*), and bliss (*ānandamaya*), also appears in the *Taittirīya Upaniṣad*.[19] The *Chāndogya Upaniṣad* mentions a series of channels of the heart (*hṛdaya-nāḍī*) in which contemplative processes take place, a subtle inner body accessible to a skilled practitioner.[20] The syllable *oṃ*, which appears early, but briefly, in the *Bṛhadāraṇyaka Upaniṣad*, becomes a major focus of discussion throughout the Upaniṣads.[21] The first chapter of the *Chāndogya Upaniṣad*, for example, is dedicated to the representation of *oṃ* as the encapsulation of the truth of the Vedic literature.[22] The Upaniṣads are also populated with sages whose namesakes, such as Yājñavalkya, become closely associated with yoga tradition in later eras.

Yoga appears as a formal spiritual discipline in the *Kaṭha Upaniṣad* as the "yoga of the inner self" (*adhyātmayoga*) and as a technique for the fixation of the senses (*indriyadhāraṇā*).[23] The *Kaṭha Upaniṣad* narrates a dialogue between a young *brāhmaṇa* named Naciketas and the lord of death, Yama. After Naciketas arrives in the land of the dead as a result of his *brāhmaṇa* father's careless performance of *yajña*, he receives poor hospitality and is consequently granted three wishes by Yama as atonement for the breach of etiquette. Naciketas asks for three things: release from death, knowledge and mastery of sacrifice (*yajña*) leading to exaltation, and ultimate knowledge regarding the destiny of human beings.[24] While graciously granting the first two wishes, Yama implores Naciketas to choose a different third wish, claiming that the answer is too subtle and complex for the latter to grasp. Yama insists instead that Naciketas ask for a long life, sons and grandsons, land, livestock, gold, fame, and the love of beautiful women, appealing to the slate of conventional Vedic "goods." This represents an early instantiation of a trope in Indian literature in which accomplished yogis are tempted to obtain worldly or spiritual boons at the expense of their spiritual progress.[25] Naciketas chooses, in a spirit of renunciation, to forsake the worldly goods that Yama offers and persists in his request to understand the mystery of death. Death reveals to Naciketas that the syllable *oṃ* encapsulates the collective knowledge and power of the Vedic tradition, stating that its recitation allows a practitioner to reach the underlying, immortal reality of *brahman*.[26] The self (*ātman*) is likened to a driver of a chariot made of the mind and body of person, whose purpose is to bring restraint and control of the vehicle.[27] Through control of the chariot, of mind and body, the charioteer is able to recognize the source of their manifest consciousness as the unmanifest reality of the person (*puruṣa*), the reality of *brahman*. The practice of yoga is framed as the reining-in of the senses, especially as the power to overcome distraction. The process of liberation is further represented as an ascension in which the knots (*grantha*) of the heart (*hṛdaya*) are cut and the practitioner rises through an inner channel (*nāḍī*) of the heart into a state of liberation, paralleling the structure of the subtle body (*sūkṣma-śarīra*) found in the earlier *Chāndogya Upaniṣad*.[28] At the end of the *Kaṭha Upaniṣad*, Naciketas is referred to as having received the precepts of yoga (*yogavidhi*) from Yama, and on that basis having obtained *brahman* (*brahmaprāpta*) and thus deathlessness (*amṛtyu*).[29]

In a manner parallel to the presentation of yoga in the *Kaṭha Upaniṣad*, the *Śvetāśvatara Upaniṣad* describes a yoga of meditation (*dhyānayoga*) that yields insight into the nature of divinity (*deva*), the self (*ātman*), and power (*śakti*).[30] This is understood as ultimately the realization of *brahman*, the underlying reality of all things, on the basis of knowing the self (*ātman*) and thereby becoming liberated (*mukta*).[31] The vehicle for realizing the nature of one's innermost identity is the mystical syllable *oṃ*, represented in the *Māṇḍūkya Upaniṣad* as symbolic of a mystical "fourth" (*turīya*) state of consciousness, beyond the waking, dreaming, and dreamless states. In the *Śvetāśvatara Upaniṣad*, the power of yoga is represented as the source of the power of the gods, such as Savitṛ, who brings light to the earth through his yoga, and of the poets of old, whose creative potential was realized through yoga.[32] Students are advised to hold the body steady and control the breath, senses, and mind, which are like wild horses yoked to a chariot.[33] They are also encouraged to find a place suitable for the practice, a remote and undisturbed location, and instructed to pay attention to various signs, such as visual experiences of light, that indicate proximity to success in meditation.[34] The practice of yoga is said to yield mastery of the elements; freedom from old age, sickness, and suffering; health; and physical beauty, though the ultimate goal is established as liberation from bondage through knowledge of *brahman*.[35] Later passages in the *Śvetāśvatara Upaniṣad* discuss the import of the Vedic god Rudra in his auspicious form (Śiva) as the creator and lord (*īśvara*) of creation, the cycle of rebirth (*saṃsāra*) and of liberation (*mokṣa*), paralleling the development of Śaiva theology and the intimate connection between Śiva and yoga in the Purāṇa literature of classical Hinduism.[36] The ultimate reality is said to itself manifest the yoga of power (*śaktiyoga*).[37] Several passages suggest a connection to the *yoga darśana* with respect to the utilization of the philosophical language of *sāṃkhya* dualism and the practice of dedication to the lord (*īśvarapraṇidhāna*) as a means of accelerating yogic progress in meditation (*dhyāna*).[38] The reader is admonished that Vedānta should not be taught to those who are disturbed, and only to one's sons (*putra*) and disciples (*śiṣya*), suggesting a *brāhmaṇa*-centered mode of transmission of the teachings, and that the one should have devotion (*bhakti*) to one's *guru* on a level akin to one's devotion to god.[39]

A number of concepts and practices of yoga are consolidated in detail in the *Maitrī* or *Maitrāyaṇīya Upaniṣad*, one of the last of the early

Upaniṣads. The *Maitrī Upaniṣad* introduces a concept of five forms of *prāṇa*, which are represented in the text as critical to biological processes and to the spiritual nature of embodiment.[40] In association with this, the text discusses utilizing the sacred mantra *oṃ* and pressing the *prāṇa* into the central channel (*suṣumṇā*) as a means to enter into a state of isolation (*kevala*).[41] This process is framed as depending on the use of a six-limbed (*ṣaḍaṅga*) system of yoga, including breath control (*prāṇāyāma*), withdrawal (*pratyāhāra*) of the senses, meditation (*dhyāna*), concentration (*dhāraṇā*), inquiry (*tarka*), and contemplation (*samādhi*).[42] Bondage and release is discussed in terms of the principles of nature (*prakṛti, pradhāna*) and the spiritual self (*puruṣa, ātman*), akin to the later Sāṃkhya-Yoga system, and the isolation of the self (*ātman*) is further subsumed within a Vedāntic notion of union with *brahman*.[43] As such, the *Maitrāyaṇīya Upaniṣad* provides a template for the development of "limbed" (*aṅga*) systems of yoga and for the bridging of Vedāntic and Sāṃkhya-Yoga philosophical positions in describing the liberated state.

In addition to the common focus on *mokṣa* or *kevala*, the Upaniṣads also provide numerous prescriptions for obtaining worldly power, success, and prosperity.[44] The *Bṛhadāraṇyaka Upaniṣad*, for example, offers instructions in obtaining a range of the goods of Vedic society, including the satisfaction of worldly desires (*kāma*) and obtaining sons (*putra*).[45] The *Kauṣītaki Upaniṣad* includes rites and rituals for obtaining wealth, romantic success, and protection of one's wealth and progeny.[46] Such passages demonstrate the fluidity, but also the tension, between the world of Vedic sacrifice and renunciation. This tension between worldly and other-worldly goals is demonstrated clearly in *Kaṭha* and *Muṇḍaka Upaniṣad* passages that view the goals of *vaidika brāhmaṇa* traditions as inferior to liberation. However, the recognition that ritual and ascetic acts yield power runs through the Upaniṣad literature alongside the theme of obtaining liberating knowledge of *brahman*. The concepts of *ātman*, *deva*, and *brahman* in the Upaniṣads link together the human, divine, and ultimate cosmological levels. The early and late Vedic views are also linked by the practice of approximation (*upāsanā*), a technique of internal worship and embodiment of deities developed in the Āraṇyakas and which appears frequently alongside yoga in the Upaniṣads.[47] In addition to linking the contemplation of Vedic deities in *vaidika* tradition to the contemplative traditions of Brāhmaṇical asceticism, the notion of *upāsanā* exemplifies the numinous aspect of yoga in which a practitioner assimilates the capacities of a deity through contemplation of their form and powers.

Emergence of the Śramaṇa Traditions

The fifth-to-sixth century BCE in India witnessed the emergence of a range of *śramaṇa* or "striver" traditions that challenged Vedic orthodoxy, including the Jain, Buddhist, Ājīvika, and Lokāyata traditions. Although it is difficult to determine to what degree these traditions were outgrowths of Vedic thought and practice or independently developed systems, it is clear that they aimed to set themselves apart from the Vedic tradition through polemical argument and by reinterpreting the meaning of Vedic concepts. Jainism and Buddhism developed a range of influential ascetic and yogic practices and established long-standing monastic traditions that have survived to the present. Other major *śramaṇa* groups of the late Vedic era included the Ājīvika tradition of Maskarin Gośāla (Pāli Makkhali Gosāla), associated with asceticism and fatalism, and the Cārvāka or Lokāyata tradition, which criticized moral law and doctrines of rebirth as having no basis in experienced reality. The practice of nakedness (*nagna*) was prevalent among the Jain and Ājīvika traditions, demonstrating their renunciation of householder life, and became a pervasive expression of ascetic commitments in Indian religious traditions. When Alexander entered India in 326 BCE, he is reported to have encountered what he termed "gymnosophists," literally "naked philosophers," who likely were representatives of the *śramaṇa* traditions of the time, perhaps including some *brāhmaṇa* ascetics as well.[48]

Both Vardhamāna and Siddhārtha Gautama (Pāli Siddhattha Gotama), the respective historical founders of Jainism and Buddhism, are portrayed in traditional narratives as being born into the *kṣatriya* class of Indian society. Both founders are represented as being "conquerors" or "victors" (*jina*) with respect to the religious life, and as being born with the physical marks and attributes of a universal emperor (Skt. *cakravartin*, Pāli *cakkavattin*).[49] The early Buddhist and Jain communities were, to a great extent, composed of and propagated by *brāhmaṇa* and *kṣatriya* classes, and both Jainism and Buddhism appropriate and reinterpret practical, metaphysical, and cosmological concepts from the Vedic tradition.[50] As in Brāhmaṇical asceticism, the worldview embraced by the Jains and Buddhists was of an endless cycle (*saṃsāra*) of birth and rebirth, driven by the moral quality of one's actions (*karma*). However, the Jains and Buddhists were on the vanguard of a broader critique of the efficacy and morality of the *vaidika* model of sacrifice (*yajña*) and Vedic notions of *dharma*, pressing for a more radical break from the Vedic tradition. Jainism and Buddhism offered their own models of what constitutes a *brāhmaṇa*, redefining the category in terms of the demonstration of virtue and wisdom as opposed to heredity or skill in ritual performance.[51]

Vardhamāna and Siddhārtha Gautama were likely contemporaries of the fifth-to-sixth century BCE, and though narratives suggest their disciples engaged one another, they do not indicate that the two ever met. Both founders are represented as being born under auspicious circumstances into the Vedic *kṣatriya* class of Indian society, as leaving their princely lives of luxury and pleasure to pursue renunciation, and as becoming spiritually liberated and forming a community of disciples, both monastic and lay, to propagate their teachings. Both are represented as providing teachings on spiritual liberation, framed respectively as being separated (*kevala*) from *saṃsāra* and having the passions extinguished (*nirvāṇa*). The two teachers differ, however, in their understanding of the ultimate nature of reality and the means whereby one is freed from *saṃsāra*, pain, and rebirth. The teachings and communities of these two traditions had unique durability over time and demonstrate the persistent appeal of *śramaṇa* ideas and practices. Buddhism has become one of the major world religions, having a global representation and vast following throughout Asia, and Jainism remains a regional minority religion in India, with small communities in Europe, North America, and other parts of the world.

Mahāvīra and the Jain Model of Asceticism and Yoga

The terms "Jaina," "Jain," and "Jainism" are all derived from the Sanskrit term *jina*, which means "conqueror" or "victor." This term is applied to the spiritual masters of Jainism, who are referred to as Tīrthaṃkaras, or Crossing Makers. Tīrthaṃkara and Jina are titles given to individuals who have, according to tradition, reached perfect knowledge (*jñāna*) and liberation (*kevala*). A Jina is one who has won the spiritual battle over the problem of suffering (*duḥkha*) in the form of the cycle (*saṃsāra*) of birth and rebirth. The term *jina* demonstrates the metaphorical linkages between worldly sovereignty, the domain of the Vedic *kṣatriya* or *rājanya*, and spiritual sovereignty, as exemplified by the Tīrthaṃkaras, appealing to the Vedic ideal of the universal emperor or "wheel turner" (*cakravartin*). The Tīrthaṃkaras, as such, discover the means of crossing over the ocean of *saṃsāra* to the other side, and thus liberation, in the form of separation or isolation (*kevala*) from the processes of embodied existence, particularly *karma*. The Jina or Tīrthaṃkara associated with the present historical era is Mahāvīra Vardhamāna, literally The Great Hero (*mahāvīra*) who is The Prosperous One (*vardhamāna*). It is possible that the early Jain community was a combination of a new movement associated with Mahāvīra and an older movement associated with a previous Jain teacher, Parśva.[52] Mahāvīra is considered by Jains to be the twenty-fourth in a line of Tīrthaṃkaras, or Crossing Makers, of Jainism with Parśva or Parśvanātha being the previous one, the twenty-third in the spiritual lineage. Vardhamāna's parents are sometimes represented as having been lay devotees of Parśva.[53]

The Life of Mahāvīra Vardhamāna

According to Jain tradition, as codified in the Jain Prakrit and Sanskrit *sūtra* and *āgama* literature, Mahāvīra Vardhamāna was born as a *kṣatriya* prince who renounced his worldly claims as a prince to pursue a life of asceticism, leaving for the forest and plucking out his hair from his head to begin life as a *śramaṇa* at the age of thirty.[54] It is said he lived a life of extraordinary austerity as a naked ascetic, his life punctuated by attacks by animals, insects, humans, and gods, all of which tested his ascetic self-mastery.[55] Villagers are described as cutting him, pulling his hair, throwing dirt at him, and picking him up and dropping him. He fasted assiduously, sometimes not taking water for a week or even a month, squatted in the sun, and meditated with equanimity despite the pain caused by his various ordeals. His enlightenment, as represented in the early Jain text of the *Ācārāṅgasūtra*, which came after a period of thirteen years, as he sat squatting in the mid-day sun near a tree and a river and having fasted without water for two and a half days, exemplifies the intensity of his austerities that culminated in his achievement of liberating knowledge (*kevala-jñāna*).[56] This liberating knowledge is described in the

Kalpasūtra as being omniscience of all things and their conditions, the modes of existence of humans, gods, animals, and hell-beings and their thoughts and deeds, and an understanding of the processes of bondage and liberation.[57]

Having achieved *kevala*, Mahāvīra is referred to as being a Victor (*jina*), a Worthy One (*arhat*), a Separated One (*kevalin*), and after his death is referred to as a Perfected or Accomplished One (*siddha*), a Liberated One (*mukta*), and an Awakened One (*buddha*).[58] Mahāvīra's awakening became the basis upon which a fourfold society, or conjunction (*tīrtha*) of monks (*sādhu*), nuns (*sādhvī*), laymen (*śrāvaka*), and laywomen (*śrāvikā*), was constructed (*kara*) in order to propagate his teachings.[59] According to one of the major traditions of Jainism, shortly after his enlightenment Mahāvīra gave a discourse on nonharming (*ahiṃsā*) to a group of *brāhmaṇa* engaged in the performance of sacrifice (*yajña*), which yielded the first of a series of converts from the priestly tradition referred to as the *gaṇadhara*. These would be among the first of a great number of conversions to Jainism, and by the time of Mahāvīra's death at the age of seventy-two, the community numbered in the hundreds of thousands, according to tradition.[60] Over time, the community split into two principal sectarian factions, the naked or "sky clad" (*digambara*) and the "white clad" (*śvetāmbara*), in part based on different understandings of the nature of the Tīrthaṃkara and questions regarding whether Jain monks should wear clothing. In the model established by Mahāvīra, monks and nuns are to practice an idealized mode of life, supported by a lay community that gains merit (*puṇya*) through providing for the monastic community, building temples, and constructing icons.[61] Laypeople also practice devotion toward the monastic community and toward the Tīrthaṃkaras and other sacred beings within the sphere of Jain narrative through worship (*pūjā*), thus making merit (*puṇya*) and inspiring spiritual practice.[62]

At the center of the narrative of Mahāvīra's liberation is the principle of *ahiṃsā*, "nonharm" or "nonviolence," which has an intimate relationship to the process of obtaining release from the bonds of *karma* and existence in *saṃsāra*. These are encapsulated in the three jewels (*ratnatraya*) of Jainism, namely true insight (*samyak-darśana*), right knowledge (*samyak-jñāna*), and right conduct (*samyak-cāritra*), which later becomes a basis for organizing Jain yoga practice.[63] At the foundation of Mahāvīra's realization is the view that all living things, not only animated bodies but also subtle beings dwelling in inanimate elements, possess a soul, or *jīva*, which is caught up in the fourfold world of birth (as a god, animal, human, or hell-being) due to the material burden of action (*karma*) produced in this life and previous lives. In this framework, one's *karma* leads to the accumulation of substance, and ultimately embodiment, for the *jīva*, and liberation consists in restraint of all action, especially that which results in the harm (*hiṃsā*) of living creatures. Escape from *saṃsāra* is secured by those who are able to perfectly restrain all *karma*, both good and bad, and endure pain and hardship, thereby attaining a state of complete mastery over mind and body in which liberating knowledge (*kevala-jñāna*) arises. The methods for accomplishing this include the observance of vows (*vrata*), the practice of ascetic discipline (*tapas*), and the practice of meditation (Prakrit *jhāṇa*, Skt. *dhyāna*, Pāli *jhāna*). These methods are, over time, subsumed in Jainism under the umbrella of the term *yoga* (Prakrit *joga*) in a manner analogous to the ways in which ascetic and contemplative techniques are systematized in Hindu and Buddhist traditions.

Yogic Principles and Practices in Early Jainism

A set of principles and practices inform the early Jain tradition that provide a framework of yogic discipline foundational for Jainism and broader Indian traditions of asceticism and yoga. The concept and practice of nonviolence or nonharm (*ahiṃsā*) is linked to the process whereby the cycle of rebirth (*saṃsāra*) is overcome, along with four other vows (*vrata*) that extend from the observance of *ahiṃsā*. Another major proto-yogic element in early Jainism is the systematic practice of asceticism (*tapas*), especially disciplines of self-restraint and self-mortification, which the Jain monastic tradition exemplifies in its various austerities. The practice of meditation (Pkt. *jhāṇa*, Skt. *dhyāna*) provides a link between Jainism and the Buddhist and Brāhmaṇical ascetic traditions. Later Jain philosophers establish a conception of progressive spiritual development referred to as the "stages of virtue" (*guṇasthāna*), which are linked to a systematic practice of yoga as a method of progressing through the sequence.[64]

Ahiṃsā and *Vrata*

The principle of nonharm (*ahiṃsā*), often translated as "nonviolence," roots the Jain worldview in a social and environmental ethic. As the causing of harm (*hiṃsā*) to other beings is the central karmic force behind continued misery in *saṃsāra*, the restraint of harm, especially killing, of living beings is at the forefront of Jain practice. The harm of *hiṃsā* is not only of others, but ultimately of oneself in the inhibition of one's capacity to achieve *mokṣa*.[65] Two of the principal expressions of *ahiṃsā* in Jainism are vegetarianism and the avoidance of occupations involving the harm of living creatures. Vegetarianism is observed strictly in Jain traditions, requiring the abstinence from the consumption of meat and from sweet, fermented, and multiple-seed fruits and vegetables, the latter group associated with higher concentrations of *jīva*.[66] Extending out of *ahiṃsā* are four other restrictions, each in turn associated with a the vow (*vrata*) to restrain oneself: truthfulness or nonlying (*satya*), nonstealing (*asteya*), sexual restraint (*brahmacarya*), and nongreed or nonpossessiveness (*aparigraha*). This set of five vows are developed into a twofold system of observance, in which monastic practitioners observe a "great vow" (*mahāvrata*) and laypeople observe a "lesser vow" (*aṇuvrata*), that condition the application of the vows to different modes of living. This parallels, if not prefigures, the discussion of the five restraints (*yama*) in Patañjali's system, in which the *mahāvrata* signifies an ideal mode of practicing self-restraint, not limited by situation.[67] The fivefold structure of *vrata* in Jain and Hindu traditions also parallels the Buddhist Five Precepts (*pañcaśīla*), which act as a Buddhist *śramaṇa* ethic applicable to lay and monastic life. The practice of *ahiṃsā* has a reflexive role in all of these traditions as facilitating the development of insight into the nature of the world and being supported by the understanding of the world that is the result of such insight.

Tapas

The practice of asceticism (*tapas*) in Jainism demonstrates the fluidity of the boundary between Vedic and *śramaṇa* worldviews and the manner in which *śramaṇa* traditions transformed Vedic ideals. Passages in Jain literature indicate that they viewed the *tapas* or "heat" of austerity to be greater than the *tapas* of the sacrificial fire, adapting the Vedic language of sacrifice to interpret, but also elevate, the ascetic model of self-transformation.[68] Among various practices that exemplify Jain asceticism are extended periods of fasting and self-mortification, embodied by the so-called "practitioner of the extended penance" (Pāli *dīgha-tapassī*, Skt. *dīrgha-tapasvin*), the extraordinary intensity of which distinguishes Jain practices from those of Hindu and Buddhist traditions.[69] The Jain repertoire included the use of uncomfortable postures (Pkt. *āsaṇa*, Skt. *āsana*), such as the squatting position that Mahāvīra is represented as having utilized in pursuit of liberation, and the immobile standing posture commonly depicted in representations of the Jinas, as well as the observance of vows of silence (*mauna*). As an expression of world-renunciation, Tīrthaṃkaras are portrayed as being naked, a practice emulated among monastic practitioners of the Jain Digambara sect. Jain *tapas* is said to be uniquely productive, and is contrasted in its superior quality to that of even esteemed Hindu ascetics such as Vasiṣṭha.[70] External forms of *tapas* in Jainism are complemented by the development of inner attitudes and formal meditation (*jhāṇa*) practice as methods of disciplining of mind. As with the Vedic tradition, *tapas* is viewed in Jainism as a basis for the attainment of extraordinary powers. These powers are illustrated in narratives of Mahāvīra's life that portray him as engaged in magical battles with Brāhmaṇical ascetics and his former disciple, Makkhali Gosāla (Skt. Maskarin Gośāla), the founder of the Ājīvika tradition.[71]

Jhāṇa

The Prakrit term *jhāṇa* (Skt. *dhyāna*, Pāli *jhāna*) refers to the cultivation of meditative states in service of the process of liberation. Early Jain scriptural references to a "bright" or "pure" meditation (Pkt. *sukka-jhāna*, Skt. *śukla-dhyāna*) indicate notions of a purified state of mind accessible through the practice of meditation.[72] *Śukla-dhyāna* is presented in some contexts as being preceded by *dharma-dhyāna*, meditation on the nature of reality (*tattva*) that provides the foundation for *śukla-dhyāna*.[73] Mahāvīra's experience of enlightenment is described in the *Uttarapurāṇa* an achievement of perfect knowledge (*jñāna*) and (*darśana*) within deep meditation (*jhāṇa*) supported by the external austerities of fasting, exposure, and posture. *Jhāṇa* is characterized by an inner stillness that arises at the culmination of the release of mental and physical *karma* and withdrawal from sensory experience.[74] *Jhāṇa* is an excellent example of the continuity between practices of *tapas* and those understood within the rubric of "yoga." *Jhāṇa*, as such, represents an inwardly focused disciplining of the senses and the mind as a counterpart to the outer disciplining of the body.

The Development of Buddhism and the Buddhist Path (*mārga*)

As with the terms *jina* and *tīrthaṃkara* in the Jain tradition, the term *buddha* is a title given in Buddhism to a person who knows the true nature of the world, achieves liberation, and proceeds to teach the truth to others. *Buddha* literally means "Awakened One," and more figuratively "Enlightened One." As an Awakened One, the Buddha is represented as having achieved liberating insight through overcoming ignorance and mistaken views, the former being likened to the lack of awareness of the world during sleep and the latter comparable to the fantasies and illusions of dreaming. As an Enlightened One, the Buddha has overcome the darkness of ignorance through attaining the light of knowledge (*jñāna*) or wisdom (*prajñā*). Gautama Buddha (Pāli Gotama Buddha), who is also referred to as the Sage of the Śākyas (Skt. Śākyamuni, Pāli Sakkamuni), is considered the historical founder of Buddhism. However, he is not unique in his spiritual achievements, having been preceded by previous Buddhas and to be succeeded by those of the future. The state of Buddhahood is viewed as the summit of spiritual accomplishment in Buddhism, as a Buddha possesses unexcelled spiritual capacity. Gautama Buddha is referred to in Buddhism as a Victor (*jina*), as a Worthy One (Skt. *arhat*, BHS *arhant*, Pāli *arahant*), as the Blessed One (*bhagavat*), and as Thus Gone (*tathāgata*) and Well-Gone (*sugata*), terms used to refer to other Buddhas as well. A person striving toward Buddhahood, such as the prince Siddhārtha Gautama before his awakening, is referred to as an Awakening Being (*bodhisattva*). Disciples of the Buddha who have realized the truth of the Buddha's teachings and have achieved freedom from the cycle (*saṃsāra*) of rebirth are also given the title of *arhat*, even if they have not achieved the spiritual capacity characteristic of a fully awakened *buddha*. Buddhist traditions recognize three principal levels of attainment, that of a Fully Awakened One (*samyaksaṃbuddha*), a nonteaching or Solitary Awakened One (*pratyekabuddha*), and a Hearer (*śrāvaka*) or disciple who achieves liberation through receiving a Buddha's teachings. As with Mahāvīra, the representation of the historical Buddha is connected to the symbolism of the universal emperor (*cakravartin*), and symbols of royalty such as the umbrella, the chariot wheel, and elongated earlobes (a result of adornment with heavy jewelry) are associated with the Buddha in his capacity as a "spiritual monarch." Buddhist traditions differ in their degree of focus upon human (*manuṣyaka*) characteristics of the historical Buddha versus the transcendent (*lokottara*) capacities associated with the state of Buddhahood. Narratives of the life of the historical Buddha, found in Pāli *sutta* literature (3rd–5th century BCE) and in later Sanskrit narratives, such as the *Divyāvadāna* (1st–2nd century CE), the "Divine Achievements," and the *Buddhacarita*, the "Acts of the Buddha," of Aśvaghoṣa (1st–3rd century CE), portray the historical Buddha's life as both human and extraordinary in nature.

The Life of the Buddha

The Buddha's conception is marked by his mother Māyā having an auspicious dream that featured a white elephant, a symbol of fortune and royalty.[75] His mother subsequently gives birth to Siddhārtha Gautama while standing up and supported by the branch of a tree, upon which he emerged from her side, echoing miraculous births of previous heroes. After his emergence, he is said to have taken seven strides, with lotuses blossoming under his footsteps, and declared that he had been born for the last time and would achieve liberation.[76] Other narrated events in the early life of Siddhārtha Gautama include a prediction by a sage, Asita, that he would either become a great king or a great sage, based on markings on his body; his mother Māyā dying and his being raised by his aunt, Prajāpatī; his mastery of various sports; his marriage to the princess Yaśodharā; and his father Śuddhodana's shielding of him from the miseries of the world inside his palaces. The turning point in his life narrative takes place when Siddhārtha travels outside the palace on a chariot ride and sees the so-called Four Sights (*caturnimitta*): a sick man, an old man, a corpse, and a *śramaṇa*. This formative experience with the truth of suffering (Skt. *duḥkha*, Pāli *dukkha*) is said to have motivated Siddhārtha to follow the *śramaṇa* path in hopes of finding a solution to the problem of suffering. He leaves the palace and his wife and, in some versions, his newborn son, cuts off his hair, and takes on the garb of a *śramaṇa*. In some variants of the story, the gods are portrayed as ensuring the exposure of Siddhārtha to *duḥkha* and assisting him in escaping the confines of the palace upon his renunciation.[77]

Siddhārtha is said to have proceeded to study meditative practices of withdrawal from worldly experience, cultivating the states of nothingness (*ākiṃcanyāyatana*) and neither-perception-nor-non-perception (*naivasaṃjñānāsaṃjñāyatana*) with teachers Ārāḍa Kālāma (Pāli Aḷāra Kālāma) and Udraka Rāmaputra (Pāli Uddaka Rāmaputta). He quickly mastered these states, ultimately being asked by the teachers to assist in propagating their systems, but Siddhārtha identified such achievements as only a temporary reprieve from suffering (*duḥkha*) and not a solution to it. He subsequently turned to asceticism (*tapas*), joining a group of five ascetics (*pañcavargika*), his body withering away due to his intensive fasting, forceful breath control, and exposure to the elements. Upon reaching the threshold of death, he comes to the conclusion that his death through ascetic austerities will not secure the goal of release from suffering (*duḥkha*). Instead, he turns toward the Middle Way (Skt. *madhyamā-pratipad*, Pāli *majjhimā-paṭipadā*), recognizing the relationship between physical health and mental acuity, turning away from self-mortification. This can be interpreted as a rejection of the intense austerities of the Jains and Ājīvikas, where such intense self-mortification, including fasting unto death, were a part of ascetic culture.[78]

Turning away from the practice of self-mortification, Siddhārtha took a bowl of rice porridge from a cowherd named Sujātā or Nandā, and with a nourished body and revitalized spirit continued his quest. Sitting down at the foot of a tree and having vowed to not leave the spot until he reached liberation, he entered into a succession of states of meditation (Skt. *dhyāna*, Pāli *jhāna*), utilizing his breath in a manner he had discovered as a child. As the full moon rose, he entered into deep contemplation (*samādhi*), and on that basis achieved a sequence of extraordinary perceptions, including his former lives, the coming and going of beings throughout *saṃsāra* in accordance with their *karma*, and the causal processes that undergird *saṃsāra*. In some versions of the narrative, Siddhārtha was also forced to overcome the god of death and desire, Māra or Yama, who attempted to prevent Siddhārtha from achieving liberation through force and temptation. In one variant, Siddhārtha defeated Māra by touching the earth, which testified to the merit he had accrued over the course of lifetimes, a gesture codified in the common representation of Gautama Buddha in earth-touching gesture (*bhūmisparśamudrā*). Siddhārtha is said to have achieved liberation (*nirvāṇa*) as the sun rose on a new day, becoming the Awakened One (*buddha*), a Worthy One (*arhat*), a Victor (*jina*), and a Thus-Gone One (*tathāgata*), having reached a noetic confidence that he had achieved his goal.

Following his awakening, the Buddha is said to have traveled throughout northern India for approximately forty years propagating his teaching and building a community of followers, using demonstrations of his extraordinary powers and didactic methods to inspire faith and wisdom. Around the age of eighty, he achieved final liberation (*parinirvāṇa*), entering into meditation and passing away. His body was cremated, and his remains were divided and distributed, some preserved in relic domes (*stūpa*). The relics of the Buddha and his disciples continue to be among the principal material objects of veneration in Buddhist traditions throughout the world today and are often enshrined in Buddhist domes (*stūpa*) and temples (*vihāra*).

The *Dharma* and *Saṃgha*

As was the case for Vardhamāna Mahāvīra, Gautama Buddha quickly established a community of monks, nuns, laymen, and laypeople, beginning with his teaching to pious householders and the five ascetics he had previously associated with. The foundation of Buddhist society was the community (*saṃgha*), of monks and nuns, the ideal (*ārya*) subcommunity being those who have achieved the status of *arhat* (Pāli *arahant*). The Buddha's first discourse, which encapsulates the basic principles of his teaching, is referred to as the "Discourse of the Turning of the Wheel of the Dharma" (Skt. *dharmacakrapravartanasūtra*, Pāli *dhammacakkappavattanasutta*). The Buddha's teaching, doctrine, or law (Skt. *dharma*, Pāli *dhamma*) is represented by the paradigmatic Four Noble Truths (*caturāryasatya*): the truth of suffering (*duḥkha*); the truth of the origination of suffering (*samudaya*); the truth of the cessation of suffering (*nirodha*); and the truth of the eight-limbed or eightfold path (*aṣṭāṅgamārga*) to the cessation of suffering. The Noble Eightfold Path provides a step-like, but recursive, methodology for obtaining spiritual progress and ultimately cessation (*nirodha*), which includes correct (*samyañc*) view (*dṛṣṭi*), resolve (*saṃkalpa*), speech (*vāc*), action (*karmānta*), livelihood (*ājīva*), effort (*vyāyāma*), mindfulness (*smṛti*), and contemplation (*samādhi*).[79] The term *dharma* encapsulates both the sense of the Buddha's teaching or doctrine as reflective of the law, order, or truth of the universe and the idea that the teaching is a call to action, toward both what is to be known and what is to be done.

The Eightfold Path is a method for obtaining cessation (*nirodha*) and liberation (*nirvāṇa*), but also is a basis for a mode of living in which a practitioner gains merit (*puṇya*) and avoids demerit (*apuṇya*), the former of which ripens (*vipāka*) and comes to fruition (*phala*) as favorable life experience and rebirth in fortunate realms of rebirth. Like the Jain and Brāhmaṇical ascetics, the early Buddhists viewed *saṃsāra* as having numerous modes of rebirth. These included rebirth as a high *brahmā* deity in remote realms (*loka*) of subtle form (*rūpa*) and formlessness (*ārūpa*), or as a more tangible form in the realm of desire (*kāma*), including the realms of the gods (*deva*), demigods (*asura*), humans (*manuṣya*), animals (*tiryañc*), hungry ghosts (*preta*), and hell-beings (*nāraka*). Among the forms of rebirth in the desire-realm (*kāmaloka*), the first three were considered fortunate and the others unfortunate modes of rebirth, though birth as a demigod (*asura*) was sometimes considered unfortunate as well. In the paradigm of early Buddhist practice in India, monastic practitioners lived an idealized life of study and meditation, while laypeople provided the material support necessary for them to do so, as well as offering their devotion and reverence to the Buddha and his followers. As in Jainism, monastic practitioners accumulate merit through meditation, teaching, moral restraint, and providing opportunities for laypeople to serve them, and laypeople earn merit through their generosity (*dāna*), pious behavior, and moral restraint. Additionally, the practice of meditation (*dhyāna*) serves as a vehicle for monastics and pious lay practitioners to obtain merit (*puṇya*) as well as having the function of purifying the mind and facilitating liberating insight (Skt. *prajñā*, Pāli *paññā*).

The entirety of the Buddhist tradition is often summed up in the concept of the Three Jewels (*triratna*) of Buddhism, which represents a triad at the heart of Buddhist practice, namely the Buddha, the Dharma, and the Saṃgha (Pāli *saṅgha*). Over time, the Buddhist community divided into a number of sects and schools, of which two primary sectarian traditions have survived to the present, the "Teaching of the Elders" or Theravāda tradition, sometimes referred to as "Southern Buddhism," geographically represented in Sri Lanka, Burma, Thailand, Cambodia, and Laos, and the

"Great Vehicle" or Mahāyāna tradition, which correlates as "Northern Buddhism" and is geographically represented in Nepal, Tibet, Mongolia, China, Vietnam, Korea, and Japan.

Yoga in the Early Buddhist Tradition

The term "yoga" appears infrequently in the early strata of Buddhist literature, so it is important to be cognizant of the ways in which the term is being applied retroactively.[80] The terms *yoga* and *yogin* appear more frequently in later Theravāda literature such as the *Milindapañha* and *Visuddhimagga* and in the emergent literature of Mahāyāna Buddhism. Yoga as "yoking" can refer to bondage, in the sense of being yoked to "unwholesome" mental or physical states, and to spiritual application, in the sense of being yoked to the "wholesome."[81] With respect to the latter, the *Dhammapada* refers to paths of wisdom and loss of wisdom, the first being the path of yoga and the other of non-yoga (*ayoga*), contrasting a commitment to worldly distractions with commitment to yoga.[82] A verse from the Theragāthā, the "Songs of the Elders," refers to the application of yoga as the practice of concentrative (Skt. *śamatha*, Pāli *samatha*) and insight (Skt. *vipaśyanā*, Pāli *vipassanā*) meditation.[83] In the *Buddhacarita*, yoga is referenced as a restraining of sense activity and a calming of the mind, echoing the Upaniṣadic formulation of yoga.[84] Those focused on applying the teaching of the Buddha, or examining its principles, are referred to in Pāli by the term *dhammayogin*, in contrast to those whose focus is deep concentration (*jhāyin*), both exemplifying aspects of yogic practice.[85] The idea of yoga as intellectual application may further be connected to the notion of yoga in the larger philosophical traditions of India, such as the Nyāya, where *yoga* refers to an intellectual focus or contemplation of ideas.[86] The concept of yoga, however, is most typically applied to those meditators who are actively pursuing direct and liberating insight through the practice of *bhāvanā*, or mental cultivation, specifically practices that calm (*śamatha*) and concentrate the mind and those that cultivate insight (*vipaśyanā*).

As with Jainism, Buddhist contemplative practices are situated within a framework of ethics (*śīla*) as integrated into the Buddhist path (*mārga*) in the form of the Three Trainings (*triśikṣā*) of wisdom (*prajñā*), ethics (*śīla*), and contemplation (*samādhi*). The development of the Buddhist path is associated with the five faculties (*pañca-indriya*) of faith (*śraddhā*), vigor (*vīrya*), mindfulness (*smṛti*), contemplation (*samādhi*), and wisdom (*prajñā*). Faith or confidence (*śraddhā*) in the teachings of the Buddha are the basis for developing the vigor (*vīrya*) necessary to pursue the cultivation of mindfulness (*smṛti*), contemplation (*samādhi*), and wisdom (*prajñā*).

Mārga, Vrata, Triśikṣā

The Noble Eightfold Path provides a structured mode of living that aims to secure liberation, favorable rebirth, and communal harmony. The three trainings in wisdom (*prajñā*), ethics (*śīla*), and contemplation (*samādhi*) encapsulate the idea of embodying the Buddha's wisdom through restraint of action and purification the mind. This is in line with a popular passage from the *Dhammapada* that states the Buddhist path can be summed up as "not doing evil, enjoining the good, and purifying of one's mind."[87] In Theravāda Buddhism, monks and nuns can also choose a deliberately austere life as an option in Buddhist monasticism, a practice formalized as the "limbs of removal" (Pāli *dhutaṅga*, Skt. *dhūtaguṇa*), which consist of thirteen additional observances to monastic life, including control of diet and posture.[88] The Threefold Training and Eightfold Path contain a principle of mutual relationship, in which the strengthening of one member of the series is said to strengthen the others. A calm mind makes it easier to realize the truth and to abstain from harmful actions, for example. As training in wisdom (*prajñā*), the first two members of the Eightfold Path, right view (*dṛṣṭi*) and right resolve (*saṃkalpa*), are the foundation of the Buddhist path, a baseline orientation to the world and to practice. The training in ethics (*śīla*) encompasses speech (*vāc*), action (*karmānta*), and livelihood (*ājīva*), and is exemplified by the five precepts (*pañcaśīla*), which include nonkilling, nonstealing, nonlying, not performing sexual misconduct, and not consuming intoxicants. These vows are founded on the principle of *ahiṃsā*, sharing a foundation with the Jain and Hindu yoga traditions. The training in contemplation (*samādhi*) includes the three factors of effort (*vyāyāma*), mindfulness (*smṛti*), and concentration (*samādhi*), which aim to cultivate skillful states of mind and to uproot unskillful ones. The cultivation of states of meditation (Skt. *dhyāna*, Pāli *jhāna*), which leads to deep contemplation (*samādhi*) and serenity (*śamatha*), is complemented by examination of the nature of mind, body, and world through the cultivation of insight (*vipaśyanā*). Though having different applications, *śamatha* and *vipaśyanā* utilize similar processes, such as mindfulness (*smṛti*) and recollection (*anusmṛti*).

Paritta

In Theravāda Buddhism, monastic practitioners perform a formalized style of chanting or recitation referred to as "protection" (Pāli *paritta*, Skt. *paritrāṇa*). *Paritta* recitation serves as one of the primary ritual activities performed by monastic communities in Southeast Asian Theravāda communities, marking special occasions from festival observances and public ceremonies such as weddings and funerals to the consecration of temples and rituals of healing and exorcism.[89] The texts chanted as *paritta* are largely drawn from the Theravāda Buddhist canon, especially the Nikāya literature, with some common examples being the *Aṅgulimālasutta*, the *Mettāsutta*, and the *Maṅgalasutta*, along with specific *Jātaka* stories.[90] *Paritta* recitation demonstrates a parallelism with the performance Vedic *mantra*, especially as prescribed in the *Atharvaveda*, in that it is seen as having a powerful effect in averting evil and creating auspicious circumstances. It is also viewed as a means of gaining spiritual merit (Skt. *puṇya*, Pāli *puñña*). *Paritta* may be used to empower physical objects, such as amulets, through the contact between sound and the item.[91] Though not conceived as soteriologically efficacious, the use of *paritta* is understood to enliven the mind with the energy of the particular *paritta* used. The recitation of the *Mettāsutta*, for example, is said to charge the mind with a divine power of "loving-kindness" or "friendliness" (Pāli *mettā*, Skt. *maitrī*), transforming the practitioner and the environment around them.[92]

Bhāvanā and *Śamatha*

The practice of mental cultivation (*bhāvanā*) in Buddhism is systematized in early Buddhism as a dialectic between the development of a concentrated and serene mind (Skt. *śamatha*, Pāli *samatha*) and the development of reflective insight (Skt. *vipaśyanā*, Pāli *vipassanā*) into the component factors (Skt. *dharma*, Pāli *dhamma*) of mind and body. Both forms of meditation have at their root the practice of mindfulness (*smṛti*), which supports both the one-pointed practice of *śamatha* and the reflective and analytical process of *vipaśyanā*. Mindfulness reins in awareness, whether it be directed toward one object, such as the breath, or as an observation of or reflection on the moment-by-moment transformations of mind and body. *Śamatha* was organized into a system of practices that aimed to reduce mental affliction and develop increasingly subtle states of meditation (*dhyāna*), absorption (*samāpatti*), and contemplation (*samādhi*). Some objects were understood to serve as powerful antidotes (*pratipakṣa*) for specific unskillful cognitive and emotive states.[93] Meditation on the breath, for example, might be prescribed for those with an over-sabundance of conceptual thought, and meditation on friendliness or loving-kindness (Skt. *maitrī*, Pāli *mettā*) might be prescribed for those afflicted by anger. The principal set of forty *śamatha* meditation objects, "action-bases" (Skt. *karmasthāna*, Pāli *kammaṭṭhāna*), found in early Buddhist configurations of *śamatha* included ten earth and color devices (Skt. *kṛtsna*, Pāli *kasiṇa*); ten forms of foulness (*aśubha, asubha*); ten recollections (*anusmṛti, anussati*), including those of the Buddha, Dharma, Saṃgha, ethics (*śīla, sīla*), generosity (*dāna*), deities (*deva*), death (*maraṇa*), body (*kāya*), breathing (*ānāpāna/prāṇāpana, ānāpāna*), and peace (*śānti, santi*); the four immeasurable (*apramāṇa, appamāṇa*) states of loving-kindness (*maitrī, mettā*), etc.; four immaterial meditation subjects (*ārūpa*); the loathsomeness of food (*āhāre pratikūla-saṃjñā, āhāre paṭikkūla-saññā*); and the four elements (*caturdhātuvyavasthāna, catudhātuvavaṭṭhāna*). Practices such as the recollection of the Buddha (Skt. *buddhānusmṛti*, Pāli *buddhānussati*) and of deities (*devānusmṛti, devānussati*) aimed to cultivate faith in the power of virtuous beings and to facilitate the assimilation of their spiritual capacities. The practice of the four altruistic attitudes, referred to as the immeasurable (Skt. *apramāṇa*, Pāli *appamāṇa*) states or as the divine abodes (*brahmavihāra*), facilitated the cultivation of four principal emotive states, friendliness or loving-kindness (Skt. *maitrī*, Pāli *mettā*), compassion (*karuṇā*), sympathetic joy (*muditā*), and equanimity (*upekṣā, upekkhā*). The cultivation of these four altruistic emotive attitudes is common to Jain and Hindu yoga traditions as well, demonstrating the pervasive significance of the practice in Indian contemplative traditions.[94]

Meditation (*dhyāna*) and Absorption (*samāpatti*)

Meditation (*dhyāna*) is framed as requiring the overcoming of five chief hindrances (*nīvaraṇa*) or obstacles to concentration in the untrained mind, which include doubt (*vicikitsā*), sloth and indolence (*styānamiddha*), restlessness and remorse (*auddhatyakaukṛtya*), and fantasies of pleasure (*kāmacchanda*) and violence (*vyāpāda*). With the suppression of these hindrances, the factors of meditation (*dhyāna*) arise and the meditator is said to enter into access concentration (*upacāra-samādhi*), establishing pliancy (*praśrabdhi*) of mind that makes it more serviceable for the sake of meditation and virtuous life.[95] The progression of development concentration is viewed in terms of a succession of subtle and powerful *dhyāna* states. The root factors of *dhyāna* include applied thought (*vitarka*), sustained thought (*vicāra*), bliss (*prīti*), happiness (*sukha*), and one-pointedness (*ekāgratā*). As the first *dhyāna* is mastered, the mind becomes increasingly quiet and focused, eventually giving way to successively deeper states of concentration, namely the second, third, and fourth *dhyāna* states. These are characterized by moving from highly blissful but unstable early *dhyāna* states toward more peaceful, stable, and equanimous later *dhyāna* states, the latter exemplified by the *dhyāna*-factor of equanimity (*upekṣā*) that appears in the fourth *dhyāna*. Some schools of Buddhism postulate a series of states of subtle immaterial (*ārūpya*) absorption (*samāpatti*) that can be contrasted with the material (*rūpya*) attainments of the four *dhyāna* states, and an additional state of complete meditative cessation (*nirodha*) of all mental functioning in addition to the eight *dhyāna* and *samāpatti* states. The immaterial attainments reflect the assimilation of practices associated with the Buddha's former teachers, Ārāḍa Kālāma and Udraka Rāmaputra, into the Buddhist system.[96] The function of *śamatha* as defined in Buddhist literature is to purify the mind of defilements and thereby facilitate the cultivation of liberating insight. This is exemplified by the Buddha's attainment of the powerful, serene, and unwavering mind of the fourth *dhyāna* as a basis for his meditative insight into the root causes of the cycle (*saṃsāra*) of rebirths, namely dependent co-origination (*pratītya-samutpāda*), that led to his awakening.

Abhijñā

Śamatha meditation is closely connected in Buddhism to the development of forms of "higher knowledge" (*abhijñā*), which are extraordinary powers of action and perception obtained through mastery of *dhyāna* and *samādhi*. The view that *dhyāna* leads to heightened capacities is illustrated in the narrative of the Buddha's awakening, in which he attains knowledge of his former lives, knowledge of the structure and nature of the cosmos, and knowledge of the causal processes of *saṃsāra* on the basis of achieving the fourth *dhyāna* state. Buddhist sources list six *abhijñā* capacities: the divine eye (*divyacakṣus*), the divine ear (*divyaśrotra*), knowledge of other's minds (*paracittajñāna*), knowledge of former lives (*pūrvanivāsānusmṛti*), preternatural accomplishments (*ṛddhi*), and knowledge of the destruction of the outflows (*āsravakṣayajñāna*). The first two point to the numinous aspect of yogic practice, as they explicitly represent the attainment of the perceptual capacities of a divine (*divya*) being. Knowledge of others' minds and magic-like abilities (Skt. *ṛddhi*, Pāli *iddhi*), which include creating multiple images of oneself and flight, similarly correlate with divine forms of agency. The meditator in higher *dhyāna* states is also said to achieve mental states characteristic of the *brahmā* deities in the form and formless realms.[97] The Buddha and his disciples are portrayed in narrative literature as utilizing various powers in service of propagating the *dharma*, though within monastic practice such demonstration was restricted due to the potential to confuse audiences about the goals of Buddhist practice.[98] Buddhist literature suggests that only Buddhist practitioners are able to accomplish the final *abhijñā*, the ending of the outflows (*āsrava*), which requires insight into the nature of bondage and affliction.[99]

Vipaśyanā and *Smṛtyupasthāna*

Unlike *śamatha*, which is viewed as used by both Buddhists and non-Buddhists as a means to bring about serenity and concentration, *vipaśyanā* is viewed as capable of leading to cessation (*nirodha*) and the extinction (*nirvāṇa*) of the fire of the passions.[100] *Vipaśyanā* is practiced for the sake of experientially validating the Buddha's teaching through insight into the nature of mental and physical objects of awareness.[101] The meditator is said to come to know the three marks (*trilakṣaṇa*) of phenomena, namely suffering or unsatisfactoriness (*duḥkha*), impermanence (*anitya*), and non-self (*anātman*) and that there are three poisons (*triviṣa*) or great afflictions (*mahākleśa*) that are the unskillful roots (*akuśalamūla*) of suffering (*duḥkha*), namely, desire (*rāga*), aversion (*dveṣa*), and delusion (*moha*). One of the key formulations of *vipaśyanā* as represented in the early Pāli *Satipaṭṭhānasutta* focuses on four categories or "foundations" of mindfulness (Skt. *smṛti*, Pāli *sati*), namely, body (*kāya*), feelings (*vedanā*), mind (*citta*), and mental objects (Skt. *dharma*, Pāli *dhamma*). The functioning of mindfulness (Skt. *smṛti*, Pāli *sati*) in the context of the practice of insight (*vipaśyanā*) is augmented by the utilization of clear comprehension (Skt. *saṃprajanya*, Pāli *sampajañña*), an attitude of self-reflection that complements the more intensive work in seated or walking meditation. The conception that *vipaśyanā* is a necessary part of the Buddhist soteriological vehicle demonstrates its focus on the development of liberating insight as opposed to simply the suppression of thought and action. Liberating knowledge and wisdom (*jñāna, prajñā*) is understood to effect a moral as well as a spiritual transformation, in that the roots of affliction that produce harmful behavior are destroyed. One who has reached the level of Arhat or Buddha becomes an exemplar of wisdom and virtue, one in whom spiritual and ethical transformation are inseparable.

Ārya-pudgala

The Theravāda tradition holds that the attainment of liberating insight into mind and body yields four successive states of spiritual attainment among Hearers (*śrāvaka*) of the teachings of the Buddha, who are referred to as "noble persons" (*ārya-pudgala*). The first level of attainment is that of the Stream Winner (*srotāpanna*), whose insight is so great they will no longer be reborn into lower destinies and will achieve the state of *arhat* within seven lives. The second level of attainment is that of the Once Returner (*sakṛdāgāmin*), who will be reborn as a human once before obtaining *arhat* status. The Non-Returner (*anāgāmin*) will be reborn in a divine realm inhabited by virtuous deities, where they will attain *arhat* status. Lastly, the Worthy One (*arhat*) cultivates liberating insight within his or her lifetime and will not be reborn again. Beyond the *śrāvaka* level of attainment, some will reach the level of a Buddha's knowledge but not teach others, becoming a Solitary Buddha (*pratyekabuddha*). Other practitioners may become an Awakening Being (*bodhisattva*), vowing to achieve a state of complete Buddhahood (*samyaksaṃbuddha*), the highest attainment. In the Buddhist discourses, Gautama Buddha predicts the coming of a future Buddha named Maitreya (Pāli Metteyya), "The Friendly One," who is described as currently residing in the Tuṣita heaven where Buddha Śākyamuni lived in his penultimate life. Maitreya will thus be reborn in the human realm, reach awakening, and teach the *dharma* in a future age. Gautama is portrayed as one in a series of Buddha figures, alternately as seventh or as twenty-fourth, the former enumeration being parallel to the Vedic conception of the Seven Ṛṣi (*saptarṣi*) and the latter to the twenty-four Tīrthaṃkara.[102]

The Politics of *Śramaṇa* Asceticism: The Mauryan Empire

The founders of the Jain and Buddhist traditions are represented in narrative literature as having received support and patronage from many of the political leaders of the time among the *kṣatriya* class of Vedic society. These include such notable figures as the kings Bimbisāra, Ajātaśatru, and Presenajit, who were represented in traditional accounts as becoming avid supporters of these traditions. The transformation of Jainism and Buddhism from grassroots regional movements to politically powerful pan-Indian traditions accelerated during the period of the Mauryan Empire (321–185 BCE), particularly under the emperors Chandragupta Maurya (340–298 BCE) and his grandson Aśoka (302–232 BCE). Though considerable scholarly debate persists regarding the personal religious commitments of these two Mauryan emperors, the Jain and Buddhist traditions view them as having brought the *śramaṇa* ethos into the mainstream of Indian society. In the wake of Alexander the Great's invasion of the Indus valley in 326 BCE, Chandragupta Maurya unified northern India into the first large-scale Indian empire, perhaps under the tutelage of Kauṭilya, the author of the *Arthaśāstra*, the Sanskrit "Treatise on Politics," a work often compared to Machiavelli's *The Prince*.[103]

Jain tradition holds that Chandragupta Maurya was a great patron of Jain art and culture, ultimately abdicating his throne to become a Jain monk and passing away through the practice of *saṃlekhanā*, or fasting unto death.[104] His grandson, Aśoka, is represented in Buddhist literature as having converted to Buddhism after a series of bloody battles in the region of Kaliṅga in eastern India that were critical in his consolidation of the Mauryan empire.[105] In the wake of his conversion to Buddhism, he is held to have embraced the principle of *ahiṃsā*, setting up edicts throughout India on pillars in which he encouraged his subjects to embrace the values of the Buddhist *dharma*, and to have built numerous monuments (*stūpa*) to entomb the relics of the Buddha and Buddhist saints. He is also credited with sending a Buddhist mission to Sri Lanka and for convening an important Buddhist council at the city of Pāṭaliputra that established orthodoxy within the Indian Saṅgha. The Mauryan empire left a profound impact on the legacy of India's religious heritage through the elevation of *śramaṇa* traditions to a central place in Indian society and through the propagation of Buddhism beyond India in the early centuries BCE. The *śramaṇa* practice of renunciation and the social ethic derived from it became a core component of the Indian worldview, as did notions of *saṃsāra* and of *mokṣa*, framing the way that religious life was understood in the centuries, if not millennia, that followed.

Chapter 4

The Classical Hindu Model of Yoga

Pātañjala Yoga and *Aṣṭāṅgayoga*[1]

The Vedic period of Indian civilization (1500–500 BCE), gave way to the rise of *śramaṇa* traditions and a sociopolitical order that led to the expansion of Jainism and Buddhism to the scale of pan-Indian traditions. During this latter period, the priestly traditions of Hinduism shifted from the Vedic (*vaidika*) model of religious practice toward a model focused on religious narrative tradition (*paurāṇika*) and a larger body of "remembered" (*smṛti*) literature, notably *sūtra* and *śāstra* works. The *paurāṇika* or *smārta* (*smṛti*-based) model of *brāhmaṇa* culture shifted Hindu practice toward a theism of personal gods, such as Śiva, Viṣṇu, and Devī, and away from the Vedic pantheon, which was assimilated within the narratives and theologies of the "great" gods and goddesses represented in the *smṛti* literature. The *smārta* model also developed elaborate textual traditions of narrative, ritual, law, and contemplation, with *vaidika* concepts and practices being absorbed into, or reinterpreted, within *smārta* practice, providing continuity within the *brāhmaṇa* model. In the elaborate *itihāsa-purāṇa* (epic and narrative) literature, in the "*dharma* discourse" (*dharmasūtra*) and "*dharma* treatise" (*dharmaśāstra*) literature, and in the *sūtra and śāstra* literature of yoga, a new model of priestly practice emerged that integrated theism, emergent social ideologies, and renouncer techniques and traditions. By the early centuries of the Common Era, the *smārta brāhmaṇa* model was being championed by powerful regimes such as the Guptas and Vākāṭakas, who built their political structures within a priestly religious and ideological framework.[2] Though these empires were pluralistic, in the sense of tolerating a diversity of traditions including Buddhists and Jains, they nonetheless signaled the elevation of Hindu priestly traditions to a privileged position in the machinations of political and cultural life.[3] *Vaidika* traditions of *brāhmaṇa* practice continued to be patronized as well, though their influence continued to fade over the course of the early centuries of the Common Era, relegating them to a limited regional representation over time. Among the priestly texts characteristic of the *sūtra* literature of the early centuries of the Common Era is the influential *Yogasūtra* attributed to Patañjali (3rd–5th century CE), which serves as the foundation of a larger textual tradition referred to as the *Pātañjalayogaśāstra*. Patañjali's work consolidates ideas and practices of yoga that extend out of Brāhmaṇical asceticism, the *śramaṇa* traditions, and the emerging *smṛti* literature, signaling the emergence of classical Hindu narrative, thought, and practice with respect to yoga. Patañjali's *Yogasūtra* provides one of the first dedicated attempts to define and systematize the theory and practice of yoga in Hindu literature, and its presentation of the eight-limbed yoga (*aṣṭāṅgayoga*), in particular, provides one of the most coherent and influential models of yoga in India's history, becoming one of the chief expressions of the authoritative practice of yoga throughout the Indian tradition.[4]

The *Yoga Darśana*

The *yoga darśana*, or "yoga view," also called Yoga Philosophy, Pātañjala Yoga, Sāṃkhya-Yoga, or simply Yoga, is commonly represented as one of the principal Indian and Hindu philosophical systems. The Indian *darśana* systems are sometimes counted as six in number, especially with respect to the Hindu systems of philosophy that emerged in the late Vedic and early classical era, out of the Vedic and *smṛti* literature. The term *darśana* literally means "view" or "viewpoint," as derived from the verbal root √*dṛś*, "to see," and is often translated into English as "philosophy" or "philosophical system." The Indian *darśana* systems were focused on the nature of the truth or principles (*tattva*) of reality and the nature of valid knowledge (*pramāṇa*) and the means to it, the latter including direct perception (*pratyakṣa*), inference (*anumāna*), and verbal authority (*śabda*), among others.[5] The viewpoints included within a commonly cited "six system" (*ṣaḍdarśana*) set included the philosophy of Vedic ritual, termed Examination (*mīmāṃsā*) or Prior Examination (*pūrva-mīmāṃsā*); the philosophy of the Upaniṣads, termed the End of the Vedas (*vedānta*) or Later Examination (*uttara-mīmāṃsā*); Enumeration (*sāṃkhya*); Discipline (*yoga*); Logic (*nyāya*); and Categories (*vaiśeṣika*). In this scheme, the six schools are linked together in dyadic pairs, given the import of the principles of the former in the formulation of the latter, as *mīmāṃsā-vedānta*, *sāṃkhya-yoga*, and *nyāya-vaiśeṣika*. Though yoga is typically thought to be particularly relevant to the first two pairs, the term *yoga* as a "discipline" or an "application" of mind to a subject has also had relevance within the contexts of *nyāya-vaiśeṣika* and may have appeared as a technical term in those systems very early on. The concept of the *ṣaḍdarśana* is one among a number of classification systems of Indian philosophy, as the field in India has historically been highly varied and complex. Schools of philosophy are additionally categorized whether they affirm (*āstika*) or reject (*nāstika*) the authority of the Vedas. Medieval and modern philosophical traditions accepted a wide range of different viewpoints. The Vedānta philosopher Mādhava analyzed sixteen *darśana* traditions, including schools of grammatical philosophy and Śaiva sectarian traditions.[6]

Patañjali and the *Yogasūtra*

The *yoga darśana* is often referred to as being "Patañjali's Yoga" (*pātañjala-yoga*), due to the long-standing association between the author-compiler Patañjali and the philosophical framework and practical instruction on yoga given in the *Pātañjalayogaśāstra*, which is composed of the *Yogasūtra* and its principal commentary, the *Yogabhāṣya*. The *Yogasūtra* is also referred to as the "Instruction on Yoga" (*Yogānuśāsana*), in part based on its self-referencing of that rubric in its opening verse. According to some of its commentators, the Pātañjala Yoga system is also linked to a figure known as Hiraṇyagarbha, "The Golden Embryo," a name associated with the Hindu creator deity, Brahmā, and with conceptions of a primordial deity that precedes or transcends creation, such as *brahman*.[7] In the *Mahābhārata*, the formulation of the Yoga system is associated with Hiraṇyagarbha, and Sāṃkhya with the sage Kapila.[8] The text of the *Yogasūtra* itself suggests that

"The Lord" (*īśvara*) is a special or distinct (*viśeṣa*) self or soul (*puruṣa*) that is free from bondage, having been the *guru* of yoga since time immemorial, thus providing a divine origin to the system. The primary commentary (*bhāṣya*) to the *Yogasūtra* mentions a *guru* of yoga taking the form of the "Highest Ṛṣi" (*paramarṣi*) in order to teach a figure named Āsuri. This links yoga to Āsuri's teacher, the sage Kapila, who is, in turn, linked to Hiraṇyagarbha and to the Hindu deity Viṣṇu.[9] The first verse of the *Yogasūtra*, "now, instruction on yoga" (*atha yogānuśāsanam*), is commonly interpreted as indicating that Patañjali was a codifier or compiler of an existing yoga tradition and not the creator of the system.

Patañjali's background outside of the *Yogasūtra* is largely unknown, though some scholars have theorized he may have been a Sāṃkhya philosopher aiming to integrate Brāhmaṇical ascetic and Jain and Buddhist *śramaṇa* practices within the framework of the Sāṃkhya philosophy.[10] It is also possible that Patañjali was a *yogin* himself and the head of an order of *brāhmaṇa* ascetics, though textual and archeological evidence of a lineage of Pātañjala-yogis is limited at this time.[11] Patañjali as the author or compiler of the *Yogasūtra* has been traditionally identified with the Hindu grammarian Patañjali, the author of the *Mahābhāṣya*, which is the principal commentary to the Sanskrit grammar (*vyākaraṇa*) of Pāṇini, the *Aṣṭādhyāyī*. Patañjali has also been traditionally identified as the author of the *Carakapratisaṃskṛta*, a commentary on Caraka's work on *āyurveda*, linking together a larger theme in which Patañjali is associated with treatises on *yoga*, *vyākaraṇa*, and *āyurveda*.[12] These connections are represented in invocatory verses associated with the *Pātañjalayogaśāstra*, in which Patañjali is lauded as the author of treatises on yoga, grammar, and medicine. Though scholars have often dismissed the identification of Patañjali the grammarian with Patañjali the philosopher on text-historical grounds, it is nevertheless worth noting the import of the notion of the polymath as an Indian scholastic ideal.[13] This ideal frames the representation of Patañjali as a master of the ancient Indian "sciences" of mind (*citta*), language (*śabda*), and medicine (*cikitsā*).[14]

Hindu tradition further identifies Patañjali as an incarnation or manifestation (*avatāra*) of the "Serpent-King" (*nāgarāja*) known as Ādiśeṣa, "Primordial Remainder," or Ananta, "Endless One," a deity intimately associated with the god Viṣṇu.[15] The narrative of the *Patañjalicarita* (17th century CE), or "Acts of Patañjali," relates a story in which Patañjali descends from heaven to answer the prayers of the daughter of a sage (*munikanyā*) named Goṇikā, ultimately falling (*pat*) from her prayerfully folded hands (*añjali*).[16] Material representations of Patañjali, many of which resemble a well-known representation of Patañjali at the Chidambaram temple in Tamil Nadu, portray Patañjali in the form of a *nāga*, with a serpentine lower half, a human head and torso, multiple arms, and flanked by a many-headed cobra hood.[17] An association between contemplation and the figure of the *nāga* is not unique to Pātañjala yoga, as Buddhist and Jain narratives also associate ascetic mastery and the manifestation of *nāga* figures, the latter of which represent mastery over the elements and hidden knowledge.[18] Like those of Patañjali, Buddha and Tīrthaṃkara figures are often flanked by the hoods of a many-headed *nāga*, as are those of popular Hindu deities, such as Śiva and Viṣṇu.

Patañjali's audience appears to have been *smārta brāhmaṇa* practitioners of either limited or varied sectarian affiliation, given the lack of sectarian indicators in the text and commentaries. The expansive commentarial tradition associated with the *Pātañjalayogaśāstra* and the referencing of the *aṣṭāṅgayoga* system in the Purāṇa literature and medieval Vedānta and *haṭhayoga* systems demonstrate that the principles and practices developed in Pātañjala Yoga were adapted to fit various sectarian and philosophical molds. The *Yogasūtra* can be viewed as an expression of a genre of Hindu texts centered on a pithy narrative or thread (*sūtra*) of a discourse, intended to be explicated through oral and textual commentary, like the thread of a necklace or of a rosary might be adorned with beads or flowers. As such, the *Yogasūtra* can be compared to other examples of *sūtra* discourse such as the *Kāmasūtra*, the discourse on pleasure (*kāma*), which aims to elucidate the pursuit of *kāma* as a goal of human life (*puruṣārtha*). The *Yogasūtra*, similarly, might be considered to elucidate the *puruṣārtha* of liberation (*mokṣa*) as represented by the Pātañjala Yoga notion of liberation as separation (*kaivalya*). The root text (*sūtrapāṭha*) of the *Yogasūtra* is 195 verses, broken down into four parts (*pāda*), dealing with contemplation (*samādhipāda*), practice (*sādhanapāda*), powers (*vibhūtipāda*), and liberation (*kaivalyapāda*). There is considerable scholarly disagreement as to whether the *sūtrapāṭha* is a unitary single-author text or a compilation of texts from either one or several authors developed over time.[19]

The *Yogabhāṣya*, the "Explanation of Yoga," or simply the *Bhāṣya*, "Explanation," attributed to Vyāsa is the principal commentary to the

Yogasūtra. Given that the *Yogasūtra* does not appear to be represented in manuscripts independent of the *Yogabhāṣya*, and textual colophons refer to them as a unit, the two texts together are often designated as the *Pātañjalayogaśāstra*.[20] It is unclear how proximate the composition of the *Yogabhāṣya* was in time to the *sūtrapāṭha*. Some scholars believe that the *Yogabhāṣya* may have been an autocommentary composed at the same time that the *sūtra* verses were authored or compiled.[21] The name associated with the *Yogabhāṣya*, Vyāsa, can be interpreted as a generic term meaning "compiler" or as designating an appeal to the authority of the Indian sage Veda-Vyāsa, the revered compiler of the Vedas and the Indian epic of the *Mahābhārata*, whose name bears considerable weight. Other scholars have suggested that the Vyāsa of the *Yogabhāṣya* might have been a Sāṃkhya philosopher, such as Vindhyavāsin, who aimed to frame the yoga discourse as an expression of Sāṃkhya philosophy in order to compete with contemporaneous Buddhist and other non-Vedic traditions, such as Jainism.[22]

In addition to the *Yogabhāṣya* of Vyāsa, important commentaries to the *Yogasūtra* include the *Yogasūtrabhāṣyavivaraṇa*, "Uncovering the Commentary on the *Yogasūtra*" (9th century CE) attributed to Śaṅkara, also referred to as the *Pātañjalayogaśāstravivaraṇa*, Vācaspati Miśra's *Tattvavaiśaradī*, "Clarity on the Truth" (9th century CE), Bhoja Rāja's *Rājamartaṇḍa*, "Royal Sun" (11th century CE), and Vijñānabhikṣu's *Yogavārttika*, "Exposition on Yoga" (16th century CE). Translations and commentaries of the *Yogasūtra* have historically appeared in diverse linguistic and cultural contexts, including in Arabic and Persian literary worlds and in Southeast Asia, in addition to numerous modern editions, with variations in the English language playing a critical role in the development of the discourse of anglophone yoga in global and cosmopolitan traditions.[23]

Foundations of Pātañjala Yoga

The connections between Pātañjala Yoga and Vedic *brāhmaṇa* traditions are evident in common practices such as physical and mental cleanliness (*śauca*), ascetic self-discipline (*tapas*), and the performance of self-recitation (*svādhyāya*). Practices of posture (*āsana*), breath control (*prāṇāyāma*), and sense withdrawal (*pratyāhāra*) similarly demonstrate linkages between Patañjali's work and the late Vedic literature of the Upaniṣads. A number of concepts and practices found in the epic and narrative (*itihāsa-purāṇa*) literature significantly predate their development in the formal yoga literature, perhaps even the notion of an eight-part practice of yoga.[24] The practice of meditation (*dhyāna*) as described in the *Pātañjalayogaśāstra* can be connected conceptually with the concept of *dhyānayoga* found in the Upaniṣads, but also closely parallels Buddhist *śamatha* meditation practice in a number of ways. The moral commitments of Pātañjala Yoga, which are framed as forms of restraint (*yama*), parallel Jain concepts of the *aṇuvrata* and *mahāvrata* and the larger *śramaṇa* emphasis on the principle of nonviolence or nonharm (*ahiṃsā*). The formulation of suffering (*duḥkha*) and its resolution through the eight-limbed yoga (*aṣṭāṅgayoga*) that is detailed in the *Yogasūtra* parallels the relationship between the Four Noble Truths and Eightfold Path in Buddhism.[25] Patañjali's formulation of yoga represents a priestly synthesis of knowledge, especially of Hindu, Jain, and Buddhist philosophy, which was a part of an emerging *smārta brāhmaṇa* paradigm in which various fields of knowledge were consolidated into *sūtra* literature in order to establish priestly authority over them.[26]

The *Yogasūtra* draws heavily upon the Sāṃkhya tradition of philosophy, its counterpart within the six-system (*ṣaḍdarśana*) framework of Hindu philosophy, and manuscript colophons refer to the *Pātañjalayogaśāstra* as an "explanation of Sāṃkhya" (*sāṃkhyapravacana*). Elements of Sāṃkhya thought appear in the early Upaniṣads, including the *Bṛhadāraṇyaka*, *Chāndogya*, and *Kaṭha Upaniṣad*, and it is linked to the practice of yoga in its early appearances in the Itihāsa-Purāṇa literature, especially in the Mokṣadharma section of the epic *Mahābhārata*.[27] Drawing on the metaphysics of Sāṃkhya, Pātañjala Yoga philosophy proposes a basic ontological duality between person (*puruṣa*) and nature (*prakṛti*) as the basis for bondage to and liberation from *saṃsāra*. The *puruṣa* is known as the perceiver (*draṣṭṛ*), consciousness (*citi*), and master (*svāmin*) in relationship to *prakṛti*, which is what is perceived (*dṛśya*) and the basis (*pradhāna*) of material reality. *Prakṛti* is viewed as existing in a process of flux or change (*pariṇāma*), in which its three primary characteristics or qualities (*guṇa*) of luminosity (*sattva*), energy (*rajas*), and inertia (*tamas*) shift dynamically. The levels of the *guṇa* factors within *prakṛti* extends from an unmanifest or unmarked (*aliṅga*) state, through a manifest state (*liṅgamātra*), to an indistinct state (*aviśeṣa*), and finally to a distinct state (*viśeṣa*). Out of the movement from subtle (*sūkṣma*) to gross (*vyakta*) states of *prakṛti* emerge the mind (*manas*), sense organs (*indriya*), and gross or concrete elements (*bhūta*). Sāṃkhya and Pātañjala Yoga share the conception that nature (*prakṛti*) is the source of mental and material reality but distinct from consciousness, which is the unique power of the spiritual person (*puruṣa*).[28] The root of bondage in *saṃsāra* is an ignorance (*avidyā*) of reality that leads to misidentification of *prakṛti* as *puruṣa*, which results in the rise of afflicted (*kliṣṭa*) and unafflicted (*akliṣṭa*) modes of action (*karma*) that plant the seeds of future existence. These seeds are the residue (*āśaya*) of karmic impressions (*saṃskāra*) left in the mind that form the basis for future life conditions. Ignorance (*avidyā*) is the root cause of the other afflictions, which include egoism (*asmitā*), attachment (*rāga*), aversion (*dveṣa*), and clinging-to-life (*abhiniveśa*). These afflictions manifest in the form of emotive states (*vāsanā*) that color experience and instigate further afflictive action. Liberation (*mokṣa*), conceived of as isolation or separation (*kaivalya*), consists in the discernment of the difference between *prakṛti* and *puruṣa*, which is facilitated by the meditative refinement of the cognitive faculties. The goal is cognitive cessation or suppression (*nirodha*) in which the *puruṣa* dwells in its own nature, no longer bound by the conflation of *puruṣa* and *prakṛti* by the mind.

Practices of Pātañjala Yoga

Patañjali states in the second verse of the *Yogasūtra* that yoga is the "cessation of the fluctuations of mind" (*cittavṛttinirodha*). When this is accomplished, the person (*puruṣa*) or seer (*draṣṭṛ*) abides in its own-form (*svarūpa*), which is distinct from body and mind.[29] Yoga is defined in terms of two disciplines, the first being the yoga of action (*kriyāyoga*), which is comprised of ascetic discipline (*tapas*), self-recitation (*svādhyāya*), and dedication to the lord (*īśvarapraṇidhāna*), which are prescribed to support the cultivation of contemplation (*samādhi*) and to attenuate affliction (*kleśa*).[30] The components of *kriyāyoga* are, in turn, subsumed within the rubric of the eight-limbed yoga (*aṣṭāṅgayoga*), which includes the factors of restraint (*yama*), observance (*niyama*), posture (*āsana*), breath control (*prāṇāyāma*), sense withdrawal (*pratyāhāra*), fixation (*dhāraṇā*), meditation (*dhyāna*), and contemplation (*samādhi*).[31] *Yama* is broken down into five factors: nonharm (*ahiṃsā*), truthfulness (*satya*), nonstealing (*asteya*), sexual restraint (*brahmacarya*), and nongreed (*aparigraha*). Likewise, *niyama* has five factors: cleanliness (*śauca*), contentment (*saṃtoṣa*), asceticism (*tapas*), self-recitation (*svādhyāya*), and dedication to the lord (*īśvarapraṇidhāna*).[32]

Kriyāyoga

The section on practice (*sādhanapāda*), part two of the *Yogasūtra*, begins with a presentation of the Yoga of Action (*kriyāyoga*), which includes *tapas*, *svādhyāya*, and *īśvarapraṇidhāna*, which represent the successive purification of body, speech, and mind.[33] *Kriyāyoga* is portrayed as attenuating affliction (*kleśa*) and as supporting the cultivation of *samādhi*. The rootedness of *tapas* in the Vedic and *śramaṇa* contexts is evident in its role in physical and mental purification and its use as a preparation for the internal limbs of practice. In the *Yogabhāṣya*, Vyāsa describes *tapas* in terms of bearing hunger and thirst, environmental extremes, the use of standing postures (*sthānāsana*), and restraint (*mauna*) of speech and gesture.[34] It is also associated with the observance of ascetic vows (*vrata*).[35] *Svādhyāya* has roots in Vedic practices of mantra recitation that facilitated the *brāhmaṇa* practitioner's mastery and embodiment of a particular aspect of the Vedic corpus. *Svādhyāya* is said in the *Yogasūtra* to result in union (*saṃprayoga*) with one's chosen deity (*iṣṭadevatā*), paralleling both Vedic conceptions of vision and approximation (*dhī*, *upāsanā*) and classical notions of devotion (*bhakti*) toward a deity with attributes (*saguṇa*).[36] In the *Yogabhāṣya*, *svādhyāya* also includes a commitment to the study of treatises on liberation (*mokṣaśāstra*) and the recitation (*japa*) of *praṇava* (*oṃ*).[37] In the *sūtrapāṭha*, Patañjali links the recitation of *praṇava*, the mantra *oṃ*, to the practice of *īśvarapraṇidhāna*, as the "word" (*vācaka*) that expresses the nature of the Lord (*īśvara*), a *puruṣa* who has never been caught up in the process of *saṃsāra* who serves as an impetus and archetype for the aspiring yogi.[38] Īśvara is referred to as unbound by time and the *guru* of time immemorial, containing the seed (*bīja*) of omniscience (*sarvajñā*), a concept familiar within *śramaṇa* traditions. *Īśvarapraṇidhāna* is akin to later conceptions regarding devotion (*bhakti*) to a formless deity without attributes (*nirguṇa*), as opposed to *bhakti* oriented to deity with attributes (*saguṇa*), which could be likewise correlated with *svādhyāya*. In later centuries, the presence of Īśvara in Pātañjala Yoga was a point used to distinguish it from Sāṃkhya, with Pātañjala Yoga being understood as Sāṃkhya-with-Īśvara (*seśvara-sāṃkhya*).[39] Some modern scholars have argued that the presence of Īśvara in Patañjali's system may have been a concession to the emerging popular theistic traditions of Hinduism.[40] However, given that *īśvarapraṇidhāna* is seen as uniquely efficacious as a practice in the *Yogasūtra* and is a prominent part of later, particularly the Purāṇic, accounts of *aṣṭāṅgayoga*, this is a thesis that deserves critical scrutiny.[41] Similarly, the view of Sāṃkhya as an exclusively atheistic system may be, in part, a more recent and revisionist view of its past.[42]

Aṣṭāṅgayoga

The *Mahābhārata* contains a reference to an eight-virtue yoga (*aṣṭaguṇayoga*) that may predate *aṣṭāṅgayoga* of the *Yogasūtra*, but the passage itself does not clearly indicate what the eight *aṅga* are.[43] The *Carakasaṃhitā*, an important early text of *āyurveda*, includes an eight-aspect program of mindfulness (*smṛti*) in its section on the discipline of yoga, and medical texts more broadly used the terminology of *aṣṭāṅga* quite extensively.[44] Perhaps the most direct association that can be made with respect to the use of the *aṣṭāṅga* rubric is between Patañjali's system and the Buddhist conception of the eight-limbed or eightfold path (*aṣṭāṅgamārga*). Verses 2.15–29 of the *Yogasūtra* appear to paraphrase the Four Noble Truths of Buddhism, culminating in a discussion of the *aṣṭāṅgayoga*.[45] It is also possible that the use of the term "eight" (*aṣṭa*), as with "four" (*catur*), simply served a heuristic purpose as a mnemonic device for remembering oral teachings.

The *aṣṭāṅgayoga* framework may have also been preceded by the development of the *ṣaḍaṅgayoga* of the *Maitrāyaṇīya Upaniṣad*, which bears a strong resemblance to Patañjali's system. Variations on this *ṣaḍaṅgayoga* system appear in a variety of Indian sources, including the Purāṇas, mainstream sectarian literature, Hindu and Buddhist tantric literature, *haṭhayoga* texts, and the Yoga Upaniṣads. The larger concept of "yoga limbs" (*yogāṅga*) clearly served as a common device used to frame yoga systematically in terms of its component parts.[46] The *aṣṭāṅgayoga* paradigm became, over time, the most influential paradigm for the theory and practice of yoga, evident in its pervasive presence in the literature of yoga from the classical era to the present.

The eight limbs of the Pātañjala yoga system begin with the sphere of external behavior through restraint (*yama*) and religious practice through observance (*niyama*), then proceed to disciplining the physical and energetic processes of the human organism by means of *āsana* and *prāṇāyāma*, shifting away from external stimuli through withdrawal (*pratyāhāra*) of the senses, culminating in a contemplative process (*dhāraṇā*, *dhyāna*, and *samādhi*). Despite significant focus on the role of meditation, the *aṣṭāṅgayoga* system represents the process of liberation as demanding mastery in all spheres of human activity, not just the mind. Every limb of yoga, and each part of each limb, yields a particular perfection (*siddhi*) that is of benefit in the development of yoga practice. The practice of yoga, according to Patañjali, is a dialectic between practice (*abhyāsa*) and dispassion (*vairāgya*), in which what is to be done is taken up with discipline, and what is to be abandoned is abandoned fully and without any lingering attachment. The practice of the *aṣṭāṅgayoga* is said to be cultivated in order to destroy impurity and for the illumination of knowledge up to the point of discriminative discernment (*vivekakhyāti*), which effects the process of liberation.[47]

Yama

As mentioned earlier, the five factors of *yama* include nonharm (*ahiṃsā*), truthfulness (*satya*), nonstealing (*asteya*), sexual restraint (*brahmacarya*), and nongreed (*aparigraha*). Their presentation in the *Yogasūtra* parallels, if not duplicates, that of the lesser vow (*aṇuvrata*) and greater vow (*mahāvrata*) system in Jainism, as one verse introduces the five *yama* factors and another specifies that their universal application is characterized as the *mahāvrata*.[48] The conception that *yama* is to be observed in a manner consistent with one's mode of life, whether as householder or renouncer, is evident in later representations of *aṣṭāṅgayoga*.[49] The foundation of *yama* is the observance of *ahiṃsā*. In its most explicit form, it refers to restraint from killing living things, but it can also refer to harmful speech and thought. *Satya* is coherence in thought and in speech, and is often interpreted as including the restraint of injurious, though truthful, speech. In the commentarial literature, *asteya* is described as not taking what belongs to others and *brahmacarya* as restraint of the urges arising from the sexual organ and senses that give rise to sexual desire. *Aparigraha* is described as the restraint of greed, hoarding, and the acceptance of gifts. The mastery of each *yama* factor leads to an associated accomplishment or perfection (*siddhi*). In the case of *ahiṃsā*, it is the absence of animosity in the presence of the practitioner; *satya* brings coherence to thought and deed, making language powerful; *asteya* leads to the achievement of wealth, either spiritual or material; *brahmacarya* results in vigor (*vīrya*); and *aparigraha* in knowledge of the "how" or "why" of the process of birth.[50] In each case, the mastery of a *yama* factor leads to enhanced powers of action and perception, laying a foundation for the development of successive limbs of yoga.

Niyama

The five factors of *niyama*, as listed above, move from the sphere of social relationships, and especially the cultivation of moral restraint (*yama*), to personal observances. The practice of cleanliness (*śauca*) situates Patañjali's yoga within the paradigm of *brāhmaṇa* traditions. Priestly notions of the relationship between cleanliness (*śauca*) and purity (*śuddha*) are central to both *vaidika* and *smārta* traditions. The factor of contentment (*saṃtoṣa*) is a deliberate cultivation of simplicity in one's mode of existence, and *tapas* encourages the undertaking of ascetic austerities such as fasting as an accessory to yoga practice. *Svādhyāya* is the recitation of religious texts or mantras, drawing upon the Vedic model of oral performance, and *īśvarapraṇidhāna* posits a formal practice of dedication to the Lord (*īśvara*). The factors of *tapas*, *svādhyāya*, and *īśvarapraṇidhāna* appear together among the *niyama* factors as well as the three factors of *kriyāyoga* mentioned earlier. As with *yama*, the practice of each *niyama* is said to yield a particular perfection or accomplishment (*siddhi*).[51] From perfection of *śauca* arises a repulsion to the body, a distancing from others, mental clarity, cheerfulness, mental focus, mastery of the senses, and a fitness for seeing the self (*ātmadarśana*). From *saṃtoṣa* comes unexcelled happiness (*sukha*) and from *tapas* the perfection of the body and senses due to the destruction of impurity (*aśuddhi*). Lastly, from *svādhyāya* comes unification with one's desired deity (*iṣṭadevatā*), and *īśvarapraṇidhāna* is said to lead to the perfection of contemplation (*samādhi*). These factors, then, rather than being simply precursors to the practice of the successive limbs of yoga, are seen to have direct influence over the yogic process, suggesting that the mastery of *yama* and *niyama* leads to the spontaneous arising of other factors.

Āsana, *Prāṇāyāma*, and *Pratyāhāra*

The yama and niyama factors of *aṣṭāṅgayoga* are succeeded by the limbs of posture (*āsana*), breath control (*prāṇāyāma*), and sense withdrawal (*pratyāhāra*).[52] With respect to *āsana*, Patañjali's chief focus appears to be in establishing stability (*sthira*) and comfort (*sukha*) so that the meditator can abide in meditation indefinitely. The resultant accomplishment (*siddhi*) of perfected posture is being unaffected by the opposites (*dvandva*) of hot and cold, etc., which would otherwise lead to physical and mental instability. On that basis, the control or extension (*āyāma*) of the breath (*prāṇa*) is established, through the control of inhalation, exhalation, and suspension of breath in accordance with time, place, and number, yielding a fourth (*caturtha*) state that is uniquely productive. The mastery of this fourth mode of *prāṇāyāma* leads to illumination (*prakāśa*) of mind and the accomplishment (*siddhi*) of fitness for fixation (*dhāraṇā*). This is followed by the withdrawal (*pratyāhāra*) of the senses from their objects, yielding the perfection (*siddhi*) of mastery of the senses. This progression provides another case for not viewing the outer limbs (*bahiraṅga*) as less significant than the inner limbs (*antaraṅga*), but rather as the building blocks of yogic practice in Patañjali's system.

Dhāraṇā, *Dhyāna*, and *Samādhi*

Fixation (*dhāraṇā*), meditation (*dhyāna*), and contemplation (*samādhi*) constitute the inner limbs (*antaraṅga*) of *aṣṭāṅgayoga* and are basis for the establishment of meditative mastery (*saṃyama*).[53] Though they are internal (*antar*) with respect to the outer limbs (*bahiraṅga*), they are said to be external with respect to the establishment of the seedless (*nirbīja*) state. *Dhāraṇā* refers to the fixation of the mind on an object, *dhyāna* to the development of continuity of focus on an object, and *samādhi* to the perfection of that concentration or focus in which the object alone shines forth. *Samādhi* is characterized as being cognitive (*saṃprajñāta*) or noncognitive (*asaṃprajñāta*), the former characterized by the factors of applied and sustained thought (*vitarka*, *vicāra*), bliss (*ānanda*), and egoity (*asmitā*), and the latter by the impression (*saṃskāra*) of cessation (*nirodha*).[54] When perfected, the three factors of *dhāraṇā*, *dhyāna*, and *samādhi* together are referred to as yogic mastery (*saṃyama*), which gives rise to the light or illumination of wisdom (*prajñāloka*). This leads to various types of accomplishment (*siddhi*) or power (*vibhūti*), including the ability to discern the distinction between *puruṣa* and *prakṛti* and thereby achieve liberation (*kaivalya*). Whatever phenomenon the meditator turns the concentrated mind toward reveals its inner nature, giving the meditator special power or agency relative to it.

Vibhūti and *Siddhi*

After addressing the final three limbs of the *aṣṭāṅgayoga* system, the third section (*pāda*) of the *Yogasūtra*, *vibhūtipāda*, deals with the various types of power (*vibhūti*) or accomplishment (*siddhi*) that emerge out of the practice of *saṃyama*, culminating in the discernment of the distinction between *puruṣa* and *prakṛti* that yields *kaivalya*. These attainments can be placed into two primary categories, one of perception and one of action.[55] The former includes knowledge of the past and future, previous births, others' minds, the mode and time of one's death, the structure of the cosmos, and the structure of the body. The latter includes such powers as invisibility, physical indestructability, possession of others' bodies, mastery of the elements, and superhuman strength, among others. This also includes a group of eight *siddhi*, which the commentary describes as smallness (*aṇimā*), lightness (*laghimā*), greatness (*mahimā*), obtaining (*prāpti*), willfulness (*prākāmya*), pervasion (*vaśitva*), lordship (*īśitṛtva*), and the suppression of desire (*kāmāvasāyitva*).[56] The arising of powers includes mastery of vitality in the form of *prāṇa*, and contemplation on various parts of the body.[57] The meditator's mental state is represented in the *Yogabhāṣya* as becoming equivalent to that of beings who dwell in higher cosmological levels of the universe, an analysis akin to Buddhist views of meditation.[58] The progression of powers in *vibhūtipāda* culminates in the achievement of virtual omniscience and omnipotence, indicating progressive signs of the meditator's success.[59] However, the *sūtrapāṭha* warns about the danger of pride in entreaties of the "established ones" (*sthānin*) or gods, and Vyāsa relates how the gods approach a yogi and offer various powers and objects of desire, including heavenly vehicles, potions, and seductive heavenly beings, trying to entice the practitioner to enjoy the fruits of their practice and abandon further progress.[60] Ultimately, the extraordinary capacities obtained through meditation are said to need to be abandoned, at least temporarily, for the sake of discerning the distinction between *puruṣa* and *prakṛti* and thereby attaining *kaivalya*.[61]

In the fourth *pāda* of the *Yogasūtra*, *kaivalyapāda*, Patañjali indicates and discusses five principal sources for the attainment of *siddhi*, which include birth (*janma*), herbs (*oṣadhi* or *auṣadhi*), incantation (*mantra*), and asceticism (*tapas*), as well as contemplation (*samādhi*).[62] This passage, which parallels a similar list in the Buddhist *Abhidharmakośabhāṣya*, represents a window to the range of techniques that were theorized as sources of *siddhi* in Patañjali's era.[63] These various modes of developing *siddhi* might be seen as a phenomenological paradigm for understanding how yoga practitioners sought to transform human embodiment and thus produce extraordinary capacities.[64] Such powers have been interpreted by scholars in a number of ways: as concrete, literal powers over the world; as compelling fantasies; as psychological phenomena indicating spiritual development; as analogous to near-death phenomena; and as metaphors for concrete physical and psychological transformations, among other possibilities.[65]

Kaivalya

Separation (*kaivalya*) or liberation (*mokṣa*) is presented in the *Yogasūtra* as the result of a process in which a practitioner cultivates detachment and insight, disciplining the mind and body as to gain the capacity to discern the true nature of the world and self. Liberation is represented as the result of the termination of the conjunction (*saṃyoga*) or misidentification of *puruṣa* and *prakṛti*. This is framed in one context as the purity of the mind becoming like that of *puruṣa*, as the result of a process of returning to the source (*pratiprasava*) of *prakṛti* through discriminative discernment (*vivekakhyāti*).[66] The nature of liberation in the yoga system is a subject of considerable debate, principally with respect to the issue of the possibility of liberation-in-life (*jīvanmukti*). One interpretation followed in traditional commentaries is that *kaivalya* can, and should, be understood as equivalent to liberation in Sāṃkhya, namely as a state of radical isolation from phenomenal reality or nature (*prakṛti*). The Sāṃkhya system posits an unlimited number of monadic *puruṣa* that are distinct from one another, and which exist in a state of isolation upon separation from *prakṛti*. The final verse of the *Yogasūtra* connects *kaivalya* with *pratiprasava*, the returning of the *guṇa* factors to their source in *prakṛti*, possibly suggesting such a separation from material existence. This view would appear, significantly, to be supported by the *Yogabhāṣya*.[67] This view is proximate to the *śramaṇa* viewpoint of Jainism, in which monadic *jīva* are freed in the process of liberation into a state of distinction or isolation (*kevala*) that is cosmologically distinct. A liberated *jīva* in Jainism is said to exist as a perfected one (*siddha*) at the top of the universe, a concept which may be obliquely referred to in a verse in *vibhūtipāda*, as well.[68]

A counterargument to this view suggests that *kaivalya* represents a radical reorientation to nature (*prakṛti*) rather than a separation from it, with the concept of the power of consciousness (*citi-śakti*) that appears in the final verse of the *Yogasūtra* indicating an active component of *kaivalya*.[69] Additionally, in the fourth *pāda*, Patañjali discusses the manner in which the perfections of *samādhi*, especially that of the created-mind (*nirmāṇa-citta*), does not lead to further bondage to the world for the practitioner of yoga.[70] Instead, the karma of the *yogin* is described as "neither black nor white" and thus not operating within the ordinary sphere of the process of *saṃsāra*. Lastly, Īśvara, the unbound *puruṣa* who represented as serving as a *guru* of yoga in the world over successive ages, provides at least one example of the possibility of worldly activity of a being not bound by *prakṛti* within the Pātañjala Yoga system.

Role and Import of Pātañjala Yoga

Some scholars have argued that the modern emphasis placed on Patañjali and the *Yogasūtra* is disproportionate with its historical importance. According to this argument, the championing of Patañjali's yoga by Orientalist scholars and by the formulators of modern Hinduism, such as Swami Vivekananda, elevated what may have been a moribund tradition from obscurity to being at the center of modern yoga discourse.[71] Similarly, the notion of a "classical yoga" associated with Patañjali and the *Yogasūtra* has been called into question as lending to a myopic understanding of yoga that obscures its breadth and historical complexity.[72] The physicality of much of modern yoga, especially postural forms, lends to the view that the meditatively focused text of Patañjali is a poor match as a philosophical framework for modern practitioners. Modern postural yoga is arguably more deeply rooted in medieval *haṭhayoga* traditions and in modern, especially Indian and European, physical cultures that are distinct in many ways from the Pātañjala Yoga tradition. The practices of *āsana* and *prāṇāyāma*, the focus of modern postural yoga traditions, each draw on only three verses in Patañjali's work.

Nonetheless, significant evidence validates viewing Pātañjala Yoga as uniquely important in understanding the history of yoga traditions. One is the extensive commentarial tradition associated with the *Pātañjalayogaśāstra*, which has been a window to the propagation of the discourse of yoga by *brāhmaṇa* scholars for over a thousand years. The *Pātañjalayogaśāstra* and its commentarial tradition provide a resource for the study of Indian and Hindu culture of yoga in a manner analogous to how the *brāhmaṇa* Dharmaśāstra literature provides insight into Hindu *dharma*. Another reason is the pervasive representation of the framework of the *aṣṭāṅgayoga* system in Indian literature, from the classical literature of the epics and Purāṇas to its representation in Jainism, Vedānta, Hindu Tantra, and in Medieval *Yoga Upaniṣad* and *haṭhayoga* texts. Although Patañjali's name is often not mentioned explicitly in association with the *aṣṭāṅgayoga* system in these other contexts, the *Pātañjalayogaśāstra* served as a chief locus for scholarly analysis and discussion of the eight-limbed system and its components for centuries, buttressing its authority and influence. To the degree to which Pātañjala Yoga is identified with the formal development of the eight-limbed yoga framework, Patañjali and the *Yogasūtra* stands out as being of unique importance in the history of yoga traditions. The elevation of Pātañjala Yoga to canonical status as one of the six orthodox systems similarly indicates its import as a classical representation of the Indian philosophical position with respect to yoga. Lastly, it is hard to overestimate the manner in which Patañjali's yoga continues to serve as a simple and coherent pedagogic model for disseminating the foundational principles of yoga in the modern era, regardless of debates over its historical impact. Academic and historical issues aside, Patañjali's yoga system as developed in the *Yogasūtra* provides a coherent philosophical framework that presents the building blocks of yoga that inform virtually every yoga system developed in India in the classical and postclassical periods. In this respect, it provides an excellent example of the broader purpose of the classical Hindu *sūtra* and *śāstra* literature, which is to provide an examination of a topic that establishes the parameters of a discourse, thereby supporting investigation of it, be that in the form of scholarly and philosophical examination or of dedicated practice.

Chapter 5

Hindu Epic, Purāṇic, and Scholastic Representations of Yoga

The philosophical presentation of yoga in the *Yogasūtra* has a counterpart in the narrative and didactic literature of the Hindu epics and Purāṇas (*itihāsa-purāṇa*). In this literature, the discourse and practice of yoga is framed within narratives that illustrate the structures of law and duty (*dharma*) within Hindu theistic and sectarian traditions. Yoga also appears in the Hindu legal and larger philosophical literature of the classical era, including the *dharmaśāstra* literature and the highly influential texts of Vedānta philosophy. During this period, one of the key features that distinguished *brāhmaṇa* from *śramaṇa* traditions was an increasing focus on domestic concerns in the case of the former and on elite monastic practice in the latter, lending toward the greater adoption of priestly traditions into Indian life at a grassroots level.[1] In concert with this, the entry of yoga into the mainstream of Indian householder life is evident in the *itihāsa-purāṇa* texts, which consciously and deliberately negotiate the tensions between world-affirming conceptions of *dharma* and the renouncer-inspired pursuit of liberation (*mokṣa*). The *itihāsa-purāṇa* tradition is a pervasive, if not the most pervasive, literary influence in the development of Hindu traditions, representing the integration of Hindu narrative and practice over the course of many centuries, from roughly 500 BCE to 500 CE and beyond, illustrating the three strata of practice in the Hindu tradition, namely, Vedic (*vaidika*), classical (*smārta* or *paurāṇika*), and tantric (*tāntrika*).[2] Of these three, the *itihāsa-purāṇa* tradition represents the flowering of the classical and theistic mode of Hindu religious practice, with the integration of *vaidika* and *tāntrika* models as accessories to the mainstream.

The two principal Indian epics (*itihāsa*, lit. "thus it was") are the *Rāmāyaṇa* and the *Mahābhārata*, which tell the stories of heroic princes who illustrate the safeguarding of law and duty (*dharma*) in the universe in the face of the forces of injustice and disorder (*adharma*). The Purāṇas (lit. "of old") tell the story of the genealogies and archetypical actions of ancient gods, sages, and kings. In addition, the *itihāsa* and *purāṇa* texts contain numerous didactic or instructional sections, which teach the principles of *dharma*, various rites and ritual processes, such as sacrifice (*yajña*) and worship (*pūjā*), and the practice of yoga. The *itihāsa-purāṇa* literature is sometimes referred to as the Fifth Veda (*pañcama-veda*) in the early Upaniṣads, in the *itihāsa-purāṇa* literature itself, and in subsequent Hindu literature.[3] The significance of this conception, of *itihāsa-purāṇa* as *pañcama-veda*, is that it sets this body of literature, which is by nature "remembered" (*smṛti*) literature, on a par with the "heard" (*śruti*), or revealed, literature. As such, for *smārta brāhmaṇa* tradition, *itihāsa-purāṇa* carries a level of authority that, at times, approaches that of the Vedas. As a nexus of priestly and popular traditions, the *itihāsa-purāṇa* literature was formative in the development of pan-Indian theistic traditions, which culminated in the elevation of three primary sectarian traditions of Hinduism, each focused on a particular deity: Śaiva (followers of Śiva), Vaiṣṇava (followers of Viṣṇu), and Śākta (followers of Devī). In some cases, a fourth sect is added to this group, the Smārta, named after the *smārta* mode of religious practice, and focused ritually on a set of five principal deities, specifically Śiva, Viṣṇu, Devī, Sūrya, and Gaṇeśa. Yoga was integrated on many levels of this emerging framework of the practice of Hinduism as a mode of religious discipline that yields power (*siddhi*) and liberation (*mokṣa*), as a mode of devotion (*bhakti*), and as a capacity that the gods themselves embody, represent, and wield in various ways.

Hindu Epic (*itihāsa*) Literature: *Mahābhārata* and *Rāmāyaṇa*

The Hindu epic (*itihāsa*) texts, like those of ancient Greece, represent the crystallization of narratives developed over a significant span of time. The *Mahābhārata*, "The Great [War] of the Bhāratas," attributed to Vyāsa, and the *Rāmāyaṇa*, "Story of Rāma," of Vālmīki, are the two principal Sanskrit epics, though additional epic literature exists in a range of vernacular languages that localize epic narratives and offer variant readings. The Sanskrit epics are among the largest literary works in the world, some 75,000 and 20,000 verses, respectively.[4] The Hindu epics were likely composed by poets, referred to by the term "bard" (*sūta*), who built up the collection of stories over time through creative retellings and the expansion of existing stories. These poets may have originally been members of the *kṣatriya* or warrior class, but at a certain point the control of these texts passed over to *brāhmaṇa* traditions.[5] The *Mahābhārata* contains several different strata of narrative that reflect the changing social and cultural environment in India during the early centuries of the Common Era, particularly the reemergence and revalorization of a model of Indian society in which Hindu priestly ideals, such as Vedic *dharma*, are at the center.[6]

An important theme in the epic narratives is the integration of *tapas* and renouncer ideology into the mainstream of Vedic householder practice, countering the *śramaṇa* model of the rejection of worldly *dharma* and the Vedic heritage. In the *itihāsa-purāṇa* literature, the boundary between concepts such as yoga and of *tapas* is often fluid, offering evidence that the development of yoga in Hindu traditions was a logical extension of Vedic conceptions of *tapas* that had been appropriated by *śramaṇa* traditions.[7] Mirroring ideas found in the Upaniṣads, *tapas* and yoga are described in epic literature as the source of the power of the gods and a basis for humans to obtain worldly powers in life and liberation at the time of death.[8] Likewise, consistent with the trope of the *kṣatriya* master of ascetic discipline found in both Brāhmaṇical asceticism and in the *śramaṇa* traditions, the *Mahābhārata* and *Rāmāyaṇa* center on heroic figures of the *kṣatriya* class who obtain power and knowledge through meditative, ascetic, and martial discipline. The connection between yoga and the *kṣatriya* class in the *itihāsa* literature exemplifies a long-running association between martial and ascetic discipline in Indian history. This link extends from the Vrātya brotherhoods of the Vedic era and the *kṣatriya* leadership of the *śramaṇa* traditions through the classical era into the Hindu traditions of warrior-ascetics in the medieval era and the use of yoga in modern military training in India and the United States.

Lastly, the vivid representations of *ṛṣi*, yogis, and various other types of ascetic virtuosos in the *itihāsa* literature provides a set of archetypal images that frame Indian, and especially Hindu, perspectives on the figure of the *yogin* and *yoginī* to the present. The deities of classical Hinduism, such as Śiva, Viṣṇu, and Devī are themselves represented as embodying the practice of yoga and demonstrating extraordinary capacities derived from the power of yoga (*yogabala*).

The *Mahābhārata*

The story of the *Mahābhārata* is centered on a war between cousins, the heroic Pāṇḍavas, the sons of Pāṇḍu, and the villainous Kauravas, the sons of Dhṛtarāṣṭra. The five Pāṇḍavas are all sons of Vedic deities born to human mothers, Kuntī and Mādrī, through the use of a *mantra*. Yudhiṣṭhira is descended from Yama or Dharma, Bhīma from Vāyu, Arjuna from Indra, and Nakula and Sahadeva from the twin Aśvin gods. Kuntī also had a previous son, Karṇa, resulting from a mantra-based union with the Vedic god Sūrya. Karṇa, a foundling, ultimately allies himself with the Kauravas. The Kauravas, Duryodhana and his ninety-nine brothers, are incarnations of an *asura* named Kali and ninety-nine demons (*rākṣasa*).[9] As such, the *Mahābhārata* parallels a late Vedic and early classical Hindu narrative of an ongoing cosmic struggle between the virtuous *deva* and unvirtuous *asura* deities. The Pāṇḍava brothers are all married to a single woman, Draupadī, who is their confidant and plays a key role in many parts of the narrative. The Pāṇḍavas are further supported by their cousin, Kṛṣṇa Vāsudeva, who, in the narrative of the *Bhagavadgītā*, reveals himself as a *guru* of yoga and, according to commentaries on the text, as a manifestation (*avatāra*) of Viṣṇu and as the eternal *brahman* of the Upaniṣads.[10] The Pāṇḍavas are trained by the celebrated warriors Bhīṣma and Droṇa, who serve as *guru* figures through their instruction in and demonstration of yogic and military mastery.[11]

The central narrative of the *Mahābhārata* focuses on the Pāṇḍavas, who lose their kingdom in a game of dice and are forced to wander for twelve years in exile and live for one year undercover before returning to reclaim their birthright. During exile, they undertake adventures that provide for narrative intrigue and didactic discourse on a variety of subjects. When the Pāṇḍavas return home, war is precipitated between the cousins, bringing to culmination the tensions in the epic between the *kṣatriya* warrior-ideology of *dharma* and the renouncer ideology of yoga and *ahiṃsā*. In the *Bhagavadgītā*, or "Song of the Lord," a narrative that describes the final moments before the battle between the Pāṇḍavas and Kauravas begins, Kṛṣṇa, serving as Arjuna's charioteer, provides a discourse on yoga and *dharma* that solidifies Arjuna's resolve to fight, effectively placing yoga in the service of *dharma*. Though the Pāṇḍavas prevail in the battle that follows, it is a bloody and destructive war, marked by dishonest tactics and revenge killings, with the Pāṇḍavas themselves resorting to deception at critical moments. The Kauravas and their allies are destroyed, as are many of the Pāṇḍavas friends, relatives, and teachers, including Bhīṣma and Droṇa. Following the war, some of the principal characters go into retreat and reach peace through yoga, and the Pāṇḍavas ultimately perform a walk-unto-death in the Himalayan mountains.[12]

The Yoga of the *Mahābhārata*

The five Pāṇḍava brothers are instructed in techniques of yoga by their *guru* Bhīṣma. One episode focuses on the practice of *dhyānayoga*, which is framed in a manner that has significant resemblance to both Buddhist and Pātañjala Yoga representations of *dhyāna* and *samādhi*.[13] Another expression of yoga in the *Mahābhārata* is as a vehicle for warriors to enter into the sun, and thus liberation, upon death, a process illustrated in the death of Droṇa.[14] More broadly, yoga is allied with *tapas* as a means to spiritual perfection and worldly accomplishment, the disciplining of mind and body being viewed as a fruitful enterprise in both respects.[15] There are ample examples of *yogin* and *yoginī* figures, such as Kāvya Uśanas, Kuvalāśva, Vipula, Vidura, Sulabhā and others, who obtain various powers through yoga, including flight, entering others' bodies, or mastery over the elements.[16] These powers are viewed with ambivalence, potentially as detriments to achieving liberation, evident in admonishment of Śuka by Vyāsa to focus on the world-negating (*nivṛtti*) aspects of yoga, but nevertheless they play important roles in the transformation of the order of the world.[17] The *Mahābhārata* contains numerous discussions of the concepts of *sāṃkhya* and *yoga*, some appearing to hint at the development of systems of practice with a distinct identity, others pointing simply to a contrast between theory and practice. The *Śāntiparvan*, "The Book of Peace," of the *Mahābhārata* refers to a Vedic eight-virtue yoga (*aṣṭaguṇayoga*, *aṣṭaguṇitayoga*), perhaps a precursor of the *aṣṭāṅgayoga* system, mentioning practices of *prāṇāyāma* and *dhāraṇā*, but not providing the complete list of eight elements.[18] Threads of yoga developed in the Upaniṣads, *śramaṇa* traditions, Sāṃkhya-Yoga, and Vedānta are evident in the *Mahābhārata*. The *Mahābhārata*, as such, provides a snapshot of the crystallization of the discourse and practice of yoga in the late-Vedic to early classical era of Hinduism.

The *Bhagavadgītā*

The *Bhagavadgītā*, which appears in part six of the *Mahābhārata*, tells a story that integrates priestly ideology, especially with respect to *dharma*, with renouncer practices oriented toward liberation (*mokṣa*) and emergent theistic and devotional traditions. As such, the *Bhagavadgītā* is often seen as the *locus classicus* for the articulation of the idea of three paths of yoga, namely a yoga of action (*karmayoga*), a yoga of knowledge (*jñānayoga*), and a yoga of devotion (*bhaktiyoga*), respectively. In referring to *sāṃkhyayoga*, *buddhiyoga*, *dhyānayoga*, and other modes of practice, the *Bhagavadgītā* further establishes the concept of yoga as a "method" or "discipline," that can be appended on to different modes of practice. The story is portrayed as taking place just as the *Mahābhārata* battle is about to begin. The Pāṇḍava warrior Arjuna, losing heart, confesses to Kṛṣṇa, who is serving as his charioteer, that he cannot bear the idea of fighting his family members and former teachers, and suggests that instead he should renounce his worldly life to seek liberation as a renouncer. Kṛṣṇa responds with a discourse on the use of an internal yoga process as a means of skillfully discharging one's duty (*dharma*) in the world, leading to the attainment of liberation (*mokṣa*, *nirvāṇa*) within the sphere of moral obligation. Yoga is described by Kṛṣṇa in various ways, as evenness (*samatva*), as skillfulness (*kauśala*) of action (*karma*), as a form of devotion (*bhakti*) in which one acts in a spirit of renunciation, and as a realization of extinction in the ultimate reality underlying all things (*brahmanirvāṇa*) realized by meditation on the syllable *oṃ*.[19]

Kṛṣṇa depicts the heavenly rise and fall of *brāhmaṇa* ritualists observing the Duty of the Three [Vedas] (*trayīdharma*) in a manner that parallels the critique of the Vedic sacrificial model found in the *Muṇḍaka Upaniṣad*.[20] Sāṃkhya categories that inform the Yoga system are invoked by Kṛṣṇa as well, including the distinction between *puruṣa* and *prakṛti* and the powers of the *guṇa* factors, integrating the dualism of Sāṃkhya-

Yoga into its overarching theistic and proto-Vedāntic framework. The *aṣṭāṅgayoga* system is approximated, if not implicitly invoked, in passages that emphasize self-control of behavior, body, and mind.[21] Yoga is referred to as a means to the restraint of mind (*cittaniruddha*), an expression akin to the *cittavṛttinirodha* of Pātañjala Yoga, and as cultivated through *abhyāsa* and *vairāgya*.[22] Kṛṣṇa tells Arjuna that he first passed the knowledge of yoga onto Vivasvat, a Vedic sun god portrayed as the progenitor of the human race, who taught it to his son Manu, who in turn propagated it for further generations via the Royal Ṛṣis (*rājarṣi*), paralleling depictions of Hiraṇyagarbha as the divine source of the yoga tradition.[23] This conception connects further to Pātañjala Yoga's portrayal of Īśvara as a primordial *guru* that has propagated the knowledge of yoga (*yogavidyā*) since ancient times. It also connects to passages in the *Mahābhārata* where Kṛṣṇa identifies himself with Kapila and Hiraṇyagarbha, the formulators of the Sāṃkhya and Yoga systems.[24] Kṛṣṇa identifies himself with Kapila, among other objects and persons of greatness, in the *Bhagavadgītā*.[25] At the conclusion of the *Bhagavadgītā*, Kṛṣṇa as the Great Yoga Lord (*mahāyogeśvara*) grants Arjuna divine sight, whereby Arjuna is able to view Kṛṣṇa in his ultimate form as Viṣṇu and as an expression of the universal *brahman* in all his awe- and terror-inspiring majesty.[26] As such, the *Bhagavadgītā* draws together multiple threads of religious discourse to provide a coherent, world-affirming ideology that challenges the *śramaṇa* viewpoint by subsuming renunciation within the framework of social *dharma*. With its extensive focus on the role and import of yoga in the religious life, the *Bhagavadgītā* stands out as one of the most important testaments to the impact of yoga on the mainstream of classical Hindu thought and practice. Its devotional and world-affirming rubric of yoga was instrumental in establishing a model of Hindu yoga that validated both theistic and domestic practice.

The *Rāmāyaṇa*

The *Rāmāyaṇa*, attributed to Vālmīki, documents the development of popular Hindu conceptions of worldly order and duty (*dharma*) and the establishment of the model of theistic devotion (*bhakti*) in Hinduism. The *Rāmāyaṇa* builds upon Vedic thought and narrative, developing narratives and doctrines characteristic of sectarian *smārta brāhmaṇa* traditions and classical Hindu practice and ideology. The *Rāmāyaṇa* tells the story of a prince of Kosala named Rāma who is forced into exile with his wife Sītā as a result of palace intrigue in which his father, Daśaratha, places Rāma's half-brother Bharata on the throne in honor of a boon the king had promised to his wife Kaikeyī.[27] Rāma and Sītā, along with Rāma's brother Lakṣmaṇa, retreat to the forest to live with the forest-dwelling (*vānaprastha*) sages, and for a period of time their life is pastoral and idyllic. Among other adventures, they help protect the forest sages from the attacks of marauding demons (*rākṣasa*). Sītā is eventually captured by a demon named Rāvaṇa, who takes Sītā to his castle in Laṅkā. Rāma, with the help of the monkey-god Hanumān (*hanumat*, the son of the wind-god Māruta), and an army of monkeys and bears, is able to defeat Rāvaṇa and his army and rescue Sītā. Rāma returns to the capital of Kosala, Ayodhyā, and is consecrated as king, though his relationship with Sītā is complicated by issues related to the propriety of her having dwelled in Rāvaṇa's home for some time.

The overarching narrative of the story that is revealed over time is that the battle between Rāma and Rāvaṇa is cosmic in scope. Rāvaṇa has obtained invulnerability to the attacks of the gods and great martial power from the creator deity, Brahmā, in return for his extraordinarily intense ascetic austerities (*tapas*). As a result, he has conquered the Vedic gods, and is bent on terrorizing the human world. Rāma is an incarnation (*avatāra*) of Viṣṇu that has taken on human form in order to destroy Rāvaṇa and restore *dharma*. Likewise, Sītā is viewed as an incarnation of Lakṣmī or Śrī, the consort of Viṣṇu. Though explicit language of yoga is largely absent in the *Rāmāyaṇa*, the power of ascetic discipline and the validation of the forest-dweller (*vānaprastha*) lifestyle is displayed quite prominently. Both humans and demons (*rākṣasa*) are seen as obtaining tremendous power, including the use of powerful spiritual weapons, through ascetic discipline. This numinous ascetic power is morally ambiguous in nature, as both the virtuous (Rāma and his allies) and the unvirtuous (Rāvaṇa and his allies) possess it and wield it. However, the forces of *dharma*, embodied in the form of Viṣṇu and his incarnation as Rāma, are victorious over those of *adharma*. In the Hindu traditions, Rāma serves as an exemplar of the performance of "one's own [male] duties" (*svadharma*) and Sītā as the exemplar of "women's own duties" (*strīsvadharma*) and the observance of the "husband-vow" (*pativrata*), an ascetic practice of self-discipline in loyalty to one's husband.[28] In addition, the three persons of Rāma, Sītā, and Hanumān are among the most beloved objects of Hindu devotion (*bhakti*) that emerge in classical and medieval Hinduism, especially in the emerging Vaiṣṇava sectarian traditions.

The *Yogavāsiṣṭha*

Though the *Yogavāsiṣṭha*, "Yoga of [the Sage] Vasiṣṭha," based on an earlier text, the *Mokṣopāya*, "Method of Liberation," is not a formal part of the *itihāsa* literature, it is worth mentioning here, as it is a text built upon the narrative of the *Rāmāyaṇa*.[29] The *Yogavāsiṣṭha*, which dates from the mid-to-late first millennium CE, is a narrative of the instruction of prince Rāma in the techniques of yoga by the sage Vasiṣṭha, in a manner that parallels the dialogue between Kṛṣṇa and Arjuna in the *Bhagavadgītā*.[30] Likely influenced by the development of formal schools of Hindu Vedānta, Mahāyāna Buddhism, and Śaivism, the *Yogavāsiṣṭha* represents a Vedāntic interpretation of the practice of yoga, representing liberation (*mokṣa*) in life (*jīvanmukti*) as an immediate goal and a final extinction (*nirvāṇa*) at death as an ultimate goal. Like the *Bhagavadgītā*, it portrays the spiritual path as being a balance between world-affirmation (*pravṛtti*) and negation (*nivṛtti*) effected through the yoga of action (*karmayoga*). It represents the practice of yoga in terms of a sevenfold progression of negation (*nivṛtti*), thought (*vicāraṇa*), nonassociation (*asaṃsaṅga*), dreamworld (*svapnaloka*), non-dual sleep (*advaitasuṣupta*), liberation-in-life (*jīvanmukti*), and bodiless liberation (*videhamukti*).[31] Though parts of the text may have been composed relatively late, it nevertheless links the *itihāsa* tradition to the continued development and innovation of ideas and practices of yoga. The representation of the divine and heroic figure of Rāma as a student and practitioner validates the unique power and status of yoga within the Hindu narrative context. As with the *Bhagavadgītā*, the narrative places yoga at the center of a Hindu soteriology that negotiates the goals of *dharma* and of *mokṣa*. This is exemplified in one case through the story of Cūḍālā and Śikhidvaja, in which a spiritually liberated queen, Cūḍālā, utilizes various yogic *siddhi* in order to help her errant husband achieve realization.[32]

Hindu Purāṇa Literature: Sectarian Narrative and Practice

The Hindu Purāṇa literature is one of the most all-encompassing bodies of religious text in the Hindu tradition, and its importance in broader Indian and Southeast Asian culture cannot be overestimated. In many respects, the Purāṇas can be said to represent a codification of Hindu narrative and practice that is uniquely constitutive and representative of the Hindu tradition and its broader sectarian subsets. In addition to the Sanskrit Purāṇa literature, vernacular Purāṇas exist, and the Sanskrit Purāṇas themselves likely drew from vernacular sources in numerous ways over the course of their development.[33] Purāṇa narratives contain the stories of the great gods such as Śiva, Viṣṇu, and Devī as well as those of kings, heroes, and sages. They tell the stories of the universe, gods, and human beings.[34] They also relate the mechanics of a variety of modes of practice, including yoga, drawing upon and further developing the strata of *vaidika*, *smārta*, and *tāntrika* modes of priestly practice. The "major" or "great" Purāṇas (*mahāpurāṇa*) are typically listed as eighteen in number, though there is disagreement over the content of the list.[35] One oral-tradition-based variation of this list is as follows: *Bhāgavata*, *Bhaviṣya*, *Matsya*, *Mārkaṇḍeya*, *Brahma*, *Brahmavaivarta*, *Brahmāṇḍa*, *Viṣṇu*, *Varāha*, *Vāmana*, *Vāyu*, *Agni*, *Nārada*, *Padma*, *Liṅga*, *Garuḍa*, *Kūrma*, and *Skanda*.[36] In a list found in the *Viṣṇu Purāṇa*, they are organized as follows: *Brahma*, *Padma*, *Viṣṇu*, *Śiva*, *Bhāgavata*, *Nārada*, *Mārkaṇḍeya*, *Agni*, *Bhaviṣya*, *Brahmavaivarta*, *Liṅga*, *Varāha*, *Skanda*, *Vāmana*, *Kūrma*, *Matsya*, *Garuḍa*, and *Brahmāṇḍa*.[37] In addition to the great (*mahā*) Purāṇas, there are also minor (*upa*) Purāṇas, sometimes numbered as eighteen as well. One of the characteristic elements of the Purāṇic representation of yoga is that the gods and sages are knowers and expositors of yoga, as is the case with Śiva in the *Śiva Purāṇa*, for example, and yoga is homologized with the power of the gods. Though yoga is principally framed as a means of obtaining liberation (*mokṣa*) and thus freedom from worldly misery, a significant amount of discussion in the Purāṇas is dedicated to attaining spiritual accomplishments (*siddhi*), including becoming a Lord of Yoga (*yogeśvara*), and the destruction of disease.[38] It is represented as being characterized as six-limbed or eight-limbed (*ṣaḍaṅgayoga*, *aṣṭāṅgayoga*), as being threefold (*jñāna*, *bhakti*, and *karmayoga*), or as uniquely focused on devotion (*bhakti*), among other possibilities.[39] Some sections discuss the yoga practices of emergent subsects of Hinduism, such as the Pāśupatas, in which Śiva-devotion and transfiguration of the practitioner through yoga takes center stage. In one example of Purāṇic Pāśupata teaching, for example, the *aṣṭāṅgayoga* rubric is adopted as a preparatory practice for a supreme and final consummation of absorption in Śiva.[40]

Deities of the Purāṇas

The Purāṇas are the chief locus for the development of classical Hindu theism, in which a small group of principal deities, especially Śiva, Viṣṇu, and Devī, are elevated to a supreme status within their sectarian literature, for example in the *Śiva*, *Viṣṇu*, and *Mārkaṇḍeya Purāṇa*. These principal deities are, in turn, associated with a pantheon of tutelary deities, such as Pārvatī, Gaṇeśa, and Skanda for Śiva and Lakṣmī and Hanumān for Viṣṇu, and with human and animal incarnations (*avatāra*) that are worldly manifestations of these deities. One common Hindu theological frame drawn from the Purāṇa literature postulates three principal male deities, *Brahmā*, *Viṣṇu*, and *Śiva*, who are situated at the top of the hierarchy of the thirty-three Vedic gods. The three are known collectively as the *trimūrti*, or "three forms" of *īśvara* or *brahman*, and serving as creator, preserver, and destroyer, respectively, when viewed as a unit, with each deity taking on the powers of the others, such as creation and preservation, within their distinct sectarian context.[41] The *trimūrti* is, in some cases, viewed as having a composite personal manifestation as the deity Dattātreya, who appears as an idealized *yogin* and *guru*.[42] Though Brahmā plays an important role within Hindu cosmological narratives and in the dramas of the other gods, Hindu sectarian traditions associated with Brahmā disappeared over time, unlike those of Śiva and Viṣṇu. This may be partly because Brahmā, along with Indra, was critiqued and assimilated by Theravāda Buddhism.[43]

One of the major classical *brāhmaṇa* systems of Hindu practice focused on five principal Purāṇic deities: Śiva, Viṣṇu, Devī, Gaṇeśa, and Sūrya. Śiva, whose name is connected to that of the Śiva Rudra of the Vedas, the "auspicious" (*śiva*) Rudra, is often represented as a renouncer who dwells in the Himalayan mountains and practices asceticism, yoga, and meditation. Viṣṇu, the "dweller" or "pervader," is represented in the garb of royalty alongside his wife Lakṣmī or Śrī, "prosperity" or "glory." In one form, he is represented as reclining on the cosmic serpent Ādiśeṣa or Ananta in a cosmic ocean between the cycles of destruction and creation. He is said to take the form of many "descents" or incarnations (*avatāra*), the most famous of which are Kṛṣṇa and Rāma, but include other figures such as the Buddha and Mahāvīra. One common list of *avatāra* is ten in number: fish (*matsya*), tortoise (*kūrma*), boar (*varāha*), man-lion (*narasiṃha*), dwarf (*vāmana*), Rāma with an axe (*paraśurāma*), Rāma of Ayodhyā (*rāma*), Kṛṣṇa, Gautama Buddha, and Kalki. The Goddess or Devī, also known as the Great Goddess (*mahādevī*) or the Powerful One (*śakti*), is viewed as the source of power for the male gods and as the one behind the many goddesses (*devī*) of the Indian pantheon. In the Śākta and goddess-focused sub-traditions of Śaivism, Devī is represented as being equal to or superior to the great gods, resplendent in royal glory. In the *Devī Māhātmya*, the "Greatness of the Goddess," of the *Mārkaṇḍeya Purāṇa*, the goddess functions as a preserver of the world and of *dharma* in the face of demonic threat. The *Devī Māhātmya* also describes the manifestation of the fierce goddess Kālī from the body of Devī, who is able to destroy a demon named "red seed" (*raktabīja*) by drinking up its drops (*bīja*) of blood (*rakta*, lit. "red") before they can give rise to new demons. Another figure whose narratives figure prominently in the Purāṇa literature is the elephant-headed god Gaṇeśa or Gaṇapati, the "Leader of the Troops [of Śiva]" who is the son of Śiva and Pārvatī. Sūrya, the sun god, is represented as a giver of life and health, and for a period of time was the principal deity within an independent Saura sectarian tradition.[44]

These deities are known throughout India and other parts of Asia influenced by Hindu and *brāhmaṇa* thought and culture, such as Southeast Asia. The Purāṇic gods and goddesses serve as personal or chosen deities (*iṣṭadevatā*) and as family or ancestral deities (*kuladevatā*). Local gods and goddesses are often viewed as incarnations (*avatāra*) or manifestations of Purāṇic pan-Indian gods, such as Śiva, Viṣṇu, and Devī. The Purāṇa literature integrated local, tribal, and perhaps even village deities (*grāmadevatā*) into a sectarian priestly Hinduism that served as the arbiter of orthodoxy and authenticity. With the advent of *smārta* or *paurāṇika* priestly traditions that drew upon the Purāṇa literature, the focus of Hindu practice shifted away from the performance of public *yajña* focused on Vedic deities to worship (*pūjā*) directed toward Purāṇic deities, including Śiva, Viṣṇu, and Devī.

The practice of *pūjā*, in which a deity is worshipped in the form of an icon (*mūrti*), utilizing *mantra* and various offerings, including food, water, incense, and fire (in the form of a lamp), became central to priestly and popular practice. Over time the practice of *pūjā* was extended beyond the sphere of *smārta* practice into *tāntrika* traditions as well. The worship and veneration of the Purāṇic gods is coextensive with the practice of many traditions of Hindu yoga, providing a narrative, ritual, and theological framework in which the practice of yoga is situated.

Aṣṭāṅgayoga in the Purāṇa Literature

The images of the gods and goddesses in the Purāṇa literature are deeply connected to the iconography of asceticism, yoga, and tantra in the Indian tradition, and the practice of yoga is integrated into the Purāṇic texts with a distinctly theistic and sectarian flavor. Though there is reference to a *ṣaḍaṅgayoga* system, the *aṣṭāṅgayoga* paradigm is a pervasive framework for the theory and practice of yoga in the Purāṇas. The Purāṇas use the terms *Yogaśāstra* and *Yogānuśāsana*, pointing to an extant tradition of yoga literature that is a resource for its concepts and practices, with the latter term likely referring to the *Yogasūtra* or *Pātañjalayogaśāstra*. Patañjali's name is not explicitly mentioned in reference to the *aṣṭāṅgayoga* framework, though this perhaps follows a Purāṇic convention of abstraction without citation of authorship. Focused and elaborate discussions of the practice of yoga utilizing the *aṣṭāṅgayoga* paradigm appear in the *Viṣṇu Purāṇa*, *Agni Purāṇa*, *Vāyu Purāṇa*, *Kūrma Purāṇa*, *Śiva Purāṇa*, *Liṅga Purāṇa*, and *Bhāgavata Purāṇa*.[45] The representation of *aṣṭāṅgayoga* in the Purāṇas situates it within the theistic sectarian traditions, the *aṣṭāṅgayoga* of the *Viṣṇu Purāṇa* being framed within a Vaiṣṇava theology, and the *aṣṭāṅgayoga* of the *Śiva Purāṇa* and *Liṅga Purāṇa* being situated within a framework of Śaiva theology, for example. The representation of *aṣṭāṅgayoga* in Pātañjala Yoga, on the other hand, has few, if any, explicit sectarian references.[46] In the Purāṇas, meditation is often represented as a focusing on Śiva or Viṣṇu and their attributes, framed within a larger philosophical context that includes principles characteristic of both Sāṃkhya and Vedānta. Purāṇic accounts of yoga often synthesize these three frameworks (theistic, dualistic, and non-dual) together into a viewpoint in which to know the divine is to realize one's inmost identity (*ātman*) as the primordial reality (*brahman*), escaping bondage to *prakṛti* and achieving unity or identity with a personal deity such as Śiva, Viṣṇu, or Devī.[47]

In these contexts, *aṣṭāṅgayoga* is also represented as being observed in relationship to one's *svadharma*, suggesting that *ahiṃsā* and *brahmacarya*, for example, mean different things to different classes within society.[48] The limbs of yoga are elaborated using emergent models of yoga practice, most notably medieval *haṭhayoga* traditions of *āsana* and *prāṇāyāma* and a standardized set of postures. The technical terms associated with the different limbs of yoga are, in some cases, presented with variant but largely equivalent terminology to that of Pātañjala yoga, such as the substitution of *japa*, "chanting," for *svādhyāya* and *tuṣṭi*, "satisfaction," for *saṃtoṣa*.[49] With respect to the inner limbs (*antaraṅga*) of the *aṣṭāṅgayoga*, the Purāṇas often represent the culmination of the yogic process as a contemplation of Śiva or Viṣṇu leading to the deepest realization of self (*ātman*), ultimate reality (*brahman*), and god (*bhagavat*, *īśvara*). Meditative mastery (*saṃyama*) is the basis for the development of a wide range of accomplishments (*siddhi*), mirroring the range of powers and capacities described in the *vibhūtipāda* section of the *Yogasūtra*. The representation of *aṣṭāṅgayoga* in the Purāṇas also allows for the possibility of a state of liberation within life (*jīvanmukti*), indicating that a realized *yogin* can choose either to enter *kaivalya* immediately or to remain to travel about and enjoy the world.[50] In the *Liṅga Purāṇa*, for example, the liberated *yogin* is described as remaining in the world to teach others on religious matters and to produce creative work, such as poetry in sophisticated meters, before entering final liberation.[51]

The Integration of Yoga into *Brāhmaṇa* Life

Given its pervasive use in the Purāṇa texts, it is clear that the *aṣṭāṅgayoga* paradigm was widely disseminated beyond the *Pātañjalayogaśāstra* tradition. Although Pātañjala Yoga and its commentarial traditions serve as a uniquely authoritative body of texts, the Purāṇic representation of yoga has likely had considerably greater impact on popular conceptions and practices of yoga than the elite philosophical tradition. In the Purāṇas, the *aṣṭāṅgayoga* system was woven into mainstream Hindu sectarian practice, only obliquely referencing Sāṃkhya-Yoga philosophy of the *Yogaśāstra* or *Yogānuśāsana*. As such, knowledge of the *aṣṭāṅgayoga* system and its practice was the domain of *smārta* priests who studied and transmitted the texts through their traditional channels. Training in yoga would, then, not necessarily be associated with traditions of renunciation, but would rather be a significant part of the baseline of training in priestly narrative and ritual traditions, as illustrated in and drawn from the Purāṇa literature. Other genres of *brāhmaṇa* literature, including legal and philosophical texts, similarly illustrate the "mainstreaming" of yoga into legal, ritual, and philosophical culture, where yoga became a topic of considerable reflection, especially to the degree to which it was seen to augment or challenge priestly practices, ideas, and values.

Smārta Yoga and Priestly Law and Ritual

The *aṣṭāṅgayoga* of the Purāṇas is founded on a knowledge of the theory and practice of yoga as represented in its *śāstra* texts and as elucidated within the context of the lived tradition of *smārta brāhmaṇa* Hinduism and other priestly-focused Hindu sects such as the Pāśupatas. In this respect, authority over instruction in yoga is thoroughly situated within the sphere of priestly control, recognizing its utilization within the context of priestly traditions of the householder and the renouncer, as negotiated by concepts such as class (*varṇa*), stage of life (*āśrama*), and goals of life (*puruṣārtha*).[52] These concepts, central to *brāhmaṇa* ideology, relate how one's class (*varṇa*) and stage of life (*āśrama*) are linked to the goals of human life (*puruṣārtha*). They were established as such in the legal treatise of Manu, the *Manusmṛti*, by approximately the second century CE.[53] The four classes (*varṇa*) include those of the priest (*brāhmaṇa*), warrior or ruler (*kṣatriya* or *rājanya*), merchant (*vaiśya*), and servant (*śūdra*). Males of the first three levels are eligible for initiation (*upanayana*) into Hindu society as a twice-born (*dvija*) person, who is permitted to study religious texts. *Varṇa* is the foundation upon which the more complex system of birth (*jāti*), often translated as "caste," is developed, yielding an association between heredity and social identity and linking one's karma from previous lives to one's present life conditions. The stages of life include those of the celibate student (*brahmacārin*), householder (*gṛhastha*), forest-dweller (*vānaprastha*), and renouncer (*saṃnyāsin*). The goals of life (*puruṣārtha*), or four objects of life (*caturvarga*), include instruction in law and duty (*dharma*) for the *brahmacārin*, wealth (*artha*) and pleasure (*kāma*) for the householder (*gṛhastha*), and liberation (*mokṣa*) for the forest-dweller (*vānaprastha*) and renouncer (*saṃnyāsin*). The emerging legal treatises of the Hindu *brāhmaṇa* traditions, such as the *Manusmṛti* and *Vāsiṣṭha Dharmaśāstra*, demonstrate differing attitudes toward the practice of yoga, in some cases equating it with excessive austerities and the quest for power and in others acknowledging its unique soteriological value.[54] The priestly orthodoxy sought a middle ground in their discourse that validated yoga in its temperate forms that neither destroyed the body nor contradicted the goal of obtaining liberation (*mokṣa*) and invalidated those focused on the pursuit of power, especially through self-mortification.[55]

Examples of the integration of yoga into the performative ritual life of *smārta brāhmaṇa* traditions can also be found in the priestly manuals of the *Sāmavidhāna* and *Ṛgvidhāna* and in the *Vaikhānasasmārtasūtra*, among others.[56] In the *Vaikhānasasmārtasūtra*, an early priestly text that documents various traditions of renunciation, the *aṣṭāṅgayoga* system is lauded as particularly important among a wide range of documented ascetic practices. The *Vaikhānasasmārtasūtra* is associated with the Vedic school of the *Kṛṣṇa* (black) *Yajurveda*, incorporating teachings previously outside the Vedic fold, including some proto-tantric elements that may have been influential on later traditions.[57] The priestly manuals of the *Sāmavidhāna* and *Ṛgvidhāna* include references to various yogic accomplishments (*siddhi*), and the *Ṛgvidhāna* contains a passage that summarizes the progression through *āsana*, *japa*, *prāṇāyāma*, and *dhyāna* in a manner that parallels *aṣṭāṅgayoga* and Purāṇic descriptions of the performance of yoga. The integration of asceticism and yoga into priestly practice was clearly part of the larger paradigm of the emerging *smārta* traditions, evident in the framing of such practice as part of larger ritual observances in these priestly manuals.

Yoga and Vedānta Philosophical Systems

Among the different schools of thought in India, the tradition of Vedānta is possibly the most influential expression of Hindu philosophy, pervading Hindu discourse from the classical era onward. As a philosophical *darśana*,

Vedānta is focused on the teachings of the end (*anta*) of the Veda (*veda*), namely those of the Āraṇyakas and Upaniṣads, especially as they were concerned with the process of achieving liberation (*mokṣa*), though a recognition of the underlying reality of things (*brahman*). In one key formulation, this ultimate reality (*brahman*) is qualified as being (*sat*), consciousness (*cit*), and bliss (*ānanda*).[58] Based on the Upaniṣadic commentary of Bādarāyaṇa's (3rd century CE) *Brahmasūtra*, the "Discourse on *Brahman*," also known as the *Vedāntasūtra*, and other primary texts that expand on the philosophy of the Upaniṣads, such as the *Bhagavadgītā*, Vedānta traditions analyze the nature of bondage and liberation. The philosopher and reformer Śaṅkara (8th century CE), typically represented as a Śaiva or a Smārta *brāhmaṇa*, is the foremost representative of the non-dual (*advaita*) school of Vedānta, and the Vaiṣṇava philosopher Rāmānuja (11th century CE) the principal figure in the qualified-non-dual (*viśiṣṭa-advaita*) school of Vedānta. A third major system of dualist (*dvaita*) Vedānta is associated with the philosopher Madhva (13th century CE).

Śaṅkara argues that all things that appear to exist separate from *brahman* exist only through the force of *māyā*, or illusion, as part of conventional (*vyavahāra*) and not absolute (*paramārtha*) reality, whereas Rāmānuja argues that *brahman* and the world are both real, thus qualifying (*viśiṣṭa*) the "internal" nature of the non-dual ultimate reality (*brahman*).[59] Madhva's position, in turn, can be viewed as moving beyond Rāmānuja's qualification toward one in which relationship prevails over identity, in that the supreme being, represented as Viṣṇu, is viewed as a transcendent reality radically distinct from the human soul (*ātman*). Śaṅkara's view is often represented as aligned with *jñānayoga*, while those of Rāmānuja and Madhva incrementally toward *bhaktiyoga*. Śaṅkara postulates that *brahman* must be understood without form (*nirguṇa*), but that theistic worship of personal deities with form (*saguṇa*) may facilitate the movement toward *nirguṇa brahman*. Rāmānuja and Madhva, on the other hand, emphasize the centrality of devotion (*bhakti*) to Viṣṇu as a means of achieving liberation (*mokṣa*). These philosophical orientations map, to some degree, onto different theological positions in which either identity or relationship with an ultimately deity is expressed. Śaṅkara is often formally identified with the Smārta Brāhmaṇa Hindu sect, Rāmānuja with Śrī Vaiṣṇavism, and Madhva with Sad Vaiṣṇavism.

Śaṅkara and Rāmānuja both reject the Sāṃkhya dualism that frames Pātañjala Yoga but accept the utility of yoga as a discipline that can facilitate spiritual practice. It has been argued that Śaṅkara may have himself been a practitioner of the Sāṃkhya-Yoga system before abandoning it for Vedānta, as his name is associated with an important commentary to the *Pātañjalayogaśāstra*, the *Yogasūtrabhāṣyavivaraṇa* or *Pātañjalayogaśāstravivaraṇa* (9th century CE).[60] Śaṅkara's viewpoint on yoga is clearly articulated in his commentary to the *Brahmasūtra*, the *Brahmasūtrabhāṣya*, where he validates the limbs of yoga of the *aṣṭāṅgayoga* system and the spiritual accomplishments (*siddhi*) of yoga as of value in the soteriological process and as augments to the capacities of an enlightened being.[61] With regards to the value of the latter, popular narrative in the Hindu tradition recounts Śaṅkara's ability to enter into the bodies of others through his yogic power.[62] Where Śaṅkara draws the line, however, is in his firm rejection of the dualistic assumptions of the Sāṃkhya-Yoga system and its non-Vedic pedigree.[63] Śaṅkara's mode of spiritual discipline is commonly referred to as *jñānayoga*, appealing to the goal of the realization of knowledge of *brahman* that leads to liberation (*mokṣa*) from *saṃsāra*, where yoga serves as a systematic discipline in which body and mind are purified and prepared for *jñāna*. For Rāmānuja and for Madhva, in contrast, the rubric of spiritual discipline is instead *bhaktiyoga*, the yoga of devotion. For Rāmānuja, the *aṣṭāṅgayoga* system serves as a preparatory discipline that builds a foundation for the soteriological process of *bhaktiyoga*. Similarly, the Śrī Vaiṣṇava and Viśiṣṭādvaita figures of Nāthamuni (10th century CE) and Yamunācārya (11th century CE) are linked in narrative traditions to the practice of *aṣṭāṅgayoga*, giving a sense of the cache the system had within Vaiṣṇava sectarian traditions.[64]

Yoga also plays a central role in the Vedānta philosophy articulated by the Vedāntic philosopher Vidyāraṇya (14th century CE), who in his *Jīvanmuktiviveka*, "Investigation into Liberation-in-Life," situates the *aṣṭāṅgayoga* paradigm within a Vedāntic framework, presenting the Pātañjala Yoga system as a means to realization of *brahman*.[65] Another influential late Vedāntic thinker, Vijñānabhikṣu (16th century CE), wrote a commentary on the *Pātañjalayogaśāstra* entitled the *Yogavārttika*, the "Exposition on Yoga," which is infused with the Vedāntic philosophical doctrine of "difference and non-difference" (*bhedābheda*). The concept of *bhedābheda* may be one of the earliest and most pervasive doctrines of Vedānta philosophy, sometimes ascribed to Bādarāyaṇa's viewpoint as articulated in the *Brahmasūtra*.[66] As with Vidyāraṇya, Vijñānabhikṣu articulates a viewpoint in which Pātañjala Yoga and Vedānta are seen as complementary practices, and his integration of the metaphysics and cosmology of Vedānta and Sāṃkhya extends beyond that of his predecessor.[67] Vijñānabhikṣu, like many of his contemporaries, utilizes the Purāṇa literature extensively in his commentarial work on Sāṃkhya-Yoga and Vedānta, including the *Viṣṇu*, *Kūrma*, and *Bhāgavata Purāṇa*.

The Classical Hindu Representation of Yoga

In the *itihāsa-purāṇa* literature and its accessories, in works of Hindu law and ritual, and in the major philosophical schools of Vedānta, yoga is a primary religious praxis facilitating the pursuit of *dharma*, the pursuit of liberation (*mokṣa*) from worldly miseries, and the achievement of extraordinary powers and capacities. Yoga is integrated into the scope of classical Hindu models of religious thought and practice, and the *aṣṭāṅgayoga* model and Pātañjala Yoga are preeminent models adapted to fit new paradigms of *smārta brāhmaṇa* practice. The narratives of emergent theism in Hinduism, the *Mahābhārata*, the *Rāmāyaṇa*, and the Purāṇas, document the theory and practice of yoga and its embodiment by its human practitioners and by gods and goddesses. Yoga is woven into the narrative and philosophical fabric of classical Hinduism, sharing common ground with sectarian ritual observances such as worship (*pūjā*), and its iconic status in the Indian religious imagination extends to the present. Classical conceptions of yoga draw upon the earlier Vedic literature and endorse elements of the *vaidika brāhmaṇa* model while establishing a mode of Hindu practice accessible to all levels of Hindu society. They emulate, parallel, and anticipate further developments of yoga in the non-Vedic traditions of Jainism and Buddhism, and serve as the foundation upon which later formal traditions of devotion (*bhakti*) and the various tantric (*tāntrika*) modes of religious practice develop in the medieval era.

Chapter 6

Classical *Śramaṇa* Traditions of Yoga

During the early centuries of the Common Era, Hindu, Buddhist, and Jain traditions all sought to cultivate popular support at the grassroots level and patronage by the Gupta Dynasty and other ruling powers in the upper echelons of Indian society. Within this competitive and diverse social and religious context, the *śramaṇa* traditions of Jainism and Buddhism developed extensive scholastic traditions, which were in conversation with one another and with the formal systems of philosophy emerging out of the Hindu literature. Jain traditions systematized their path to liberation (*mokṣa*, *kevala*), consolidating pan-Indian techniques of asceticism and contemplation and drawing upon non-Jain frameworks, such as the *aṣṭāṅgayoga* system of Pātañjala Yoga. The two major sectarian traditions of Jainism, the Sky-Clad (*digambara*) and White-Clad (*śvetāmbara*), both developed sophisticated conceptions of a religious path (*mārga*) that was to be traversed in a step-like progression of stages of virtue (*guṇasthāna*), through the use of ascetic and yogic techniques.

In the Buddhist tradition, scholastic analysis of Buddhist doctrine, referred to as Higher Dharma (Skt. *Abhidharma*, Pāli *Abhidhamma*) grew rapidly during the early centuries of the Common Era, yielding a range of interpretive schools of Buddhist thought and a growing body of Buddhist philosophical literature. These developments helped pave the way for the emergence of the Mahāyāna or Great Vehicle tradition of Buddhism, sometimes referred to as "Northern Buddhism" due to its geographic representation in Nepal, Tibet, China, Korea, Japan, and Vietnam. Over time, Mahāyāna became one of the two most important sectarian traditions of

Buddhism, along with the Theravāda, the Elder's Tradition or "Southern Buddhism," which consolidated in Sri Lanka, Thailand, Burma, Cambodia, and Laos. With the development of various schools of Indian Buddhist thought, enumerated as eighteen in number or more, doctrinal and path (*mārga*) systems developed that integrated Buddhist contemplative practice into elaborate cosmological and psychological frameworks. Buddhist practitioners dedicated to the development of meditative practices, especially *dhyāna* (Pāli *jhāna*), were increasingly referred to as utilizing methods of yoga, as evident in the explicit titles given to meditators, such as *yogin* and "practitioner of yoga" (*yogācāra*).[1] Theravāda Buddhist traditions developed meditation manuals that framed Buddhist practice in light of yogic and ascetic practice, often focusing on the development of *dhyāna* (Pāli *jhāna*). Similarly, over the course of the early centuries of the Common Era, Mahāyāna Buddhist traditions developed sophisticated meditative and visionary practices that were integrated under the rubric of yoga into Mahāyāna path (*mārga*) structures.

Jain Sectarian Traditions and the Path to Liberation

The two principal sectarian traditions of Jainism, the Digambara and Śvetāmbara, share a foundation of early scripture and practice but have distinct textual, philosophical, and performative traditions. Digambara and Śvetāmbara traditions are distinguished by their divergent accounts of the story of Mahāvīra, but their division may have, in part, been related to the splitting of the Jain community during a famine near 300 BCE.[2] One group, which had traveled south, came to view the northern community as heretical, due to differences in their scriptural recensions and their abandonment of nudity in favor of white (*śveta*) clothing. There are, however, variant understandings among both sects of the cause and the nature of this schism that favor one or the other.[3] Though each sect developed a unique textual tradition, some texts are shared between the two traditions, a notable example being the *Tattvārthasūtra* of Umāsvāti (4th–5th century CE), which may have predated the Digambara-Śvetāmbara schism and is accepted as canonical by both sects.[4] Later Jain texts, such as Haribhadra's *Yogadṛṣṭisamuccaya* (8th century CE) and Hemacandra's *Yogaśāstra* (12th century CE), build on the foundation of the *Tattvārthasūtra* and expand the language and categories of Jain yoga practice extensively.

The *Tattvārthasūtra* of Umāsvāti

The *Tattvārthasūtra*, or "Discourse on the Nature of Reality," (4th–5th century CE) of Umāsvāti provides a systematic overview of Jain philosophy and practice, establishing a foundation of shared concepts and practices used by the two traditions.[5] It details, among other things, the nature of the world, the sources of bondage, the process of liberation, and the nature of liberation, as reflected in the Jain Three Jewels (*ratnatraya*) of correct view (*samyag-darśana*), correct knowledge (*samyag-jñāna*), and correct action (*samyak-cāritra*).[6] The *Tattvārthasūtra* was one of the first Jain texts composed in Sanskrit, mirroring the broader development in Indic traditions of the *sūtra* mode of discourse.[7] In some respects, it can be compared to the *Yogasūtra* in its terse representation of the Jain path and its prescription of ascetic and yogic techniques.[8] Its ten chapters deal with the path to liberation (*mokṣa-mārga*), existence (*bhāva*), hell and human realms (*naraka, dvīpa*), gods (*deva*), lifeless substances (*ajīva-dravya*), inflow of *karma* (*āsrava*), virtuous and unvirtuous (*śubha-aśubha*) *karma*, bondage (*bandha*), and liberation (*mokṣa*).[9]

The *Tattvārthasūtra* codifies the practices of vows (*vrata*), ascetic discipline (*tapas*), and of meditation (*dhyāna*) that connect Jain practice to broader yoga traditions. Umāsvāti outlines the nature of the five vows (*vrata*) as the restraint of harm (*hiṃsā*), falsehood (*anṛta*), stealing (*steya*), nonchastity (*abrahma*), and greed (*parigraha*), and qualifies them as being either small (*aṇu*) or great (*mahā*). These factors are supported by the observance of the altruistic attitudes of friendliness (*maitrī*), sympathetic joy (*pramoda*), compassion (*kāruṇya*), and equanimity (*mādhyastha*) toward beings of various kinds.[10] These factors are described as facilitating the influx of virtuous or wholesome (*śubha*) karma, and are aided by asceticism (*tapas*), which blocks the influx of karma and destroys accumulated karma. There are six external austerities, including fasting and self-mortification, and six internal austerities, the latter of which includes the study of religious scripture (*svādhyāya*) and the practice of meditation (*dhyāna*), along with penance, service, and renunciation.[11] Two kinds of meditation (*dhyāna*) result in liberation (*mokṣa*), namely, discursive (*dharma*) and white or pure (*śukla*), the former a contemplation of teachings and principles, and the latter a realization of truth and omniscience.[12] The description of *śukladhyāna* is followed by a discussion of the factors of thought (*vitarka* and *vicāra*), which are components of contemplation in both Hindu and

Buddhist meditative schema.[13] The *Tattvārthasūtra* provides a list of ten stages of spiritual accomplishment, from the beginning learner to the victor (*jina*), which anticipate the later development of the *guṇasthāna*, or "stages of virtue."[14] The last section of the *Tattvārthasūtra* details the liberation of the soul (*jīva*) upon the destruction of all *karma* and the ascension of the *jīva* to the summit of the universe.[15] The final verse classifies liberation as being various types, depending on whether it is by oneself or with the help of others, and whether one becomes a teacher after liberation or not, paralleling the *śrāvaka-pratyekabuddha-buddha* distinction found in Buddhism.[16]

The *Yogadṛṣṭisamuccaya* of Haribhadra and the *Yogaśāstra* of Hemacandra

The *Yogadṛṣṭisamuccaya*, "Compilation of Views on Yoga," (8th century CE) of Haribhadra, also known as Haribhadrasūri, presents a Śvetāmbara Jain attempt to engage and synthesize the views of Jains with those of Hindus and Buddhists. Some scholars have suggested that Haribhadra himself might have been a Hindu *brāhmaṇa* who converted to Jainism.[17] In the *Yogadṛṣṭisamuccaya*, Haribhadra analyzes various yogic practices in light of the *aṣṭāṅgayoga* and *guṇasthāna* systems and critiques practices that he deems heretical, particularly goddess worship and tantric practices.[18] In the process, he synthesizes the *aṣṭāṅgayoga* factors with the names of various female deities (Mitrā, Tārā, Balā, Dīprā, Sthirā, Kāntā, Prabhā, and Parā), attaching them to *yama* and the other limbs of yoga, respectively.[19] Haribhadra also provides a larger framework of a threefold yoga of the wishful (*icchā*), precept (*śāstra*), and effort (*sāmarthya*), which may correlate to a tantric framework that was gaining prominence.[20]

The *Yogaśāstra*, or "Treatise on Yoga," (12th century CE) of Hemacandra, another influential Śvetāmbara text, similarly reframes classical and popular practices of yoga within a scholastic Jain orthodoxy. The significance of the *Yogaśāstra* as a Jain discourse is evident in that it was one of the principal sources for Mādhava's representation of the Jain system in his *Sarvadarśanasaṃgraha*.[21] Centered on the Three Jewels (*ratnatraya*) as presented in the *Tattvārthasūtra*, namely, correct view (*samyag-darśana*), correct knowledge (*samyag-jñāna*), and correct action (*samyag-cāritra*), the *Yogaśāstra* presents a uniquely Jain perspective on the *aṣṭāṅgayoga* and on broader conceptions of *karma-*, *jñāna-*, and *bhaktiyoga*.[22] Hemacandra presents the twofold doctrine (*dvidharma*) of world-affirmation (*pravṛtti*) and world-negation (*nivṛtti*), correlating to the Hindu division of *karma* and *jñāna*, especially in the form of the *karmakāṇḍa-jñānakāṇḍa* distinction, and the Buddhist view of the twofold nature of the Noble Eightfold Path as applied to monastics and laypeople.[23] The *Yogaśāstra* contains a nexus of practices shared among *śramaṇa* traditions and *brāhmaṇa* asceticism, including vows, precepts, and observances (*vrata*, *yama*, *niyama*), disciplines of posture (*āsana*) and breath control (*prāṇāyāma*, influenced by *haṭha* and *tantra*-based yogas), and meditation (*bhāvanā*, *dhyāna*). The cultivation of altruistic emotions is said to purify the mind in preparation for meditation, akin to its presentation in the *Yogasūtra*, and the practice of meditation is described as rooted in evenness (*samatva*), a term used in the *Bhagavadgītā* to define yoga.[24] Various powers or accomplishments (*siddhi*) are described as arising from yogic practice, particularly from the practice of *prāṇāyāma*, and the end of the *Yogaśāstra* describes the culmination of the perfection of *dhyāna*, the achievement of *mokṣa*, and the final liberation of the *jīva*.[25]

Buddhist Scholasticism and Path (*mārga*) and Abhidharma Literature

According to Buddhist narrative, shortly after the death of the Buddha, the early community of disciples met for the first Buddhist council at Rājagṛha and consolidated the teachings of the Buddha into a twofold division of discourse (Skt. *sūtra* or *sūkta*, Pāli *sutta*) and code (*vinaya*), sometimes referred to jointly as *dharmavinaya* or the "teachings and code" of the Buddha. The oral tradition of the *dharmavinaya* became the basis for the development of the Pāli Nikāya literature and later Buddhist narrative and philosophical literature. Over time, a third member was added to the *dharma* and *vinaya* of Buddhism, the *abhidharma* (Pāli *abhidhamma*), meaning "concerning the *dharma*" or "higher *dharma*," referring to analysis and commentary on the *sūtra* and *vinaya* literature.[26] The three, *sūtra*, *vinaya*, and *abhidharma*, together are referred to as the Three Baskets (Skt. *tripiṭaka*, Pāli *tipiṭaka*) and are the canonical scriptural foundation of Buddhism. Over the course of several hundred years, under the influence of royal patrons that included emperor Aśoka, Buddhists convened a series of councils, including important meetings at Vaiśālī and Pāṭaliputra, that marked the division of the Buddhist community into various sectarian groups. The council of Pāṭaliputra, in particular, is understood to have been the point of separation between two principal sects, the Sthaviravāda (Pāli Theravāda, "Teaching of the Elders") and the Mahāsāṃghika, or "Great Assembly," which anticipated the division between Theravāda and Mahāyāna Buddhism that persists to the present.

Following Pāṭaliputra, numerous schools of Buddhism developed, which were classified in the polemical rubric of later Mahāyāna tradition as the eighteen schools of the so-called Hīnayāna, or "lesser vehicle," Buddhism.[27] Among the influential schools were the Distinctionalist Teaching (*vibhajyavāda*, foundational for Theravāda) school, the All Exists Teaching (*sarvāstivāda*) school, the Near Discourse (*sautrāntika*) school, and the Supramundane [Buddha] Teaching (*lokottaravāda*) school. Contemporary Theravāda traditions of Buddhism are a descendent, via the Vibhajyavāda tradition, of the Sthaviravāda branch of the original community. Though all of the other schools died out in India over time, they nonetheless contributed to the rise of the Theravāda and Mahāyāna traditions, and many of them were subsumed within the Mahāyāna hierarchy of views. Just as Theravāda philosophy is characterized by a conservative impulse to preserve the teachings and mode of living of the historical Buddha, Mahāyāna has been marked by its adaptability and as conceiving Buddhahood and the Buddhist path in expansive, if not cosmic, terms. Drawing upon the systematic articulations of Buddhist philosophy in Sarvāstivāda, the early Middle Way (*madhyamaka*) school, and formulations of the transcendent nature of Buddhahood developed in the Lokottaravāda and other subschools of the Mahāsaṃghika, Mahāyāna is representative of a Buddhism transformed during the classical era of Indian religion and philosophy. Whereas Theravāda focused on the Pāli Nikāya literature developed in early Buddhism, Mahāyāna shifted toward a classical Sanskrit and Buddhist Hybrid Sanskrit literature that included existing literature and new, emergent discourses and philosophical texts. However, like the Theravāda, the Mahāyāna developed systematic presentations of the path (*mārga*) to liberation that incorporated practices of yoga, especially meditation, into a pragmatic framework for attaining successive states of spiritual accomplishment that culminated in awakening as a *śrāvaka*, *pratyekabuddha*, or even as a *samyaksaṃbuddha*.

The *Vimuttimagga* and the *Visuddhimagga*

Theravāda Buddhism has historically been most successful in South and Southeast Asia, most notably in Sri Lanka, Burma, Thailand, Cambodia, Laos, and parts of Vietnam. In the early centuries of the Common Era, it was in competition with other sects of Buddhism, but by approximately the tenth century CE, it became the dominant expression of Buddhism throughout the region. Theravāda Buddhism has historically utilized the scriptural and liturgical language of Pāli. The Pāli language is closely related to Sanskrit, but less grammatically and phonetically complex, a formal language but one closer to spoken vernaculars. In the early centuries of the Common Era, Theravādins developed texts that sought to distill the practical essence of an increasingly voluminous Buddhist canonical literature. One important representation of this literature is the *Vimuttimagga* of Upatissa, the "Path to Liberation," (1st–3rd century CE), a terse and pragmatic guide to the pursuit of liberation in the Theravāda Buddhist tradition.[28] Biographical information regarding Upatissa is limited, though it is theorized that he was born in India or Sri Lanka.[29] The text is divided into parts that detail the three trainings (Pāli *tisikkhā*, Skt. *triśikṣā*) in higher ethics (*adhisīlasikkhā*), higher thought (*adhicittasikkhā*), and higher wisdom (*adhipaññāsikkhā*), correlating to the cultivation of ethics (*sīla*, Skt. *śīla*), contemplation (*samādhi*), and wisdom (*paññā*, Skt. *prajñā*). These, in turn, lead to purity of virtue (*sīlavisuddhi*), purity of mind (*cittavisuddhi*), and purity of view (*diṭṭhivisuddhi*).[30] The training in ethics (*sīla*) consists in the discernment of the nature of virtue, the practice of renunciation (*dhuta*, literally "shaking off") and austerities, represented by a list of thirteen factors or limbs (*aṅga*) that include restrictions on clothing, food intake, place of residence, and body posture that parallel broader Indian conceptions of *tapas*.[31] The training in contemplation (*samādhi*) consists in the discernment of the nature of contemplation, the qualities of a teacher, behavior and its relation to states of mind, subjects of meditation and their practice, and the higher knowledge (*abhijñā*) that arises from the perfection of meditation. The training in wisdom (*pañña*) begins with discernment of the nature of wisdom, the structure of the compositional factors or aggregates (*khandha*) that make up the human organism, their contemplation, the methods of obtaining insight, and the different stages of attainment culminating in the state of Worthy One (*arahant*, Skt. *arhant* or *arhat*). Throughout the text, Upatissa utilizes a rubric of the "practitioner of yoga" (*yogin* or *yogāvacara*), to illustrate the ways in which Buddhist contemplative practice is to be observed and embodied.[32]

Buddhaghosa's *Visuddhimagga*, or "Path of Purification" (5th century CE), presents a complete path (*magga*) to liberation using the framework of the threefold training (*tisikkhā*), paralleling Upatissa's work. Buddhaghosa was an Indian monk who achieved considerable esteem in Sri Lanka as a translator of and commentator on Pāli Buddhist literature. According to Buddhist tradition, Buddhaghosa was an Indian *brāhmaṇa* who had converted to Buddhism, and as a result his writing was sophisticated and his Pāli vocabulary informed by his knowledge of Sanskrit.[33] Over time, Buddhaghosa's *Visuddhimagga* became a manual for Buddhist contemplation and, much like the *Yogaśāstra* of Hemacandra for Jains, a source for establishing orthodoxy. The *Visuddhimagga* appears to be an expansion of the *Vimuttimagga*, and the two texts serve as representative examples of the development of Pāli path (*magga*) literature during the early centuries of the Common Era. Buddhaghosa's work is significantly larger, as he uses canonical quotations throughout the work to illustrate and support his presentation of the Buddhist path (*magga*) and engages in sophisticated discussions of *Abhidhamma* topics and issues beyond the focus of praxis found in the *Vimuttimagga*.

Buddhaghosa outlines a systematic path to liberation, beginning with the cultivation of the threefold training (*tisikkhā*) in ethics (*sīla*), contemplation (*samādhi*), and wisdom (*pañña*). The various aspects of *sīla* are discussed with a particular focus on ascetic observances characteristic of monastic practitioners falling under the rubric of the Limbs of Removal (*dhutaṅga*). The *Visuddhimagga* deals at length with the development of *jhāna* (Skt. *dhyāna*) and its technical aspects, providing elaborate schemata for the establishment of contemplation (*samādhi*). Buddhaghosa discusses the manner in which the forty meditation subjects or "action bases" (*kammaṭṭhāna*, Skt. *karmasthāna*) serve to counter afflictive emotional states, indicating the manner in which meditative practice on particular subjects can serve as an antidote to particular unwholesome mental states.[34] Buddhaghosa's teachings on *pañña* conform to the emphasis in Theravāda Buddhism and the Nikāya literature on the causal process of dependent co-origination (*paṭiccasamuppāda*) that at base has three marks (*tilakkhaṇa*) of impermanence (*anicca*), unsatisfactoriness or suffering (*dukkha*), and selflessness (*anatta*). As with the *Vimuttimagga*, the focus of the *Visud-*

dhimagga is on the attainment of the four Hearer (*sāvaka*, Skt. *śrāvaka*) states of the Noble Person (*ariyapuggala*), including the Stream Winner (*sotāpanna*), Once Returner (*sakadāgāmin*), Non-Returner (*anāgāmin*), and Worthy One (*arahant*). This again reflects the common division of attainments into that of Śrāvakas, Pratyekabuddhas, and Buddhas that runs through Theravāda and Mahāyāna soteriology. A colophon attributed to Buddhaghosa at the end of the *Visuddhimagga* indicates that he hoped at death to be reborn in the Tāvatiṃsa (Skt. Trayastriṃśa) heaven so that he could see the future Buddha Metteyya (Skt. Maitreya) in his heavenly domain before the *bodhisattva* is born for the last time in the human realm.[35]

The *Vimuttimagga* and *Visuddhimagga* may have been utilized by Theravāda traditions of meditator-monks referred to as the "engaged in yoga" (*yogāvacara*) that are evident in late Pāli and Singhalese texts.[36] Though the question of the historical relationship between *yogāvacara* traditions and mainstream Theravāda is complex one, the *yogāvacara* traditions appear to have also used mantra practices, tantric or proto-tantric elements of visualization, and the use of *prāṇāyāma* techniques, drawing on elements from Mahāyāna Buddhism and Hindu yoga traditions.[37] These *yogāvacara* traditions, represented in small numbers throughout the Theravāda world, may have contributed to the rise of modern meditation movements, among them the highly popular and influential Dhammakaya meditation tradition in Thailand.

The *Abhidharmakośa* and *Abhidharmakośabhāṣya*

Along with the development of Pāli Abhidhamma traditions in South and Southeast Asia, elaborate systems of Abhidharma analysis developed in the Sanskritized traditions of Indian Buddhism. One of the most important examples is Vasubandhu's *Abhidharmakośabhāṣya*, "Explanation of the Collection of the Abhidharma (*Abhidharmakośa*)" (4th–5th century CE), a survey and analysis of the cosmological and ontological framework of Sarvāstivāda Buddhism. The *Abhidharmakośa* extended out of a tradition of Abhidharma literature linked to the *Mahāvibhāṣā*, or "Great Commentary" (2nd century CE), a seminal Sanskrit text that articulated the Vaibhāṣika-Sarvāstivāda system of thought and helped establish a scholastic framework for Buddhist philosophy in Sanskrit.[38] Vasubandhu, who was later associated with the Yogācāra school of Mahāyāna Buddhism, argues from a Sautrāntika viewpoint in the *Abhidharmakośabhāṣya*.[39] The composers of the contemporaneous *Pātañjalayogaśāstra* tradition were familiar with Abhidharma analysis, as many terms, concepts, and theories in Pātañjala Yoga, such as that of processes of change (*pariṇāma*), are parallel to, or perhaps even direct borrowings from, Buddhist literature.[40] As with much of Buddhist scholastic literature, particular attention is paid in the *Abhidharmakośabhāṣya* to the refutation of the Sāṃkhya viewpoint and little to critiques of the practice of yoga itself.[41] The *Abhidharmakośabhāṣya* and other Sanskrit Abhidharma treatises played an important role in the rise of the Mahāyāna tradition, which drew in important ways upon the Sanskrit traditions of Abhidharma. Although Sanskrit Abhidharma works are largely scholastic in nature and provide little practical instruction, they provide psychological and metaphysical frameworks for understanding and interpreting contemplative practice.

Rise of the Mahāyāna Tradition

In the early centuries of the Common Era (1st–3rd century CE), a new Buddhist sect emerged, referred to by its adherents as the "Great Vehicle" (*mahāyāna*), in contrast with other sects of Buddhism that were designated as the "Small Vehicle" (*hīnayāna*). The formulators of Mahāyāna argued that its teachings had superior soteriological capacity as framed in terms of securing the welfare of all beings in *saṃsāra*. *Hīnayāna* is a pejorative term, and traditions labeled as such by the Mahāyāna neither accepted nor approved of the label. Mahāyāna is characterized by an emphasis on the dual values of wisdom (*prajñā*) and compassion (*karuṇā*), the latter of which is sometimes contrasted to the emphasis on the value of generosity (*dāna*) characteristic of other Buddhist sects. The rise of the Mahāyāna was linked to an expanded Buddhist Sanskrit literature representing teachings of the Buddha and of Bodhisattvas that were held to have been revealed in secret to select disciples or received through visionary experiences. These new *sūtra*, and later *tantra*, texts, were commented on extensively in a new wave of Mahāyāna philosophical and scholastic treatises. The expanded literature of the Mahāyāna gave rise to new philosophical schools of Buddhism, most notably the Middle Way school (*madhyamaka*) school and the Yoga Practice (*yogācāra*) school. These Mahāyāna schools transformed Buddhist philosophy in significant ways, notably developing influential ideas regarding emptiness (*śūnyatā*) and mind-only-reality (*citta-mātra*), respectively. The Indian Mahāyāna tradition emphasized the aspiration to achieve complete Buddhahood as opposed to obtaining the state of the *arhat*, and as a result Mahāyāna is also referred to as the Vehicle of the Bodhisattva (*bodhisattvayāna*). The emphasis on the career of the Bodhisattva was accompanied by an expansive cosmology in which the universe was viewed as inhabited by innumerable fully enlightened Buddhas and by powerful Bodhisattvas striving for perfection, all of whom work compassionately and untiringly for the liberation of beings in *saṃsāra* from suffering (*duḥkha*).

Mahāyāna Monasticism and Householder Traditions

Mahāyāna may have represented, in part, the bridging of Buddhist monastic and householder traditions through the validation of the ideal of the householder-*bodhisattva* in Mahāyāna texts such as the *Vimalakīrtinirdeśasūtra*, bringing the *bodhisattva*-ideal to a larger popular audience. However, evidence suggests that Mahāyāna was, in the beginning, principally an organic development within Buddhist monastic traditions, which housed followers of various philosophical orientations, and that the lay-monastic split was not initially a determinative factor.[42] The rise of Mahāyāna coincided with the reemergence of *brāhmaṇa* scholarship and literature in the early centuries of the Common Era and the development of Buddhist scholasticism. Mahāyāna traditions were in conversation with classical Hindu traditions of narrative and philosophy and drew heavily on the Sanskrit literature of the Sarvāstivāda and other schools of Buddhism. The use of Sanskrit, particularly what is referred to as "Buddhist Hybrid Sanskrit," for the representation of the Mahāyāna texts signaled a shift toward a more sophisticated cultural and linguistic framework for Buddhism. This association between Buddhism and an elite, learned culture is evident in the establishment of the Mahāyāna Buddhist universities of Nālandā (6th–12th century CE) and Vikramaśīla (9th–12th century CE), which served as two of the most important institutions of higher learning in India for centuries, teaching both Buddhist and Brāhmaṇical subjects. Mahāyāna also induced the development of a range of traditions of Buddhist devotionalism that met with great success in India and throughout Asia, particularly the worship of Amitābha Buddha, who, along with key *bodhisattva* figures, is the focus of many contemporary devotional traditions collectively referred to as "Pure Land" Buddhism.

Madhyamaka

The Buddhist Middle Way school (*madhyamaka*) is strongly associated with the early Mahāyāna literature of the *Prajñāpāramitāsūtra*, "Perfection of Wisdom Discourse," and the work of the philosopher Nāgārjuna and his intellectual descendants, including Bhāvaviveka and Candrakīrti, the former of which wrote a notable critique of contemporaneous Hindu, likely Śaiva, yoga practices.[43] Nāgārjuna is represented in some Buddhist traditions as having descended into the world of the serpents (*nāga*) to retrieve the hidden Buddhist texts of the *Prajñāpāramitā*.[44] At the heart of the *Prajñāpāramitāsūtra* and Nāgārjuna's philosophy is the principle that all categories of existence are at their foundation empty (*śūnya*) of self-existence (*svabhāva*). For Nāgārjuna, even the doctrines of the Buddha himself, such as the Four Noble Truths, are viewed as ultimately empty of a final reality or absolute mode of existence. They are instead viewed as means to achieving insight and are to be abandoned once they have fulfilled their purpose, rather than becoming objects of clinging or attachment. This view, according to Nāgārjuna, is an explication and expansion on the truth of dependent co-origination (*pratītyasamutpāda*), the view that all things arise conditionally and without any permanent or abiding essence. Reality can be thus understood through two types of truth, conventional (*saṃvṛtti*) and ultimate (*paramārtha*), which designate the appearance of an existent object and the true nature of existent objects, respectively.[45] Nāgārjuna's view is non-dualist, but unlike the non-dual (*advaita*) and monistic Vedānta, he does not postulate a transcendent unity that stands beyond duality. Later commentators postulate that his aim was to move beyond language toward a mode of direct perception that represents a rejection of all views.[46] Nāgārjuna's formulation of emptiness (*śūnyatā*) pervades Mahāyāna Buddhist philosophy and serves as a subject and basis of conventional and tantric forms of meditation in Mahāyāna Buddhism.

Yogācāra

With the rise of Abhidharma schools and the Mahāyāna over the course of the early centuries of the Common Era, the concepts of *yogācāra/yogācārā* and *yogācāra bhikṣu/bhikṣunī* emerge in Buddhist literature to designate practitioners dedicated to contemplative practice, especially meditation.[47] The use of these terms, equivalent to and interchangeable with *yogin/yoginī*, demonstrate that by this time period, the rubric of yoga referred to the practice of a spiritual discipline set apart from scholarly and other pursuits. In its early stages, the Yogācāra philosophy in Mahāyāna was an extension of these contemplation-focused traditions of Buddhist practice, providing a practical epistemological framework that elucidated the nature of cognitive processes. Yogācāra is also known as Vijñānavāda or the "Consciousness Way" school, and draws from a range of Mahāyāna discourses, two of the most prominent being the *Laṅkāvatārasūtra*, "Discourse on the Descent into Laṅkā" (4th–5th century CE), which, incidentally, references a fairy (*yakṣa*) king of Laṅkā named Rāvaṇa, and the *Saṃdhinirmocanasūtra*, "Discourse on Unlocking the Connections" (4th–5th century CE). Yogācāra philosophy was articulated by third- to fifth-century CE authors Maitreyanātha (sometimes identified as the future Buddha Maitreya), Asaṅga, and Vasubandhu, in treatises such as the *Abhisamayālaṃkara*, "Ornament on Clear Understanding," the *Madhyāntavibhāga*, "Division of the Middle and Extremes," and the *Yogācārabhūmi*, "Stages of the Practice of Yoga." Yogācāra epistemology was further explicated by philosophers and logicians, two of the most notable being Dignāga and Dharmakirtī, the authors of the *Pramāṇasamuccaya*, "Collection of Valid Knowledge," (6th century CE) and the *Pramāṇavārttika* (7th century CE), "Exposition on Valid Knowledge," respectively.

Yogācāra doctrines include those of mind-only (*cittamātra*) reality, three natures (*trisvabhāva*) or levels of reality, and the three bodies (*trikāya*) of a *buddha*, namely, the manifestation body (*nirmāṇakāya*), the enjoyment body (*saṃbhogakāya*), and the truth body (*dharmakāya*). Other important concepts are of the storehouse consciousness (*ālayavijñāna*), a repository of karmic impressions, the "womb of the thus-gone [*buddha*]" (*tathāgatagarbha*), which is the potential for realization within all beings, and the concepts of "thusness" (*tathatā*) and "*buddha*-nature" (*buddhadhātu*), which refer to the empty (*śūnya*) nature of all things. The Yogācāra path to liberation is characterized by stages (*bhūmi*) of successive spiritual attainments, illustrated in texts such as the *Yogācārabhūmi*, which shares a wide range of concepts and practices, if not a genealogical relationship, with the *Pātañjalayogaśāstra*.[48] The *Yogācārabhūmi* and its commentaries identify the term *yoga* in its primary sense as the application of spiritual discipline and in a secondary sense as referring technically to the practice of *samādhi*.[49] Yogācāra, as is the case with much of Mahāyāna Buddhist philosophy, subsumes so-called Hīnayāna practices into a larger hierarchical framework of ideas and practices.

The *Lotus Sūtra* and the *Ekayāna*

The Mahāyāna emphasis on attaining the status of a fully enlightened *buddha* is illustrated in the *Saddharmapuṇḍarīkasūtra*, the "Lotus of the True Law Discourse" or simply the *Lotus Sūtra* (1st–2nd century CE). The *Lotus Sūtra* is associated with the One Vehicle (*ekayāna*) view, namely, that among the three classical Buddhist goals of the *buddha*, *pratyeka-buddha*, and *śrāvaka*, only one true goal exists, that of the attainment of full and complete Buddhahood, accomplished through the Vehicle of the Buddha (*buddhayāna*).[50] Different Buddhist paths are presented as a form of skillful means (*upāya-kauśalya*) utilized by the Buddha to adapt to the needs of his audience. This is illustrated in the *Lotus Sūtra* by the allegory of a father promising different types of carts according to the predilections of his various children to persuade them to leave a burning house. Gautama Buddha's enlightenment is represented as a drama presented by an already awakened being for the sake of those in need of such an example. The principle that the Buddha gives teachings to his disciples that are appropriate for their capacity through *upāya-kauśalya* extended existing Buddhist notions of the Buddha as a supreme teacher who used his extraordinary capacities, such as mind-reading, to best adapt the teaching to his audience. It also connects to the Mahāyāna view that the diversity of Buddhist teachings reflects the Buddha's efforts to make his message relevant to multiple audiences. In this spirit, Mahāyāna subsumed various non-Buddhist and Hīnayāna schools under the Mahāyāna aegis, a process exemplified in late Indian Buddhist works such as the *Bodhipathapradīpa*, or "Lamp for the Path to Awakening," of Atiśa Dīpaṃkara Śrījñāna (11th century CE).[51] Atiśa's work postulates that levels of the path span from non-Buddhist traditions to Hīnayāna and Mahāyāna Buddhism based upon degrees of understanding, concern for self, and concern for others.[52] The path of the *bodhisattva*, pursuing full Buddhahood for the sake of liberating beings from suffering in *saṃsāra*, stands above all other paths, as it embodies the compassionate principle of the pursuit of the liberation of others as well as oneself.

The Bodhisattva Path

The concept of the *bodhisattva* is developed extensively in the Theravāda and pre-Mahāyāna Sanskrit tradition in reference to Gautama Buddha's former lives and with respect to the nature and status of the future Buddha Maitreya (Pāli Metteyya). The extensive *Jātaka*, "[Previous] Birth," literature of Buddhism details many of Gautama's lives prior to his final birth. Buddhist narratives relate how Gautama, in a previous life as a young *brāhmaṇa* ascetic named Sumedha, made the vow to achieve Buddhahood before the Buddha Dīpaṅkara.[53] The future Buddha Maitreya is represented in various Buddhist traditions as currently residing in the Trāyastriṃśa heaven of the "Thirty Three," an oblique reference to the thirty-three Vedic gods, that was Gautama's penultimate abode before reaching full awakening, having accumulated extraordinary merit and wisdom over the course of many previous lives.

The *bodhisattva* in its principal representations is not represented as forestalling awakening (*bodhi*) and the development of wisdom (*prajñā*), but as rejecting awakening as an *arhat*.[54] The *bodhisattva* is, as such, compassionately dedicated to achieving Buddhahood in order to benefit all beings, as opposed to obtaining self-liberation as a *pratyekabuddha* or an *śrāvaka*. The Bodhisattva Path (*bodhisattva-mārga*), illustrated in Buddhist texts such as Śāntideva's *Bodhicaryāvatāra*, "Embodiment of the Acts of Awakening" (8th century CE), is marked by the development of the Bodhisattva vow (*bodhisattva-praṇidhāna*), which is the basis for the development of the mind of awakening (*bodhicitta*), an altruistic intention to obtain Buddhahood for the sake of all beings. This vow approximates the vow of the *bodhisattva* Sumedha and those of other Bodhisattvas before him who had achieved Buddhahood. As such, the cultivation of *bodhicitta* is, in principle, to be done in the presence of a Buddha, who in turn provides a prediction of the Bodhisattva's future success. Given the import of this process, Mahāyāna developed visualization practices that allow a Bodhisattva to do so when no Buddha is physically present in the world.

The Bodhisattva Path is also marked by the achievement of spiritual virtues or perfections (*pāramitā*), one permutation of these being the six perfections (*ṣaḍ-pāramitā*) of generosity (*dāna*), ethics (*śīla*), patience (*kṣānti*), vigor (*vīrya*), meditation (*dhyāna*), and wisdom (*prajñā*). A list of ten perfections that adds skillful means (*upāya*), dedication (*praṇidhāna*), strength (*bala*), and knowledge (*jñāna*) to the list of six also appears in Mahāyāna literature.[55] According to the system articulated in Kamalaśīla's *Bhāvanākrama*, or "Stages of Cultivation" (8th century CE), a Bodhisattva traverses a series of ten stages or levels (*bhūmi*) and five connected paths (*mārga*) of spiritual accomplishment, thereby attaining the various *pāramitā* and achieving Buddhahood.[56] In the *Bodhisattvabhūmi* section of the *Yogācārabhūmi*, the stage and path system is represented as a cumulative process whereby the Bodhisattva cultivates virtue, meditative mastery, and insight into emptiness (*śūnyatā*) leading up to liberating knowledge (*prajñā*). The Bodhisattva is portrayed as being transformed through this process into a being of great power, developing a range of capacities of manifestation (*nirmāṇa*), including the various *abhijñā* and the ability to take on various physical and spiritual forms in the pursuit of removing the suffering of beings in *saṃsāra*.[57] The final stage of the Bodhisattva path in the *Yogācārabhūmi* is referred to as the "cloud of *dharma*" (*dharmamegha*) and is closely related to the term *dharmamegha* that appears near the end of the *Yogasūtra* in reference to the perfection of *samādhi* and the "precipitation" of the liberating process.[58]

Mahāsattva Bodhisattvas

The Bodhisattva Maitreya serves as an exemplar of the Bodhisattva path for both Theravāda and Mahāyāna traditions, and a thread of continuity in the greater cosmology and soteriology of the two traditions. With the elevation of the Bodhisattva path in the Mahāyāna, however, a pantheon of Bodhisattva figures emerges, referred to as Mahāsattvas, or "Great Beings," who embody and exemplify the virtues and qualities of the Bodhisattva Path and serve as objects of reverence and devotion for Buddhist practitioners.[59] Among them, some of the most important are Maitreya, Avalokiteśvara, Mañjuśrī,

Tārā, Mahāsthāmaprāpta, Vajrapāṇi, and Kṣitigarbha.[60] Maitreya, beyond his import for the Theravāda, has historically been the focus of Mahāyāna cultic movements, and his identification with the Chinese Buddhist monk *Budai Heshang*, "Hemp Bag Carrying Monk," known as the "Laughing Buddha," is one of the most iconic and popular representations of a Bodhisattva figure in East Asia. Mañjuśrī and Avalokiteśvara are particularly important in the contexts of Mahāyāna contemplation and devotion as representing, respectively, the dual Mahāyāna virtues of wisdom and compassion. The Dalai Lama of Tibet is viewed by the Gelukpa Buddhist sect as being a human manifestation (Skt. *nirmāṇakāya*, Tib. *tulku*) of the Bodhisattva Avalokiteśvara. The Bodhisattva Avalokiteśvara is substituted with a female equivalent in East Asia, Guanyin, who is the object of intense devotionalism throughout the region. Another female Bodhisattva, Tārā, was important in the development of Mahāyāna in India and is particularly prominent in Tibetan Buddhism. Tārā is portrayed as manifesting in a plurality of forms, represented by different colors such as white, blue, and green, signifying her ability to manifest skillfully in different situations. Mahāyāna Bodhisattvas are the object of both identification and veneration, as they embody the spiritual capacities that practitioners cultivate, but also serve as intercessors who protect devotees from calamities and grant them various boons.

Mahāyāna Buddhas

Just as the pantheon of Bodhisattvas is extended from that of the singular Maitreya to a pantheon of Mahāsattvas, the Mahāyāna Buddhist cosmos is represented as filled with fully enlightened Buddhas from various eons and world systems that are continuously working for the benefit of those in *saṃsāra*. The Mahāyāna conception of Buddhahood, likely a further development of the earlier Lokottara school, is that of a being that is both fully liberated from *saṃsāra* and yet participating in it, having one foot in *nirvāṇa* and the other in *saṃsāra*. Unlike Theravāda conceptions of Buddhahood that view the *parinirvāṇa* as an end to the story of the historical Buddha, the Mahāyāna tradition views the physical body of the Buddha as a temporary projection, the end of a human Buddha's life being the end of only one chapter in a much larger story. The three body (*trikāya*) doctrine developed in the Yogācāra provides a conceptual framework for this view, in which the truth body (*dharmakāya*) or ultimate nature of a

Buddha takes on spiritual forms as an enjoyment body (*saṃbhogakāya*) and physical forms as a manifestation body (*nirmāṇakāya*). In other words, out of the *dharmakāya*, a Buddha can manifest in an apparitional form or as a physical body for the sake of the welfare of beings in *saṃsāra*. With the achievement of Buddhahood, the merit from the Bodhisattva's lifetimes of effort comes to fruition in the form of a Buddha-field (*buddhakṣetra*), forming a celestial heaven-like abode in which a Buddha manifests, a locus for the propagation of the *dharma* to all beings that inhabit it, especially Mahāsattva Bodhisattvas.[61]

The concept of the *dharmakāya* suggests the idea of a universal Buddha identity, as do later conceptions such as that of the primordial Buddha (*ādibuddha*). In addition to Śākyamuni or Gautama Buddha, different branches of the Mahāyāna tradition focus on various Buddha figures. One of the most well-known groupings of Mahāyāna Buddhas is the "Five Buddhas" (*pañcabuddha*), "Five Tathāgatas" (*pañcatathāgata*), or "Five Victors" (*pañcajina*), typically represented as Amitābha/Amitāyus, Akṣobhya, Vairocana, Ratnasambhava, and Amoghasiddhi. Among these five, the Buddha Amitābha, "unlimited light," or Amitāyus, "unlimited life," is of particular significance as the focus of "Pure Land" (Chn. *Jingtu*, Jpn. *Jōdo*) Buddhism in East Asia. Amitābha is a paragon of Mahāyāna virtue and an object of intense devotion to his followers. The *Sukhāvatīvyūhasūtra* details his uniquely purified (*pariśuddha*) Buddha-field (*buddhakṣetra*), referred to as the "Place of Bliss" (*sukhāvatī*), a paradise-like world of great beauty inhabited by Mahāsattvas like Avalokiteśvara and an ideal locus for *dharma* instruction, in which no beings are reborn in the lower forms of rebirth. Another important Mahāyāna Buddha figure is the so-called "Medicine Buddha" (*bhaiṣajyaguru*, lit. "teacher of remedies"), who represents the healing potency of the Buddha's teaching and the spiritual roots of all illness.[62] In Nepalese and Tibetan traditions of the Mahāyāna tradition, primordial Buddha (*ādibuddha*) figures that, like the broader conception of the *dharmakāya*, represent an ultimate Buddha figure or nature become prominent, examples being Vajrasattva, Vajradhara, and Samantabhadra. Some Mahāyāna traditions, particularly those that develop tantric systems, organize the various groupings of Buddhas into systems of families (*gotra*, *kula*) of Buddhas that correlate to the various stages of practice and to practice lineages.

Mantra and *Maṇḍala*

In addition to traditions of ritual worship (*pūjā*) of Śākyamuni Buddha common to both Theravāda and Mahāyāna, the Mahāyāna tradition developed traditions of invocation and visualization of a range of Buddha and Bodhisattva figures. These included mantra-based practices referred to as support (*dhāraṇī*), knowledge (*vidyā*), seed (*bīja*), and heart (*hṛdaya*). These mantras, which often focus on a particular Buddha or Bodhisattva, are used to evoke the benevolence of awakened beings for the purpose of accelerating spiritual development, for obtaining magical powers, and for gaining merit.[63] These practices parallel, in a number of respects, the mantra-like practice of the Pāli *paritta* tradition. Over time, Mahāyāna Buddhist practice progressed from simple "spells," to worship of deities using an icon (*mūrti*) and the representation of symbolic abodes of deities (*maṇḍala*, literally "circle" or "wheel"), marking the shift from simple worship of Mahāyāna deities toward "classical" Mahāyāna worship (*pūjā*) and esoteric, especially tantric, modes of practice.[64] One component of Mahāyāna practice that connects to other classical *śramaṇa* and *brāhmaṇa* traditions is the use of visualized images of Buddhas, Bodhisattvas, and other Buddhist deities for worship and contemplation.[65] As noted previously, the *Visuddhimagga* includes practices of visualizing the Buddha and deities, and Mahāyāna traditions of visualizing Buddhas and Buddha fields further extend such "recollection" (*anusmṛti*) practices, culminating in the elaborate visualization systems of tantric or Vajrayāna Buddhism.[66]

Śramaṇa Traditions and the Transformation of Yoga Traditions

In the first millennium of the Common Era, Jain and Buddhist traditions faced increasingly intense competition for patronage and popular support from the reemergent *brāhmaṇa* traditions of Hinduism. The rise of the Gupta Empire and the resurgence of patronage for priestly traditions undoubtedly forced Jain and Buddhist traditions to find new ways to remain relevant to both the grassroots and the political powers of India during an era of Hindu consolidation.[67] Both traditions increasingly framed their religious paths in the language of the practice of yoga, first in its primary sense as relating to spiritual discipline, and secondarily with focus on the practices of meditation (*dhyāna*) and contemplation (*samādhi*). The Jain path was subsumed by some of its most important systematic thinkers into the framework of the eight-limbed yoga (*aṣṭāṅgayoga*) associated with the Pātañjala Yoga school of Hinduism. Both Theravāda and Mahāyāna traditions used the language of the *yogin*, *yogāvacara*, *yogācāra*, and so forth to describe practitioners who were focused on contemplative practice, and the Mahāyāna school of the Yogācāra represented the Bodhisattva path itself as an expression of the practice of yoga. Under the influence of the emerging *sūtra* literature of the *smārta* or *paurāṇika brāhmaṇa* traditions of Hinduism, the framing of soteriological technique within the rubric of yoga had become part of the mainstream of *śramaṇa* scholarship. Pātañjala Yoga, however, bears the mark of considerable influence from Jain and Buddhist traditions, perhaps stemming from the influence of texts such as the Jain *Tattvārthasūtra* and from the Buddhist Abhidharma literature and the early Mahāyāna philosophical treatises of the Yogācāra.[68] Within the larger framework of yoga as a discipline, the classical era was particularly marked by the application of yoga as meditation (*dhyāna*), augmented by its various accessories, such as those represented by the members of the *aṣṭāṅgayoga* system and the spiritual perfections (*pāramitā*) acquired on the path of the Bodhisattva (*bodhisattvamārga*).

Chapter 7

The Medieval Transformation of Yoga

Bhakti, *Tantra*, and *Haṭhayoga*

The late centuries of the first millennium of the Common Era in India saw the consolidation and expansion of scholastic and monastic traditions rooted in *brāhmaṇa* and *śramaṇa* asceticism, the mainstreaming of Hindu sectarian and devotional traditions (*bhakti*), and the emergence of the tantric (*tāntrika*) mode of religious practice, which would pervasively influence Indic religions and transform the practice of yoga. Hindu traditions had developed three principal sectarian orientations in connection with three primary deities of the classical Hindu pantheon, namely, Viṣṇu, Śiva, and Devī, and Buddhist traditions had split into the branches of Theravāda and Mahāyāna, the latter with its pantheon of Buddhas, Bodhisattvas, and deities serving as objects of veneration and emulation. The Jain tradition division between the Digambara and Śvetāmbara sects was well established, and Jainism had developed its own traditions of worship (*pūjā*) toward the Jinas and toward tutelary deities who could intervene on behalf of devotees, such as the goddess Padmāvatī. All three traditions had developed a body of scholarly path-literature in which the practice of yoga played a central role in the soteriological process, both in the general sense of a spiritual discipline serving a religious path (*mārga*) and in the specific sense of the practice of meditation (*dhyāna*).

The emergence of tantra in the mid-to-late first millennium helped shape the late classical and medieval eras of religious life in India, as its techniques and ideology pervaded the religious landscape. Hindu sectarian traditions (*sampradāya*) developed monastic branches that challenged the dominance of Jain and Buddhist institutions, bridging the worlds of popular Hindu devotion and of asceticism. Both householder and renouncer traditions of *bhakti* and *tantra* flourished, giving rise to a spectrum of virtuoso religious practices that were highly influential in the religious and political spheres. From the convergence of tantric and ascetic paradigms arose the innovative modes of practice, such as *layayoga* and *haṭhayoga*, and narrative and didactic traditions of the propagators of such methodologies, such as the Nāths and Mahāsiddhas, gave rise to some of the most influential yoga systems in Indian history. Traditions of yoga and asceticism were tied to the pursuit of liberation from *saṃsāra* and to the mastery of mind and body as a vehicle for becoming a worldly master (*nātha*), accomplished one (*siddha*), or a naked warrior-ascetic (Skt. *nagna*, Hin. *nāgā*), among other possibilities. The medieval formulations of yoga that emerged out of this new synthesis, drawing strongly from *bhakti* and *tantra* as well as traditions of *tapas*, persists in the teachings of Hindu sectarian traditions and are the foundation for the modern, cosmopolitan, and often nonsectarian modern yoga traditions. Jain and Buddhist traditions were also deeply informed by the emergence of *bhakti* and *tantra*, developing extensive traditions of devotionalism and complex tantric disciplines and liturgies that aimed to accelerate spiritual development through extraordinary means.

Sectarian Traditions, Popular Devotion, and Ascetic Sampradāyas

As the *smārta-paurāṇika* traditions of *brāhmaṇa* Hinduism developed, theistic sectarian traditions multiplied, branching out on the basis of theological and liturgical variation and due to regional differentiation. Śaiva and Vaiṣṇava traditions may have originated as traditions of popular devotion to a supreme lord (*bhagavat*), the basis for the so-called Śiva-Bhāgavata and Viṣṇu-Bhāgavata traditions that appeared near the turn of the first millennium CE.[1] The Śākta tradition, the third major branch of sectarian theism, arose in conversation with the Śaiva and Vaiṣṇava traditions, and shares considerable ground with Śaiva narrative and philosophy in its classical and tantric formulations. Within the context of Hindu theism, *bhaktiyoga* encapsulates the principle of a spiritual practice centered on devoted attention to a deity, which exists alongside and is complemented by a number of other practices, including worship (*pūjā*), sacrifice (*yajña*), and *tapas*. Theism also correlates to a "geography of the sacred" of spiritual "crossings" (*tīrtha*) or "seats" (*pīṭha*), places that are held to communicate the presence of a deity, often through the linking of a particular place to a narrative of the god (*deva*) or goddess (*devī*).

Śaiva Traditions

Within Śaivism, the Hindu sectarian tradition centered on the deity Śiva, a number of different branches developed, including the Pāśupata, Lākulas, and Kālāmukha sects, which practiced ascetic austerities in emulation of Śiva, as well as the mainstream *smārta* traditions of Śiva-worship.[2] Priests associated with the formal Smārta tradition established by Śaṅkarācārya became important officiants at Śiva temples, though they were also known for the performance of a "five-altar" (*pañcāyatana*) form of worship (*pūjā*), dedicated to Śiva, Viṣṇu, Durgā, Sūrya, and Gaṇeśa.[3] The Kālāmukha sect may have given rise to the Liṅgāyat or Vīraśaiva tradition of Śiva-focused *bhakti*, a mode of practice also evident in the southern Indian tradition of the Nāyaṉmār.[4] Tantric schools of Śaivism included the mantra-focused Śaiva Siddhānta and the tantric-ascetic Kāpālika sects, the latter of which developed into the Kaula, Krama, and Trika traditions, forming the basis for the larger tradition of Kashmir Śaivism associated with the philosopher Abhinavagupta.[5] In the Sanskrit and Tamil literature of the Śaiva Siddhānta tradition, yoga is framed as a spiritual discipline, and early Siddhānta thinkers, such as Tirumūlar, placed particular value on the *aṣṭāṅgayoga* system as yielding the attainment of supernormal powers and liberation.[6] Śaiva sects have often had a strong affinity with tantric traditions, and the boundary between *smārta* and *tāntrika* practice is particularly fluid within Śaiva traditions. Śiva is often represented as the progenitor of yoga and tantric systems and as representing the ideals of their practice, both in terms of his physical appearance and his state of mind or consciousness.

Vaiṣṇava Traditions

Vaiṣṇavism, which emerged out of the confluence of traditions focused on the deities Vāsudeva, Kṛṣṇa, and Nārāyaṇa, consolidated the worship of

Viṣṇu within the priestly Bhāgavata and Pāñcarātra traditions, developing unique notions of emanation or "descent" (*avatāra*) and manifestation (*vyūha*) by which Viṣṇu appears in the world in various forms.[7] The rise of popular devotional traditions throughout the Hindu tradition in the medieval era gave rise to a number of popular devotion (*bhakti*) movements, many of which challenged priestly ideologies, in some cases critiquing caste distinctions, ritualism, and philosophical speculation. In Vaiṣṇavism, the advent of *bhakti* helped give rise to new sectarian groups, such as the Śrī Vaiṣṇava (associated with Rāmānuja) and the Gauḍīya Vaiṣṇava (associated with Caitanya) sects, which fused popular devotionalism to Viṣṇu-Lakṣmī and Kṛṣṇa-Rādhā with Hindu priestly narrative and philosophy. Caitanya was associated with the development of the practice of repetition (*kīrtana*), a mode of devotional prayer that involves the calling of the name of a deity in song, accompanied by bells, drums, and other musical instruments.[8] A closely related term, *bhajana*, communicates the idea of worship through song, being etymologically related to the term *bhakti* in the sense of enjoining in personal devotion to a god, goddess, or saint.[9] Other sects, such as the Vaikhānasa, Āḻvār, and Pāñcarātra, illustrate elements of practice drawn from the traditions of *smārta* ritual, *bhakti*, and *tantra* as adapted to Vaiṣṇava traditions. The Śrī Vaiṣṇava work of Rāmānuja validated the efficacy of Pātañjala Yoga, ultimately subsuming the *dhyānayoga* of Patañjali within Vaiṣṇava *bhaktiyoga*.[10] Later Vaiṣṇava commentators in the Gauḍīya Vaiṣṇava traditions, however, show a mixed attitude, validating the instrumental value of a Vaiṣṇava-inflected *aṣṭāṅgayoga* drawn from the Bhāgavata Purāṇa, but expressing concerns regarding the attainment of accomplishments (*siddhi*) and the potential pitfalls of renunciation.[11]

Śākta Traditions

Śākta traditions, like Śaivism and Vaiṣṇavism, encompass a wide range of practices, from Purāṇa-based *smārta* ritualism, to popular devotional (*bhakti*) and regional formulations of goddess-worship, to Śaiva- and Vaiṣṇava-related liturgies of the Śrīvidyā and other tantric sects.[12] A foundational text in the Śākta traditions is the *Devī Māhātmya*, "The Greatness of the Goddess," a section within the *Mārkaṇḍeya Purāṇa* that is a root text for the worship of the goddess as an independent deity.

The text establishes narratives of the goddess (*devī*) as a supreme being, who is referred to as Mahādevī, "Great Goddess," Ambikā, "Mother," and Caṇḍikā, "Burning One," among other names. Mahādevī slays a powerful buffalo-demon named Mahiṣāsura, and the fierce goddess Kālī, "The Dark One," manifests out of her body.[13] Mahādevī was later identified with the goddess Durgā, who became, over time, a pan-Indian deity celebrated throughout India in the yearly festival of Durgāpūjā.[14] Tantric forms of Śākta practice include the clans (*kula*) of the Kālīkula and the Śrīkula, the former focused on wrathful (*ghora* or *raudra*) forms of the goddess, including Kālī, and the latter on peaceful (*saumya* or *aghora*) forms of the goddess, such as Lalitā Tripurasundarī.[15] The goddess Tripurasundarī is worshipped in the Śrīvidyā tradition in the form of the iconic *śrīcakra*, "Wheel of the Auspicious [One]," a visual device (*yantra*) that encodes the manifestation of the goddess out of a transcendent state into emergent creation.[16] The Kālīkula has been historically linked, in part through the cult of the female Yoginī deities, to the influential Śaiva-Śākta Kaula traditions, with the boundary between Śaiva and Śākta traditions often being quite fluid if not indeterminate.[17]

Hindu Sectarian Traditions of Renunciation

A larger rubric used to identify male and female renouncers in the Hindu context is that of the "virtuous one" (*sādhu, sādhvī*). Male renouncers represent around 90 percent of membership in contemporary sectarian traditions of renunciation, with women making up the other 10 percent.[18] Renouncers may be largely solitary in nature, as in some Śaiva tantric-ascetic traditions, but many, if not most, of those identified as a *sādhu* and *sādhvī* belong to an organized communal order. Though the majority of renouncers in India have been Śaiva, Smārta, or Vaiṣṇava in orientation, parallel traditions exist in Śākta Hinduism, as well as in Buddhism, Jainism, and Sikhism.[19] They are often identifiable by particular styles of dress, body and facial markings (ash and paste), adornments (such as necklaces or earrings), hairstyles (shaven or dreadlocks), and ritual accoutrements such as a staff or water pot.[20] Some Sādhus and Sādhvīs practice intense austerities (*tapas*), including fasting, celibacy, and practices of self-mortification such as standing on one leg for an extended period of time or raising one arm until it becomes immobilized.

Indian traditions of asceticism have historically included both eremitic (solitary) and cenobitic (communal) practice, a division likely going back to the development of early traditions of *brāhmaṇa* asceticism and the *śramaṇa* traditions. Formal institutional monastic sects of Hindu renunciation developed out of the priestly sectarian traditions toward the end of the first millennium CE. These include the priestly Daśanāmī (Hin. Daśnāmī) sect of renouncers (*saṃnyāsin*), associated with Śaiva-Smārta traditions but claiming a broad influence over Hindu ideology and practice, and the Rāmānandī sect of Vaiṣṇavism, a renouncer (*vairāgin*) order built under the overarching rubric of devotion (*bhakti*) to Viṣṇu in his Rāma incarnation (*avatāra*). These two orders are held by their respective traditions to have been founded by the teachers Śaṅkara and Rāmānanda, though the historicity of such associations is disputed by some scholars.[21] The Daśanāmī sect is led by figures referred to as Śaṅkarācāryas who embody the authority of their legendary founder and are closely connected to the establishment of *brāhmaṇa* orthodoxy, in addition to being influential in politics. The Śaṅkarācāryas lead the four colleges (*maṭha*) of the Daśanāmī, namely, the Jyotir, Śāradā, Govardhana, and Śṛṅgerī, in the north, west, east, and south of India, respectively.[22] The title of Daśanāmī refers to the ten names of the orders of the Daśanāmī, including the *giri, purī, bhāratī, vana, araṇya, parvata, sāgara, tīrtha, āśrama*, and *sarasvatī*, which are also the suffixes of the names of renouncers after initiation.[23] Another renunciate order that is particularly important in the development of Hindu yoga and tantric traditions is the Śaiva Nāth (Skt. *nātha*) tradition, whose putative founders are Matsyendranātha and Gorakṣanātha. The Nāths are historically associated with the systematization of practices such as *layayoga* and *haṭhayoga* and the mainstreaming of tantric yoga and ritual in Hindu traditions. They also appear to have wielded considerable political influence in India and Nepal in broader religious, political, and economic affairs, a legacy that continues in the contemporary context.[24]

A mode of renunciation observed among the Hindu renouncer *sampradāya* sects is that of the Nāgā (from Skt. *nagna*, lit. "naked one"), whose practitioners observe ritual nudity and have, at times, populated military guilds (Hin. *akhāṛā*, Skt. *akṣavāṭa*), serving as mercenaries for rival principalities.[25] Such practice became widespread in the medieval and early modern eras in which renouncer traditions were politicized and militarized, with asceticism being intertwined with political intrigue and military action, the term *yogī* at times even being identified as a type of religious soldier.[26] The politicization and militarization of yoga during this era might be viewed as part of a thread that extends from the Vedic period (the *vrātya* mode of practice), through the classical period (the *kṣatriya-yoga* of the *Mahābhārata* and the role of the ascetic-spy in the *Arthaśāstra*), into the medieval period (warrior *sādhu* and *yogī* figures). It also echoes the powerful political influence of yoga *guru* figures and the adaptation of yoga as part of military training and nationalist physical culture in modern and contemporary India.[27]

Bhakti

The development of devotionalism (*bhakti*) in the Indian context gave rise to four primary groups of *bhakta* followers, among them those who worship Śiva, those who worship Viṣṇu (or a form of Viṣṇu such as Rāma or Kṛṣṇa), those who worship Devī, and those who worship a formless (*nirguṇa*) deity rather than one with attributes (*saguṇa*).[28] One of the primary representatives of the latter *nirguṇa bhakti* tradition was the saint-poet (*sant*) Kabīr (15th century CE), who composed songs that criticized the formalities and hypocrisies of the religiosity of his day and extolled the virtues of devotion to the one true formless (*nirguṇa*) god.[29] Kabīr is traditionally held to have been a disciple of Rāmānanda, the founder of the Rāmānandī sect of Vaiṣṇavism, and was an important figure in the development of a larger iconoclastic *bhakti* tradition that threatened the status quo of the times.[30] Mīrābāī (16th century CE), on the other hand, was an influential exemplar of *saguṇa bhakti*, in particular the Vaiṣṇava focus on Kṛṣṇa as the object of deeply personal and passionate love. The popular traditions of Sikhism and the Islamic traditions of Sufism in India were highly influenced by the rise of *bhakti*. The Sikh tradition integrated *sant* literature into its canonical corpus of texts, the "First Book" (*Ādi Granth*) or "Honorable Master Book" (*Gurū Granth Sāhib*), including the writings of Kabīr. Sikh leadership is associated with a foundational guru-disciple (*guru-śiṣya*) relationship, its formulators being the ten Sikh gurus beginning with Nānak (15th–16th century CE) and ending with the Gurū Granth Sāhib and its community referred to as "disciples" (Hin. *sikh*, Skt. *śiṣya*).

Both Kabīr and Guru Nānak challenged existing Hindu and Islamic traditions, offering especially pointed criticisms of the sectarian renouncer traditions of Hinduism, notably the Daśanāmīs, the Rāmānandīs, and the Nāths. Kabīr's teachings were centered on the spontaneous liberation of the individual through recitation of and meditation on the divine name, often in the form of *rām* (Skt. *rāma*, an abstraction from the name of the hero of the *Rāmāyaṇa*).[31] Kabīr's poetry suggests a reformulation of esoteric concepts of the subtle body drawn from Nāth techniques and principles that emphasized a heightened emotive dimension.[32] As with the followers (*panthī*) of Kabīr, the attainment of *mokṣa* for the Sikh tradition is rooted in devotion to a formless (*nirguṇa*) deity who is the agent of liberation, principally through the medium of the recitation of god's name (Skt. *nāma*, Hin. *nām*). The path of devotion, framed as "true yoga," is set apart from that of renunciation, and Sikhism critiques the Hindu renouncer model as an inferior path to that of the world-engaged Sikh.[33] However, as with Kabīr's teachings, the discourses of Nānak and the literature of Sikhism contain references to Nāth and *haṭhayoga* teachings and principles, demonstrating both continuity and discontinuity among these traditions.[34] Guru Nānak is portrayed as superseding the practices of the Nāths and as perfecting them, in the latter case achieving all of their vaunted accomplishments (*siddhi*).[35] Hindu, Sant, and Sikh narratives of the medieval era present dramatic stories of contestation between sectarian traditions in which the power of the respective systems of yoga, especially psycho-physiological techniques and devotional practices, are put to the test in battles of mind, will, and spiritual accomplishments (*siddhi*).[36] Such battles may, in part, symbolically represent the shifting tectonics of renunciation during the medieval era, in which sectarian groups were in competition for followers and for patronage.[37]

The Rise of Tantric Traditions

Two primary models of priestly practice developed over the period of the Vedic and classical eras of Hindu tradition, the *vaidika brāhmaṇa* model and the *smārta* or *paurāṇika* model of practice. These two modes of practice pervaded the broader tradition of Hinduism as it emerged in the early centuries of the Common Era, providing ritual and ideological foundations for Indian society. The Vedic model gave way to *smārta* practice at the dawn of the Common Era, though pockets of *vaidika* practice have persisted to the present in contemporary India. *Smārta* or *paurāṇika* practice, which is focused on the theism of the *itihāsa-purāṇa* literature and draws upon the *sūtra* and *śāstra* literature of law (*dharma*), politics (*ārtha*), pleasure (*kāma*), and liberation (*mokṣa*), among other subjects, continues to be the dominant paradigm for priestly practice in the Hindu tradition. *Vaidika* and *smārta* practice have significant common ground with respect to ritual and ideology, sharing a liturgical and literary foundation.

A third mode of priestly practice that builds on *vaidika* and *smārta* models but aims to supersede and encompass them is the tradition of tantric (*tāntrika*) practice. Tantra, as a mode of religious or spiritual praxis, aims to accelerate spiritual development, whether conceived of as liberation (*mokṣa*), as accomplishment or power (*siddhi*), or both, through extraordinary means. Some tantric traditions pair notions of release (*mukti*) and enjoyment (*bhukti*), indicating an ideal of spiritual development that joins liberation with worldly enjoyment and accomplishment. Tantra literally means "to stretch" or "to extend" (from the Skt. root √*tan*) and is the namesake of a class of treatises and a mode of ritual practice that expands or extends existing *vaidika* and *smārta* methodologies. One of its principal expressions is the ritual invocation, worship, and/or identification with powerful deities that are fearsome or wrathful (*ghora* or *raudra*) in character in order to rapidly obtain power and knowledge. Many of the central deities of tantra are representations of, or variations on, fierce forms of Śiva such as Bhairava, "The Terrible One," and forms of wrathful goddesses such as the Yoginīs and Kālī. The ritual practices of tantra are, in some cases, augmented through the use of dangerous and transgressive means, in particular the deliberate ritual transgression of priestly social and ideological boundaries, especially those of purity and impurity (*śuddha-aśuddha*). In its systematic formulations, tantric practice often involves yogic practices of cultivation (*bhāvanā*), meditation (*dhyāna*), breath control (*prāṇāyāma*), and other aspects of mind-body discipline.

One prominent theory regarding the widespread adoption of the *tāntrika* paradigm during the medieval era was that it provided a ritual and ideological basis supportive of individual nexuses of power in the post-Gupta political era, which was marked by political instability and a retreat to a system of regional powers.[38] Frameworks of virtuoso tantric practice were connected in important ways to the frameworks of princely governance during the medieval era, providing maps of both spiritual and social worlds during a period of upheaval.[39] The tantric emphasis on the attainment of spiritual accomplishments (*siddhi*) and on the power and authority of the embodied tantric master (*guru*, *ācārya*) or accomplished one (*siddha*) points to an environment of social and political instability in which the charismatic authority of teachers and political leaders was valued alongside, if not greater than, structural and institutional authority.[40]

Origins and Paths of Tantra

Traditional accounts of the origin of tantric practices connect them to the sacred figures at the center of sectarian practice—in the case of Hindu tantra, the progenitor of tantra is often represented as Śiva himself, as the primordial teacher or lord (*ādiguru*, *ādinātha*). Buddhist accounts represent Gautama Buddha as having practiced tantra either in another life or in a heavenly state before achieving awakening, or link the propagation of Buddhist tantric texts to primordial Buddha (*ādibuddha*) or *mahāsiddha* figures.[41] Though certain principles of tantra were present already in *vaidika* and *smārta brāhmaṇa* traditions and in Jainism and Buddhism, scholarly accounts of the origins of tantra are largely focused on the development of Śaiva traditions of asceticism, especially the antinomian Pāśupata sect, and the so-called "Yoginī Cult" of Hinduism. In the latter, the deities Rudra and Bhairava, fierce forms of Śiva, are associated with the propitiation of clans (*kula*) of fearsome female deities or sorceresses (*yoginī*) who grant spiritual accomplishments (*siddhi*) in exchange for ritual offerings of polluting substances, including sexual fluids.[42] It appears that, in some cases, women participating in such rituals would be possessed by the Yoginīs, binding the physical and spiritual world and allowing them to become channels for the divine power of goddesses to manifest in the world.[43]

Śaiva Tantra

The Śaiva traditions in which tantric methodologies were systematically developed can be categorized within two paths (*mārga*), namely, the Outer Path (*atimārga*, sometimes referred to as *raudra* rather than *śaiva*) and the Path of Mantras (*mantramārga*). These two paths respectively refer to those Śaiva ascetics concerned with liberation (*mokṣa*) and the ascetic and householder practices concerned with supernatural enjoyment (*bhoga*) as well as liberation (*mokṣa*).[44] The *mantramārga* was broken down into the two branches of the Seat of Mantras (*mantrapīṭha*) and Seat of Vidyās (*vidyāpīṭha*), emphasizing male and female deities, respectively.[45] Śaiva forms of tantra are found in a range of literature, including the Śaiva Purāṇas and a range of sectarian texts referred to as Śaiva Tantras and Āgamas.[46] Śaiva ascetic traditions, as mentioned earlier, included the Pāśupatas, Lakuliśas, and Kālāmukhas, which embraced antinomian forms of ascetic practice. These were marked in some cases by Kāpālika, "Skull Bearer," practices such as dwelling in cremation grounds, covering themselves with ashes, and carrying a skull-bowl and staff as iconic symbols of their Śaiva identity. These Śaiva practitioners emulate the appearance and behavior of Śiva himself, with Kāpālika practices being linked to a narrative of Śiva in which he performs a graveyard penance after having cut off one of the five heads of Brahmā, thereby committing the grievous sin of killing a *brāhmaṇa*. The erratic behavior of Śaiva ascetics, especially of the Pāśupatas, drew upon Vedic and Purāṇic notions of Rudra-Śiva as an outsider to Hindu orthodoxy who dwells in the forest and who breaks the purity observances of *brāhmaṇa* tradition and engages in antinomian behavior.[47] The Pāśupatas were also one of the early Śaiva sects that defined yoga in terms of union (*saṃyoga*), and, in some cases, criticized Pātañjala Yoga.[48] The practice of the Mantramārga by householders (*gṛhastha*) found expression in the literature and liturgy of the Śaiva-Siddhānta sect, which focuses on milder forms of Śiva and on an abstract goddess-force (*śakti*). Another representative was the Trika sect of Kashmir Śaivism, a sophisticated system of ritual and yoga associated with the philosopher Abhinavagupta, which focuses on the realization of one's own divine identity as a matrix of three goddess-powers (*śakti*) at the root of consciousness, subsuming Krama and Kaula sectarian elements.[49] The Kaula (lit. "of the clan") forms of Śaiva-Śākta tantric traditions, represented in texts such as the *Kubjikāmatatantra* (10th century CE) and *Kulārṇavatantra* (11th–15th century CE), provided a ritual framework for householder-practitioners to realize the transformative presence of the power of the goddess (*śakti*) through the medium of the senses, yogic practices, sexual intercourse, and the consumption of meat and alcohol.[50]

Vaiṣṇava Tantra

Within Vaiṣṇava traditions, the principal representation of tantric ideology and practice is found in the Pāñcarātra system, whose *saṃhitā* texts bear structural and ideological similarity to the Śaiva Tantras and Āgamas.[51] According to the Pāñcarātra tradition, Vāsudeva (Viṣṇu) appeared in various manifestations (*vyūha*) in order to propagate the spiritual knowledge compiled in the Pāñcarātra Saṃhitās.[52] Particularly central to Pāñcarātra tantrism, as is the case with Śaiva tantra, is the use of mantra and the concept of *mantraśakti*, the force through which the power of tantric practice (*sādhana*) yields liberation (*mukti*).[53] In the *Jayākhyasaṃhitā*, for example, the practitioner of Pāñcarātra tantra uses mantra to effect self-purification and recreate themselves in the form of the deity in a state of *samādhi*, sequentially transforming the elements, the body, and the subtle energies of the body.[54] Pāñcarātras use a number of aspects of yoga, including various *yogāṅga*, in their pursuit of liberation (*mukti*) and enjoyment (*bhukti*).[55]

Śākta Tantras

Śākta tantric traditions are typically divided into the Kālīkula and Śrīkula, focused on fierce and benevolent forms of Hindu goddesses, respectively, and like the Pāñcarātra system are similar in ideology and structure to tantric Śaivism, with the boundary between Śaivism and Śāktism often being fluid.[56] As with the Śaiva and Pāñcarātra tantras, the utilization of mantra and the involution of the cosmic process of manifestation serves as a gateway to the realization of an ultimate reality beyond the division of worldly appearances. This is represented visually in the symbolism of the *śrīcakra*, a device (*yantra*) and circular array (*maṇḍala*) that is vehicle for worship of the goddess. The cult of the goddess Tripurasundarī of the Śrīkula is a permutation of the Kaula cult of Kāmeśvarī.[57] This was adopted in a modified form by the *brāhmaṇa* Śaṅkarācāryas of Śṛṅgerī and Kāñcīpuram, demonstrating the fluidity of the boundaries between Śākta and Śaiva sects, between householder and renouncer traditions, and between *smārta* and *tāntrika* traditions.[58]

Buddhist and Jain Tantras

By the eighth century of the Common Era, Buddhist tantras had been organized into a hierarchy of systems, including Action (*kriyā*), Performance (*caryā*), Yoga (*yoga*), and Unexcelled Yoga (*anuttarayoga*), paralleling the progression of Śaiva tantric systems in the *mantramārga*.[59] *Anuttarayoga* was further divided into the categories of "Mother Tantras" (*mātṛtantra*) and "Father Tantras" (*pitṛtantra*), dependent on their relative emphasis on wisdom (*prajñā*) or method (*upāya*).[60] Tantric traditions of Buddhism were principally integrated into the Mahāyāna tradition, though tantric influences extended into other schools of Buddhism, including the Theravāda.[61] Within the Mahāyāna, the Method of Mantras (*mantranaya*), also termed the Mantra Vehicle (*mantrayāna*) or Thunderbolt Vehicle (*vajrayāna*), is contrasted with the Method of Perfections (*pāramitānaya*) of the Bodhisattva with respect to the rate of transformation of a practitioner into an enlightened being.[62] This division is also described in the Mahāyāna in terms of the development of the Sutra Vehicle (*sūtrayāna*) versus the Tantra Vehicle (*tantrayāna*). Buddhist tantric texts such as the *Guhyasamājatantra*, *Hevajratantra*, *Cakrasaṃvaratantra*, and *Kālacakratantra* demonstrate successive developments in tantric ideology and practice in the Indian context. The central deities of the Vajrayāna pantheon, such as Heruka, Cakrasaṃvara, and Kālācakra, bear the attributes of Kāpālika Śaivism and the Yoginī cult, the Cakrasaṃvara *maṇḍala* being represented in the text itself as a Buddhist subordination of a Śaiva framework.[63] Vajrayāna Buddhism is marked by a dynamic tension between ascetic and monastic traditions of tantra, akin in some respects to the *atimārga-mantramārga* division of Śaiva tantra, and its systems articulate a range of positions with respect to whether transgressive aspects of tantra were to be symbolically or literally performed. Jain traditions, in contrast, were unified in their rejection of the transgressive and antinomian aspects of tantric practice, but nonetheless developed elaborate mantra treatises (*mantraśāstra*) and *yantra* systems aimed at obtaining spiritual accomplishments (*siddhi*) resulting in various types of worldly mastery.[64] The pervasive influence of tantrism is particularly evident in the late classical and early medieval works of Jain yoga, such as the *Yogaśāstra* of Hemacandra, with tantric *layayoga* and *kuṇḍalinīyoga*-type practices being found alongside the Jain adaptations of the Hindu *aṣṭāṅgayoga* system.[65]

Principles of Tantric Practice

A practitioner of tantra (*tāntrika/tāntrikā*) is typically referred to as an adept (*sādhaka/sādhakā*) or hero (*vīra/vīrā*), in reference to the formal mode of practice (*sādhana*) and its consequent extraordinary effort. At the root of tantric practice is initiation (*dīkṣā*) by a *guru* or preceptor (*ācārya*), which grants an aspiring practitioner access, often sequentially, to different levels of ritual and yogic practice. The dynamic between external ritual and internal yogic and meditative practices is encapsulated in the Buddhist division of tantric practice into the system of actions (*kriyānaya*) and the system of yoga (*yoganaya*).[66] Tantric practices are represented in texts as esoteric traditions that are to be veiled in secrecy to non-initiates, in some cases through the use of an encoded language (*sandhyābhāṣā*) that conceals the true meaning or instructions of a teaching or text. Initiates are given a mantra or a series of mantras in the form of a process of exchange between *guru* and *śiṣya* that parallels Vedic initiation (*upanayana*), as well as undergoing a variety of ritual processes, which in some cases include spirit possession and sexual or otherwise transgressive practices. The performance of mantra is foundational in tantra, especially the recitation of seed (*bīja*) mantras that encapsulate the power of tantric deities and evoke their physical and cosmological characteristics. Practitioners use ritual seals (*mudrā*) and placement (*nyāsa*), physical gestures that have symbolic significance in invoking and embodying the power of deities, and use ritual musical implements such as the drum, pipes or flutes, and bells (*ghaṇṭa*), and ritual weapons such as the trident (*triśūla*) and thunderbolt [dagger] (*vajra*). Tantric practitioners perform worship (*pūjā*) and perform sacrifice (*yajña*, *homa*) to the deities of the various tantric pantheons, sometimes in the form of a communal circle (*gaṇacakra*), and may use both pure (*śuddha*) offerings (such as flowers and fruit) and impure (*aśuddha*) offerings (such as meat, alcohol, and bodily fluids). Tantric practice includes physical and energetic yogic techniques, notably those associated with the subtle body (*sūkṣma-śarīra*), such as *prāṇāyāma*, that manipulate the flow of vital energy and winds (*prāṇa*, *vāyu*) and vital drops (*bīja*, *bindu*) through the systems of channels (*nāḍī*) and centers or wheels (*cakra*) that link psychic and physiological life.[67] Some tantric systems feature the development of formal meditation (*dhyāna*), especially with respect to the utilization of six- and eight-limbed yoga (*ṣaḍaṅgayoga*, *aṣṭāṅgayoga*) forms within the tantric paradigm.[68]

Tantric practices also include the practice of possession (*āveśa*) and meditative cultivation (*bhāvanā*) or visualization of deities through Deity Yoga (*devatā-yoga*) as methods of establishing identity with tantric deities whose powers and capacities are to be evoked, utilized, and assimilated.

Tantric *bhāvanā* aims at developing a mental image of a deity that possesses the attributes of accomplishment that the practitioner seeks to embody. In order to facilitate the rapid transformation of the practitioner into a deity (such as *deva*, *devī*, *bodhisattva*, or a *buddha*) tantric practice may incorporate sacred diagrams (*yantra*) and circles (*maṇḍala*), which represent the abode of a central deity, sometimes with a consort, and his or her various tutelary deities, cataloging the capacities of the deity as various implements and attributes. Seed (*bīja*) mantras serve as the basis out of which deities manifest in the contemplative process of *bhāvanā*, arising from Sanskrit characters positioned on lotuses (*padma*) and populating the *yantra* or *maṇḍala*. As a performative and embodied process, tantric *sādhana* uses the medium of all of the five senses to evoke powerful physical, emotive, and cognitive experiences, homologizing the body with the elements and structures of the cosmos.

Transgression

Tantric traditions engage practices and symbolism drawn from Śaiva Kāpālika traditions, namely, the Kāpālika practice of cremation-ground asceticism, such as covering of the body in ashes and the use of bone ornaments and implements, including the skull-cup (*kapāla*) and skull-staff (*khaṭvāṅga*). Tantric practitioners may use transgressive substances and practices, epitomized by the Kaula-derived formulation of the so-called "five m [words]" (*pañcamakāra*) or "five truths" (*pañcatattva*), namely, the use of wine (*madya*), fish (*matsya*), meat (*māṃsa*), parched grain (*mudrā*), and sexual intercourse (*maithuna*) within tantric ritual practice.[69] Both Hindu and Buddhist tantra employ substances and actions considered taboo in conventional priestly and monastic practice as a vehicle to evoke psychophysical transformation and as a vehicle for transcending worldly dualisms. Examples include the mastering of the terror and disgust of encountering wrathful deities, such as Kālī, within the impure (*aśuddha*) and haunted cremation-ground, a place that is the locus of those who have "gone" (*bhūta*) or are "deceased" (*preta*) but continue to be a spiritual threat to the living. It also encompasses a process of psychological deconditioning through handling and consuming forbidden or impure substances, such as sexual fluids, urine, feces, and, in some extreme cases, human flesh. Lastly, it may involve the generation of bliss (*ānanda*) through either actual or visualized sexual intercourse in order to provide transgressive offerings to powerful deities and to effect changes in the subtle body (*sūkṣma-śarīra*) that promise to accelerate spiritual development.

Traditions of tantra that are focused on liberation (*mokṣa*) may have built on an earlier strata of practices focused primarily on obtaining spiritual accomplishments (*siddhi*) in exchange for enduring ordeals and offering vital substances such as blood and sexual fluids to powerful female deities such as the Yoginīs.[70] Some traditions of tantra differentiate between literal and actual versus visualized or substitutionary use of transgressive substances and actions, the former being referred as "left-hand" (*vāmācāra*) practice and the latter as "right-hand" (*dakṣināācāra*) practice.[71] In the contemporary context, this dynamic ranges from left-hand tantric asceticism of the Śaiva Aghori sect, a mode of Kāpālika cremation-ground practice centered on ritual impurity (*aśuddha*), to the right-hand practices of Hindu Śrīvidyā worship and of the Gelukpa sect of Tibetan Buddhism, in which tantric practice is molded to fit within orthodox *brāhmaṇa* priestly mores and Mahāyāna Buddhist monastic principles, respectively.

The Subtle Body (*sūkṣma-śarīra*)

The concept of a subtle body (*sūkṣma-śarīra*), a subphysical structure containing a series of channels (*nāḍī*) and wheels (*cakra*) or lotuses (*padma*) in which vital energy (*prāṇa*) and drops (*bīja*, *bindu*) of vitality move, in some cases inhibited by knots (*granthi*), is developed significantly in tantric traditions, providing the foundation for the emergence of the systems of *layayoga*, *kuṇḍalinīyoga*, and *haṭhayoga*. Conceptions of a subtle body and a constellation of *nāḍī* leading out of a central channel appear relatively early in Indic literature, including the *Chāndogya* and *Kaṭha Upaniṣad*. In the context of the Pātañjala Yoga philosophy and in the larger classical sphere, meditative fixation (*dhāraṇā*) or mastery (*saṃyama*) on different places in the body, such as the head (*mūrdhan*), the navel (*nābhi*), and so forth, is said to yield particular types of knowledge and expanded agency. In late medieval traditions, conceptions of the *sūkṣma-śarīra* are subsumed under the larger rubrics of *layayoga*, "the yoga of dissolution," and *haṭhayoga*, "the yoga of force," often epitomized by the ascent of *śakti* through the central *nāḍī*, known as *suṣumṇā*. The structure of the subtle body varies among Hindu, Buddhist, and Jain presentations with respect to the number and placement of *cakra* or *padma*, the use of particular mantras and phonemes, and the form and features of the deities visualized as residing within each *cakra*. One of the earliest references to a subtle-body system is found in the Buddhist *Guhyasamājatantra*, or "Secret Assembly" tantra, where the subtle body is portrayed in terms of a fourfold *cakra* system, a pattern that extends through much of the Buddhist tantric literature.[72]

Nāḍī and *Cakra* Systems

Perhaps the most widely used subtle-body model is that of the sevenfold *cakra* system associated with Kaula traditions of Hindu tantrism. In this system, the *sūkṣma-śarīra* has a foundational structure of three principal channels, a left (*īḍā*, "praiseworthy"), a right (*piṅgalā*, "radiant"), and a central (*suṣumṇā* or *mādhyama*, respectively "gracious," and "middle"), which are sometimes symbolically equated with famed Indian rivers (*nadī*) such as the Gaṅgā and Yamunā. A network of peripheral channels (*nāḍī*) extends from the central structure of the *sūkṣma-śarīra*. Within the framework of the sevenfold system, *cakra* reside along the central channel near the anus (*mūlādhāra*, *mūlasthāna*, "root support" or "root base"), the genitals (*svādhiṣṭhāna*, "own place"), the navel (*maṇipūra*, "jewel filled"), the heart (*anāhata*, "unstruck"), the throat (*viśuddhi*, "pure"), the brow (*ājñā*, "command"), and a final center referred to as the "aperture of Brahmā" (*brahmarandhra*) or as the "thousand-rayed wheel" (*sahasrāracakra*). In their more elaborate formulations, these *cakra* are represented as lotuses of various colors and numbers of petals, populated by deity-consort pairings and containing the mark of a Sanskrit character on each petal and the pericarp of the lotus. In a principal variation of this system, the latent force of *śakti* termed *kuṇḍalinī*, the "coiled one," is brought upward through *suṣumṇā* toward the *sahasrāra cakra* or *brahmarandhra*. This upward movement is homologized with an ascension through the cosmological process itself, from the gross elements to the subtle reality of consciousness, through the concentric circles on the vertical axis of the *suṣumṇā nāḍī*. The body itself is, in some cases, viewed as a microcosm of the universe, the spine being identified in tantric literature with Mount Meru, the center of the universe in Indian cosmology, and the ascension through the various *cakra* representing successive mastery and transcendence of the elements. A similar process is found in the *Hevajratantra* in Vajrayāna Buddhism, in which the peripheral channels of "sporting" (*lalanā*) and "savoring" (*rasanā*) correlate to the *iḍā* and *piṅgalā nāḍī*, the "shaking [one]" (*avadhūti*) to *suṣumṇā nāḍī*, and the "burning [one]" (*caṇḍālī*) to *kuṇḍalinī śakti*, with a primary difference being the number and locations of the *cakra* in the subtle-body system.[73] The *Hevajratantra* designates the four *cakra* as being correlates of the three bodies of a buddha (*nirmāṇa*, *dharma*, and *saṃbhoga*) and the principle of great bliss (*mahāsukha*).[74]

Yoginīs and Ḍākinīs

Tantric traditions in Hinduism and Buddhism are heavily encoded with the symbolism of Kāpālika Śaiva traditions and especially with the Śaiva-Śākta traditions of the Kula and Kaula. Of particular import in this context is the cult of the Yoginīs, a pantheon of wrathful female deities associated with Śiva in the form of Bhairava, the "Terrible One," and the related temple tradition of the propitiation of the Yoginīs in the form of a *cakra*, or wheel, of flying goddesses. The Yoginīs are often said to be sixty-four in number, one interpretation being that eight Yoginīs arose from each of eight fierce Hindu *mātṛkā*, or "mother" goddesses.[75] The cult of the Yoginīs is found in parallel scriptural collections and initiatory schemas in Hindu and Buddhist traditions, and also appears in Indian popular narratives such as the *Kathāsaritsāgara*.[76] Within the Buddhist tradition, the term *ḍākinī* is used interchangeably with *yoginī* to designate a powerful female initiatory deity associated with the *anuttarayoga*-class Yoginī Tantras. The term *yoginī*, as discussed earlier, has a wide semantic range, from that of a female practitioner of yoga to that of a human (*mānuṣya*) embodiment of a divine *yoginī* or a nonhuman (*amānuṣya*) divine (*divya*) *yoginī* goddess.[77] The divine Yoginīs are represented as being many in number, having a multifaceted relationship to human women, being organized into clans, having theriomorphic (animal and human) features, and possessing the power of flight; they are associated with danger, impurity, power, and the protection and transmission of esoteric teachings.[78]

Considerable scholarly debate persists regarding the social status of women within tantric traditions, and specifically that of the human *yoginī* and *ḍākinī*.[79] The principally male-practitioner-oriented tantric literature largely marginalizes female perspectives, portraying the *yoginī* as principally an agent or instrument serving the purpose of the transformation of the male subject. Tantric consorts are often represented as ideally being girls or young women, sixteen being a common age, and additionally of low-caste or outcaste status, suggesting an intentionally imbalanced power and purity dynamic between male and female practitioners.[80] On the other hand, the manner in which the *yoginī* or female tantric adept exists on the margins of these traditions, as a dweller on the threshold and a gateway to initiation into tantric practice, may suggest a deeper signification and perhaps greater agency among human *yoginī* figures than male-oriented philosophical and liturgical literature represents.[81]

Tantric *Aṣṭāṅgayoga* and *Ṣaḍaṅgayoga*

The conception of a limbed (*aṅga*) system of yoga, pervasive in the Purāṇas and other classical-era Hindu literature, especially the rubric of the *aṣṭāṅgayoga*, extends into tantric traditions. The tantric text of the *Śāradātilaka* of Lakṣmaṇadeśika, a twelfth-century *mantraśāstra* compendium, utilizes the *aṣṭāṅgayoga* paradigm to integrate tantric and emergent proto-*haṭhayoga* and *layayoga* techniques into classical models of yoga practice.[82] The manner in which the *Śāradātilaka* uses the *aṣṭāṅgayoga* framework, accepting the larger parameters of the system while expanding elements of *yama* and *niyama* and integrating practices such as *kuṇḍalinīyoga*, parallels the integrative approach toward the *aṣṭāṅga* system found in the Purāṇa literature. Both the *Netratantra* and the *Mṛgendrāgama* texts of Śaiva tantra present *aṣṭāṅgayoga* paradigms, though they differ in purpose and content in important ways, with the latter mentioning "investigation" (*vīkṣaṇa*), *japa*, and *yoga* as limbs.[83] Similarly, the *Ahirbudhnyasaṃhitā* of the Vaiṣṇava Pāñcarātra tradition references an *aṣṭāṅgayoga* paradigm as a framework for yoga.[84]

In addition to the *aṣṭāṅgayoga* system, a widely represented model in the context of both tantric Hindu and Buddhist practice is that of the six-limbed yoga (*ṣaḍaṅgayoga*). The *Śiva Purāṇa* represents yoga as being either *aṣṭāṅgayoga* or a *ṣaḍaṅgayoga*, though the text discusses only the *aṣṭāṅgayoga* system at length. This indicates that the *ṣaḍaṅgayoga* model was an option for practice within the Śaiva traditions at the time of the composition of the Purāṇa, though in that context it appears secondary in import to the *aṣṭāṅgayoga*. A fivefold yoga appears in the *Vāyu Purāṇa* that is quite similar to the *ṣaḍaṅgayoga* as well, indicating the broader representation of "numbered" yoga systems in the Purāṇas.[85] The *Maitrī Upaniṣad*, one of the last of the early strata of Upaniṣads, contains a description of a six-limbed yoga (*ṣaḍaṅgayoga*) that includes the elements of breath control (*prāṇāyāma*), sense-withdrawal (*pratyāhāra*), fixation (*dhāraṇā*), meditation (*dhyāna*), discernment (*tarka*), and contemplation (*samādhi*), largely paralleling the structure of later six- and eight-limbed systems. *Ṣaḍaṅgayoga* is also found in the Hindu *Amṛtabindu, Amṛtanāda*, and other Yoga Upaniṣads, the Śaiva Āgamas, the *Viṣṇusaṃhitā*, the *Vaikhānasasmārtasūtra*, the *Tantrālokaviveka*, Kṣemarāja's commentary to the *Netratantra*, the *Gorakṣaśataka-Vivekamārtaṇḍa*, and in the Buddhist *Guhyasamājatantra* and *Kālacakratantra*, among other contexts.[86] It is unclear whether the *ṣaḍ-* or *aṣṭāṅgayoga* form is primary in terms of their historical and genealogical development, as it is unknown whether the *Maitrī Upaniṣad* predates the composition of the *Yogasūtra* and the development of Sāṃkhya-Yoga.[87] It may be that the lack of reference to the *ṣaḍaṅgayoga* in the *Yogasūtra* and in the commentarial traditions, joined to the logic that later traditions sought to abstract yoga practice from its *smārta brāhmaṇa* moorings, points to the derivation of *ṣaḍaṅgayoga* from *aṣṭāṅgayoga*.[88] Another possibility would be that at least two major lines of transmission exist, one linked to an earlier six-limbed (*ṣaḍaṅga*) paradigm, and the other an adaptation of the *aṣṭāṅgayoga* system. Contemporary scholars designate three "classes" of *ṣaḍaṅgayoga* systems, characterized by the inclusion of either discernment (*tarka*), recollection (*anusmṛti*), or *āsana*, in addition to the common members of *prāṇāyāma, pratyāhāra, dhāraṇā, dhyāna*, and *samādhi*.[89] The inclusion of *tarka* is preeminent in the adoption of *ṣaḍaṅgayoga* within the context of Hindu tantrism, such as in the traditions of Kashmir Śaivism, and the use of *anusmṛti* is prevalent in Buddhist tantras such as the *Kālacakratantra*.[90] The appearance of *āsana* is prevalent within the context of the Hindu *haṭhayoga* traditions associated with Śaiva and Vaiṣṇava literature during the medieval era.

The Śaiva Āgamas have, in a common classification, four divisions, one of them being *yoga*, the others doctrine (*jñāna*), ritual (*kriyā*), and conduct (*caryā*), the inclusion of yoga in this framework indicating its overarching importance in tantric Śaiva traditions.[91] In addition to the highly influential *ṣaḍaṅga* system, Kashmir Śaiva traditions also reference three- and four-limbed systems of yoga that place emphasis on the realization of unity through contemplation of and possession (*samāveśa*) by the active consciousness of Śiva, rather than by dwelling in the passive witness-consciousness of the *puruṣa*.[92] In the *Tantrāloka*, Abhinavagupta draws upon seminal Kashmir Śaiva texts such as the *Mālinīvijayottaratantra*, in which the *tarka*-class *ṣaḍaṅga* system is articulated, and argues for the supremacy of *tarka* over other limbs of yoga.[93] He criticizes the *aṣṭāṅgayoga* system on the grounds that *tarka* is necessary for realization, that yoga discipline is unnecessarily painful, and that the *aṣṭāṅgayoga* methodology lacks spontaneity.[94] However, he suggests it may nevertheless be useful as a precursor to more sophisticated practices even if it is not soteriologically efficacious.[95] *Ṣaḍaṅgayoga* is discussed in systematic fashion by Jayaratha in the *Tantrālokaviveka*, a principal commentary to the *Tantrāloka*, setting it apart from the *aṣṭāṅgayoga* as uniquely efficacious, referring specifically to Patañjali as the articulator of the system that he is rejecting.[96]

With respect to the performance of the Vaiṣṇava tantras, the *Jayākhyasaṃhitā* prescribes a *sādhana* focused on the performance of mantra and the meditative component of yoga (*samādhi*), offering another representation of the *ṣaḍaṅgayoga* as a paradigm for tantric yoga.[97] Similarly, the Buddhist commentarial literature on the *Guhyasamājatantra* and *Kālacakratantra*, composed by renowned Buddhist scholars such as Anupamarakṣita, contains extensive discussion and analysis of the *ṣaḍaṅgayoga* system, particularly with respect to the *Kālacakratantra*, a text that received extensive commentarial elaboration in India and Tibet.[98]

Tantric Power and Enjoyment

As with yoga, the practice of tantra in some contexts is about power (*vibhūti*, *siddhi*) and enjoyment (*bhukti*, *bhoga*) as much as it is about obtaining liberation (*mukti*, *mokṣa*), though the attainment of liberation and enjoyment is, in some cases, viewed as complementary. In contemporary India, tantric practitioners are viewed principally as sorcerers who can help secure success, restore health, or harm others through the use of tantric ritual. This mode of tantric practice is sometimes referred to as "folk tantra" as opposed to "classical tantra," especially to the degree it is practiced at a non-elite, grassroots level.[99] However, "classical" tantrism highlights the achievement of power in forms such as the Eight Accomplishments (*aṣṭasiddhi*), which include the powers of smallness (*aṇimā*), lightness (*laghimā*), obtaining (*prāpti*), irresistible will (*prākāmya*), greatness (*mahimā*), lordship (*vaśitva*), mastery (*īśitva*), and suppression of desire (*kāmāvasāyitva*). Similarly, the practice of the tantric Six [Ritual] Actions (*ṣaṭkarman*), namely, appeasement (*śānti*), subjugation (*vaśya*), immobilization (*stambha*), enmity (*dveṣa*), eradication (*uccāṭa*), and killing (*māraṇa*), represents a morally ambiguous set of powers at the disposal of the *tāntrika* or *tāntrikā*.[100] The first of the six powers deals with the curing of illness, and the rest with obtaining of power over others, stopping others' activity, creating enmity between others, destroying a person's object or place, and destroying life. These powers are found in Indian Buddhist sources, such as the *Guhyasamājatantra*, and in Hindu tantric sources.[101] Tantric powers such as the *aṣṭasiddhi* and *ṣaṭkarman* are obtained through the process of tantric worship and ritual (*pūjā*, *yajña*) and through possession (*āveśa*) and meditative cultivation (*bhāvanā*) that results in the embodiment of the capacities of a deity or deities.

Tantric Liberation

The goal of liberation (*mokṣa*, *mukti*) in tantrism is typically conceived of as a state of liberation-in-life (*jīvanmukti*), in which the liberated person takes on the attributes of an awakened and liberated deity, be it in the form of a Siddha, Śiva, Viṣṇu, Devī, Bodhisattva, or Buddha. In some cases, a relationship with a deity is emphasized over identity, such as in Śaiva Siddhānta and in various Vaiṣṇava traditions. The outer mode of transformation includes the performance of mantra, the use of ritual garments, and the use of *mudrā* and *nyāsa* to emulate and embody the physical form of a deity. The inner aspects of transformation include visualization and contemplation of the structure of a *yantra* or *maṇḍala*, the manipulation of energy (*prāṇa*) and vitality (*bindu*, *bīja*) within the subtle body (*sūkṣma-śarīra*), and, in some cases, the cultivation of the bliss of tantric *maithuna*. Liberation is commonly conceived of as a non-dual state that is a realization of, or a participation in, the primordial basis of reality, framed in various ways—as Śiva and/or Śakti, as a particular Buddha or the *dharmakāya-ādibuddha*, or as Vāsudeva-Viṣṇu-Nārāyaṇa, and so forth. In Kashmir Śaivism, this attainment is connected to concepts such as those of the recognition (*pratyabhijñā*) of identity with Śiva as the ground of vibration (*spanda*) through contemplative cultivation (*bhāvanā*) and possession (*samāveśa*). In Vajrayāna Buddhism, it is associated with the realization of emptiness (*śūnyatā*) as the ground of all phenomena, referred in some sects as the Great Seal (*mahāmudrā*) of reality, which is the basis for the attainment of awakening.[102] The liberated state may be represented as a spontaneous or "co-arisen" (*sahaja*) state that represents an unmediated, primordial state of perception, free from conceptual superimposition or elaboration, and characterized by a transcendence of worldly dualisms.[103] The tantric preceptor (*ācārya*) or guru embodies the truth of these traditions, often playing the role of the enlightened deity in initiation processes that seek to catalyze the transformation of the *śiṣya*. As such, the *guru* is viewed as worthy of veneration and emulation and of being formally visualized and revered as a perfected being in tantric ritual practices such as *guruyoga*.

Nāths, Mahāsiddhas, and the Development of Medieval Yoga Systems

Śaiva and Buddhist tantric traditions, especially those that drew upon Kaula formulations of the Kāpālika mode of ascetic practice, helped precipitate Nāth, Mahāsiddha, and other traditions of tantric virtuoso practice that gave rise to a number of medieval systems of yoga, notably the set of the "Four Yogas" of *mantrayoga*, *layayoga*, *haṭhayoga*, and *rājayoga*. These traditions, which are said to be descended from the teachings of Śiva or an Ādibuddha figure, represent themselves as the transmitters of timeless methods of esoteric yoga through the vehicle of the *guru-śiṣya* relationship. The Nāths (Skt. *nātha*), literally the tradition of "The Lords," are a constellation of semi-divine (*siddha*) figures featured in Hindu narrative literature and a living sect of Śaiva ascetics who view themselves as the inheritors of a timeless lineage.[104] Similarly, the Buddhist Siddhas or Mahāsiddhas are a group, typically eighty-four in number, of male and female tantric masters who are portrayed as embodying the perfection of the tantric-ascetic practice of Buddhism as virtuosos of the Vajrayāna tradition.[105] The boundary between Nāth Siddhas and Buddhist Mahāsiddhas is fluid, and a number of figures, such as Matsyendranāth and Gorakhnāth, are common to lists of the Nāths and Mahāsiddhas.[106] This common heritage indicates that the medieval cult of tantric virtuosos extended across sectarian and geographic boundaries, whether such figures and practices were shared or borrowed. The Nāths and Siddhas were also important as religious and political figures, serving as cultic objects to devotees and aspirants and playing important roles as power-brokers in medieval India. The yoga systems that the Nāths and Mahāsiddhas propagated were characterized by the influence of ascetic and tantric practice and ideology, and often upended priestly concerns with regards to social conventions and concerns regarding purity and impurity (*śuddha-aśuddha*). The Nāths and Mahāsiddhas represent some of the fullest expressions of the conception that yoga has the capacity to transfigure a practitioner into a perfected one (*siddha*) whose power is equal to, if not surpassing, that of the deities of the Hindu, Buddhist, and Jain traditions.

The Nāths

The Nāthyogīs or Nāthjogīs (Skt. *nāthayogī*), the "Lord Yogis" or "Master Yogis," or simply "Nāths," are a Śaiva sectarian tradition that has historically extended in geographic scope from northern to south-central India. They are also known as the Gorakhnāthīs, or followers of the Nāth Siddha Gorakhnāth (Skt. Gorakṣanātha), and as the Kānphaṭa, or "split eared," Yogīs, due to their practice of wearing a large earring as their symbol (*mudrā*) in the split central cartilage of their ears.[107] For the Nāths, the *mudrā* is a symbol of initiation and is said to confer spiritual perfections (*siddhi*) upon the yogi. In addition to the earring, Kānphaṭa Yogīs carry a begging bowl, a whistle, a staff, and a crutch, and often wear a turban.[108] They may carry and adorn themselves with garlands or rosaries (*mālā*) made of *rudrākṣa*, a dried berry sacred to Śiva, or of stone, and smoke *cannabis* using a pipe called a *cilam*, a practice common among many Indian *sādhu* traditions.[109] The principal mode of Nāth practice is that of renunciation, though householder traditions exist as a derivative of the ascetic community, and most, but not all, Nāth ascetics are male.[110] The lineage of the Nāths is typically represented as having descended from Matsyendranāth (Skt. Matsyendranātha), the "Fish-Lord Master," also known as Mīnanāth (Skt. Mīnanātha), the "Fish Master," who is said to have received his teachings directly from Śiva, the "First Master" (Skt. *ādinātha*, Hin. *ādināth*). Matsyendranāth is said to have passed Śiva's teachings on to Gorakhnāth (Skt. Gorakṣanātha) and his disciples. In the *Haṭhapradīpikā*, the spiritual lineage of Nāths includes Ādinātha, Matsyendra, Śābara, Ānandabhairava,

Caurangī, Mīna, Gorakṣa, Virūpākṣa, Bileśaya, Manthānabhairava, Siddhabuddhi, Kanthaḍi, Kauraṇṭaka, Surānanda, Siddhapāda, and others.[111] In the *Kaulajñānanirṇaya*, Matsyendranāth is presented as referring to himself as a Kaula, connecting the origins of the Nāth tradition to the Kaula tantric traditions of Śaivism and Śāktism, specifically the Pūrvāmnāya sect.[112] Matsyendranāth is represented as promoting the internalization of tantric rituals in the *Matsyendrasaṃhitā*, exchanging the external performance of tantric ritual, including its transgressive elements, for a sublimation of such processes within the body.[113]

Records and tales of the Nāths, especially of a paradigmatic set of "Nine Nāths" (Skt. *navanātha*, Hin. *navnāth*), are found in various Indian vernacular languages, including Tamil and Telegu.[114] These relate wondrous stories of the acts of these Nāth Siddhas, their powers, and their often-famous disciples, which included kings and queens of high stature in medieval India, such as Bhartṛhari of Ujjain and Jālandharnāth, Maynāmati, and Gopīcandra in Bengal.[115] In some cases, Nāths are said to have assumed important roles as political leaders and counselors, especially in Rajasthan.[116] Matsyendranāth is famously portrayed in narrative as having overheard Śiva teaching Pārvatī while he was in the form of a fish, thus providing the source of his unique title as "Fish-Lord Master" (Skt. *matsyendranātha*). Another common narrative of Matsyendranāth describes his falling under the spell of powerful queen-sorceresses in Assam in northeastern India and his subsequent rescue by his disciple, Gorakhnāth.[117] Some of the Nāth narratives demonstrate antinomian themes, in which disciples are forced to perform out-of-caste duties, a trope common to narratives of the Buddhist Mahāsiddha tradition.[118]

The Nāths are often associated with the development of formal traditions of *haṭhayoga*, the "yoga of force," a set of methods for physical purification and physical and psychic discipline that provide both worldly power and liberation. However, they may be historically most intimately associated with the development of conceptions of *layayoga* practice and those associated with the rousing of *kuṇḍalinī* as drawn from Śaiva and Śākta tantrism.[119] The strong association, if not identification, of the Nāths with *haṭhayoga* may be because the relatively late but well-known *Haṭhapradīpikā* credits Nāth gurus for the formulation of *haṭhayoga*. However, the descriptions of the practices of *haṭhayoga* in the *Haṭhapradīpikā* appear to have been derived from passages in Vaiṣṇava texts such as the

Dattātreyayogaśāstra as well as from Śaiva *haṭhayoga* texts such as the *Amaraughprabodha*, suggesting a wider Hindu sectarian engagement with *haṭhayoga.*[120] The *Haṭhapradīpikā* subsumes and incorporates the Kaula-Nāth practices associated with *kuṇḍalinī* and *layayoga* under the larger rubric of *haṭhayoga*, along with a range of yogic-ascetic practices, such as *āsana*, *mudrā*, *bandha*, and *prāṇāyāma*, culled from various source materials. The practice of *layayoga* and *haṭhayoga* is limited among contemporary Nāths, who are principally known for the performance of tantric sacrifice and worship (*yajña*, *pūjā*) and devotion (*bhakti*) to Śiva and Śakti.[121] There is some indication, however, that contemporary Nāth traditions are claiming, or re-claiming, authority over *haṭhayoga* practice, including the practice of yoga *āsana*, tapping into its popular appeal and the cultural and economic capital associated with it.[122]

Haṭhayoga, *Mantrayoga*, *Layayoga*, and *Rājayoga*

The term *haṭhayoga*, or "the yoga of force," is a term that in conventional usage encapsulates a range of yogic and tantric practices that emerged in the late classical and medieval eras. A widely known etymology of this term breaks *haṭha* down into the union of the sun (*ha*) and moon (*ṭha*), especially as representing the joining of the dyadic vital energies of *prāṇa* and *apāṇa*, though textual representation of this definition is limited.[123] Some of the first known appearances of the term are found in Buddhist tantric texts, most notably the *Guhyasamājatantra* and the *Kālacakratantra*, where it involves the forcing of *prāṇa* into the central channel of the subtle body while restraining a "drop" (*bindu*) of vital essence, identified with semen, in the body, in part through the use of sound (*nāda*). In these Buddhist texts, *haṭhayoga* is described as a transformative practice of last resort, suggesting that it was peripheral to the mainstream of Buddhist tantric practice.[124] Though also appearing as a peripheral practice in Śaiva, Vedānta, and other sectarian texts of the era, *haṭhayoga* appears more centrally in early medieval texts such as the Buddhist *Amṛtasiddhi*, the Śaiva *Amaraughaprabodha*, and the Vaiṣṇava *Dattātreyayogaśāstra*, and was codified as a core method of yoga in later Śaiva and Śākta texts such as the *Gorakṣaśataka-Vivekamārtaṇḍa*, *Gorakṣaśataka*, *Haṭhapradīpikā*, *Gheraṇḍa-saṃhitā*, and *Śivasaṃhitā*.[125] Early references to *haṭhayoga* identify it as an ascetic system that sought bodily perfection and liberation through physical and energetic techniques (such as *āsana*, *prāṇāyāma*, *bandha*, and *mudrā*) that preserved and manipulated an essence or drop (*bindu*, *bīja*) of vitality within the body, the descent and expulsion of which was to be prevented.[126] However, the rubric of *haṭhayoga* was expanded over time to encompass a range of other practices, most notably *kuṇḍalinīyoga* and the larger range of practices characterized under the rubric of *layayoga*.[127]

A concept of innate (*sahaja*) perfection achieved through a *nirguṇa*-type meditation appears in Hindu, Buddhist, and Sant traditions as either an alternative to or as the perfection of *haṭhayoga* and *layayoga* methodologies. In these traditions, *sahaja* is accomplished through a variety of means, including physical yoga, mantra repetition, and the cultivation of meditation on spacious awareness or formlessness. In the *Siddhasiddhāntapaddhati*, a relatively late text attributed to the Nāth tradition, the state of having "shaken off" (*avadhūta*) is represented as the ultimate stage of yoga, and the *Haṭhapradīpikā* identifies the achievement of *samādhi* with *jīvanmukti* and the innate (*sahaja*) state, which is, in turn, equated with *rājayoga*.[128] In the *Dattātreyayogaśāstra*, *Yogabīja*, *Amaraughaprabodha*, and in the so-called Yoga Upaniṣads, the various approaches to yoga practice are organized in the fourfold division of *mantrayoga*, *layayoga*, *haṭhayoga*, and *rājayoga*, often in a hierarchical ordering. *Mantrayoga* is verbal and mental incantation (*japa*) of *smārta* and *tāntrika mantra*, and *layayoga* encompasses a range of practices of "dissolution," including reflection on inner sound (*nādānusandhāna*), resting in corpse posture (*śavāsana*), and various forms of meditation (*dhyāna*), such as *śāmbhavīmudrā*, "the seal of the goddess," or meditative gazing.[129] *Rājayoga*, the "royal yoga," in contrast, is identified primarily as a practice suited to only the most capable practitioners of yoga, being framed as a direct and unmediated achievement of the spontaneous *sahaja* state and therein the highest degree of spiritual perfection, which is free from effort or fabrication.[130]

Aṣṭāṅgayoga and *Ṣaḍaṅgayoga* in *Haṭhayoga* Literature

In its narrow sense, *haṭhayoga* refers to an ascetic discipline of yoga that has deep connections to classical, and perhaps pre-classical, traditions of *tapas* and *brahmacarya*, especially those referred to as the "raising of semen" (*ūrdhvaretas*). In its broader sense, the term *haṭhayoga* encompasses a wide range of medieval, and especially tantric, innovations in the practice of yoga, such as *kuṇḍalinīyoga* and the larger range of techniques of *layayoga*, acting as a nexus for the consolidation of range of classical and medieval practices.[131] The literature of *haṭhayoga* contains reference to both *aṣṭāṅga-* and *ṣaḍaṅgayoga* systems as frameworks for the practice of yoga. The *Dattātreyayogaśāstra*, which may contain one of the first explicit discussions of *haṭhayoga* practice in Sanskrit literature, frames *haṭhayoga* in two ways, first within the *aṣṭāṅgayoga* rubric, which it attributes to the sage Yājñavalkya, and second, as the practice of energetic seals (*mudrā*) and locks (*bandha*), which it attributes to the sage Kapila.[132] It is possible that the presentation of the *aṣṭāṅgayoga* system in the *Dattātreyayogaśāstra* that is associated with the sage *Yājñavalkya* was cognate with other presentations of the yoga system, such as the one found in the thirteenth- to fourteenth-century text of the *Yogayājñavalkya*, which similarly uses an eight-limbed system attributed to Yājñavalkya as an overarching paradigm for the practice of yoga.[133] Though there is disagreement upon its date and import in the development of *haṭhayoga*, the *Siddhasiddhāntapaddhati* attributed to Gorakṣanātha presents the tantra-derived practice of *kuṇḍalinīyoga* in the form of a nine *cakra* system, but frames the overarching practice of yoga within an *aṣṭaṅgayoga* structure.[134]

The *Yogatattva Upaniṣad* frames yoga as fourfold (*mantra-*, *laya-*, *haṭha-*, and *rājayoga*), and equates *haṭhayoga* with *aṣṭāṅgayoga*, but includes the addition of practices such as *mudrā* and *bandha*, much like the *Dattātreyayogaśāstra*.[135] Likewise, the *Yogadarśana Upaniṣad* frames the practice of yoga in terms of *aṣṭāṅgayoga*, with Viṣṇu in the form of Dattātreya serving as its progenitor, and both the *Triśikhibrāhmaṇa Upaniṣad* and *Śāṇḍilya Upaniṣad* articulate an *aṣṭāṅgayoga* framework characterized by ten *yama* and *niyama* factors.[136] Vedānta texts from roughly the same period also incorporate the *aṣṭāṅgayoga* system into its rubric, in some cases identifying Pātañjala Yoga with *haṭhayoga*.[137] Nātha texts such as the *Gorakṣaśataka-Vivekamārtaṇḍa*, also attributed to Gorakṣanātha, refer instead to a *ṣaḍaṅgayoga* paradigm, namely, that of *āsana*, *prāṇasaṃrodha* (the "arrest of *prāṇa*"), *pratyāhāra*, *dhāraṇā*, *dhyāna*, and *samādhi*, representing the so-called "*āsana*-class" of *ṣaḍaṅgayoga*. A ten-chapter version of the *Haṭhapradīpikā*, a variant on the standard four-chapter version of the text, endorses the "*āsana*-class" *ṣaḍaṅgayoga* system, and modern variations of the text sometimes include inserted descriptions of *yama* and *niyama*.[138] The *Amṛtanāda Upaniṣad* presents a *ṣaḍaṅga* system of the *tarka*-class, and the *Dhyānabindu Upaniṣad* a *ṣaḍaṅga* system of the *āsana*-class.[139]

Yogāsana

Within the broader frameworks of *haṭhayoga* traditions, be they six- or eight-limbed or otherwise, a number of features stand out as representative of the emergent medieval models of yoga. The practice of *āsana*, described as a basis for both physical health and spiritual development, draws considerably more attention than in classical presentations of yoga. In the *Haṭhapradīpikā*, four postures are described as ideal for the practice of *haṭhayoga*, namely, "accomplished posture" (*siddhāsana*), "lotus posture" (*padmāsana*), "lion posture" (*siṃhāsana*), and "fortunate posture" (*bhadrāsana*), with *siddhāsana* being the best among them.[140] Other postures include "swastika-posture" (*svastikāsana*), "cow-faced posture" (*gomukhāsana*), "hero posture" (*vīrāsana*), "tortoise posture" (*kūrmāsana*), "rooster posture" (*kukkuṭāsana*), "corpse posture" (*śavāsana*), and "Matsyendra's posture" (*matsyendrāsana*). The material culture legacy of the late medieval period includes sculptures that visually document various, and increasingly complex, forms of *yogāsana* practice and the use of a *yogapaṭṭa*, or "yoga strap," in the performance of yoga austerities in the context of Śaiva, and specifically Nāth, traditions.[141] This period saw a proliferation of yoga *āsana*, with a common trope found in the *Haṭhapradīpika* and other texts of a set of eighty-four types of *āsana* being taught by Śiva as a subset of a much larger number, indicated to be as much as eight million four hundred thousand in total.[142] Modes of *āsana* practice documented in late medieval and early modern texts such as the *Yogacintāmaṇi* (17th century CE) and *Haṭhābhyāsapaddhati* (18th century CE), included standing poses, inversions, twists, and other vigorous practices that may have provided a bridge to the gymnastic and athletic adaptations of yoga characteristic of the modern period.[143]

Prāṇāyāma and *Kriyā*

Building on the foundation of *āsana*, the *yogin* or *yoginī* observing *haṭhayoga* practices *prāṇāyāma* through alternate nostril breathing that cleanses the *iḍā* and *piṅgalā nāḍī*, leading to bodily purity, health, *siddhi*, and preparation for the state of *samādhi*. Those of particularly ill health are advised to practice purificatory actions (*kriyā*), referred to as the "six actions" (*ṣaṭkarman*), namely, cleansing (*dhauti*) the stomach and esophagus by swallowing a cloth, performing an enema (*basti*), cleansing the nose with a thread (*neti*), cleansing the eyes through water-inducing staring (*trāṭaka*), churning the abdomen through muscular contraction (*nauli*), and aggressive purificatory breathing (*kapālabhāti*, lit. "radiant skull"). Other practices added to this list include the "elephant action" (*gajakaraṇī*), the intentional vomiting of water, and "circling" (*cakri*), the cleansing of the anus and rectum with a finger. The practice of *prāṇāyāma* is characterized by achieving skill in inhalation (*pūraka*), exhalation (*recaka*), and in retention (*kumbhaka*, lit. "pot-like"), with variants such as the "cutting of the sun" (*sūryabhedana*), "victorious" (*ujjāyī*), "hissing" (*sītkārī*), "cooling" (*śītalī*), "bellows" (*bhastrikā*), "buzzing" (*bhrāmarī*), "stasis" (*mūrchā*), and "floating" (*plāvinī*) that modify the flow of the breath in various ways. In the *Haṭhapradīpikā*, the eventual attainment of *kevala kumbhaka*, "solitary" or "distinct" mode of retention, a state that may parallel the fourth (*caturtha*) mode of *prāṇāyāma* mentioned in the *Yogasūtra*, confers a spontaneous state of *samādhi* or *rājayoga*.[144] This is said to be marked by the arising of *kuṇḍalinī* and the perception of inner sound (*nāda*) in an "unstruck" (*anāhata*) form, the latter of which is sometimes identified as the primordial mantra *oṃ* and as a form of *nāda-brahman* or *śabda-brahman*.[145]

Mudrā and *Bandha*

In concert with the utilization of the three forms of energetic binding (*bandha*), specifically of the throat (*jālandhara*), the anus or "root" (*mūla*), and the abdomen in its upward movement (*uḍḍīyāna*), *prāṇa* moves in the central channel of *suṣumṇā*. This process is facilitated by the use of seals (*mudrā*), physical actions that elicit the movement of *prāṇa*. These include seals (*mudrā*) that link *āsana* and *bandha* (*mahāmudrā*) and include actions such as the pressing of the tongue in the cavity of the throat (*khecarīmudrā*), the pulling of the tongue to "rouse the [goddess of] power" (*śakticālana*), inverting the body (*viparītakaraṇī*), and aggressively dropping the pelvis to the ground (*mahāvedha*).[146] The "practice of the *vajra*" (*vajrolī*), the "natural state" (*sahajolī*), and "immortality" (*amarolī*) refer to practices that involve the retention and reabsorption of emitted bodily fluids through the urethra and through application to the body. In the *Haṭhapradīpikā*, the practice of *vajrolī* by women is said to confer upon them the status of *yoginī*.[147]

In addition to its links to *bindu*-preservation, such experimentation with bodily substances in *haṭhayoga* has both literal and symbolic connections to contemporaneous traditions of Indian alchemy (*rasāyana*) that aimed at physical and spiritual transformation through the use of potions and elixirs.[148] Similarly, the extensive use of *cannabis*, especially within Śaiva and Nāth traditions, might be considered a variant on the Indic theme of the use of psychoactive catalysts, including extracts (*soma*) and agents (*viṣa*), herbs (*auṣadhi*), and essences (*rasa*), particularly as facilitating the attainment of spiritual perfection (*siddhi*).[149]

Jīvanmukti

The culmination of the path of *haṭhayoga* is represented in the *Haṭhapradīpikā* as the spontaneous arising of *samādhi*, that is, without the need for additional formal meditative praxis. *Samādhi* is identified as the natural condition (*sahajāvasthā*) and the union of individual self (*jīvātman*) and higher self (*paramātman*). The arrest of *prāṇa* in the central channel is linked with the arising of the unstruck (*anāhata*) resounding tone (*nāda*). As such, *haṭhayoga* is presented as leading to the attainment of *rājayoga*, a state of meditative contemplation or absorption (*samādhi*) said to be identical with the *sahaja*-state, empty-and-not-empty (*śunyāśunya*), a no-mind (*amanaska*) state, and as equivalent to the attainment of *jīvanmukti*.[150]

Buddhist Mahāsiddhas and Buddhist Tantric Yoga

The Nāth Siddha narratives of Hinduism are paralleled by those of the Buddhist Mahāsiddhas, or "Great Accomplished Ones," virtuoso practitioners of tantric yoga in the Vajrayāna tradition. The traditions of these Mahāsiddhas, who appear in texts such as the *Caturaśītisiddhapravṛtti* of Abhayadatta, developed between the eighth and twelfth centuries in India, during a period in which tantra was becoming increasingly important in religious life throughout the region.[151] Many of the Mahāsiddhas, who are typically counted as eighty-four in number, are common to the Nāth Siddha tradition, indicating a shared legacy and appropriation across the boundaries of Buddhist and Śaiva practice. Matsyendranāth, for example, is both a Buddhist Mahāsiddha and a Nāth, being viewed as a manifestation of the Bodhisattva Avalokiteśvara by Buddhists in Nepal and as a Śaiva saint by Hindus in India. The Mahāsiddhas are associated with the propagation of tantric modes of the practice of yoga, especially with respect to techniques for mastering the subtle body (*sūkṣma-śarīra*), dream and death processes, and modes of spontaneous (*sahaja*) realization, the latter including the esoteric system of the Great Seal (*mahāmudrā*) that found fertile ground in Tibetan Buddhism.

The Eighty-Four Mahāsiddhas

The Mahāsiddhas are portrayed as representing a cross-section of Indian society, including royalty, merchants, prostitutes, and thieves.[152] Narratives of the Mahāsiddhas often highlight antinomian elements of tantric practice that are disruptive of caste, scholarly, monastic, and priestly mores, with the transgressive practice of tantric traditions being embodied by male virtuosos such as Tilopa, Nāropa, Saraha, Lūipa, and Ghaṇṭāpa, and by female virtuosos such as Maṇibhadrā and Lakṣmīṅkarā.[153] The Buddhist Mahāsiddhas, as with the Nāths, represent a development of the concept of the accomplished one (*siddha*), a practitioner transformed into a semi-divine being through yogic discipline. The Mahāsiddhas are, in part, an extension of larger Indian traditions of sorcerers or "knowledge holders" (*vidyādhara*), and are representative of the larger yogic and tantric quest for spiritual accomplishment (*siddhi*) characteristic of the era.[154] Within the Mahāsiddha tradition, the figures of the *yoginī* and the *ḍākinī*, fierce female deities, become especially prominent, represented in Mahāsiddha narratives as initiators into Buddhist tantric practice. Of particular import is Vajrayoginī, identified as the *ḍākinī* who initiated the Mahāsiddha Nāropa and more broadly as *sarvabuddhaḍākinī*, "The Ḍākinī of all of the Buddhas," representing the inseparable female counterpart to the Buddhas of the tantric systems.[155] This is consistent with the overarching emphasis in Mahāsiddha traditions on Vajrayāna practices of the Yoginī class, in which female initiatory deities populate the *maṇḍala* of an awakened one. It also is linked to the language of the subtle body (*sūkṣma-śarīra*) encoded in the Mahāsiddha narrative and songs (*dohā*) that highlight the importance of the *caṇḍālī-śakti*, the ultimate initiatory deity within the *nāḍī* and *cakra* system.[156]

The lineages of the Mahāsiddhas are of particular importance in late Indian Vajrayāna Buddhism and in the formation of Tibetan Buddhist traditions. The Mahāsiddha Padmasambhava is credited with removing the spiritual obstacles to the propagation of Buddhism in Tibet, specifically the opposition to Buddhism by native Tibetan deities.[157] The Mahāsiddhas Tilopa, Nāropa, Marpa, and Milarepa are of particular import in the Tibetan tradition, especially within the Kagyü sect.[158] An important root *guru* in this lineage is Saraha, an eighth-century Indian Mahāsiddha associated with Sahajiyā Buddhism and with the development of the tradition of Mahāmudrā. Mahāmudrā is cognate with other *sahajayoga* traditions in which a practitioner seeks an immediate, spontaneous experience of awakening, such as the Tibetan system of Dzogchen.[159] Such awakening is represented in some narratives as being completed by the entry of a Mahāsiddha into the heaven-like paradise of the *ḍākinī*-world.[160] Saraha and other Mahāsiddhas are credited with composing songs called *dohā* (a metrical type, but also meaning "source of gain"), which are also referred to as "*vajra* songs" (*vajragīti*) or "performance songs" (*caryāgīti*).[161] The content of the *dohā* and other Mahāsiddha songs is consistent with the overarching iconoclasm of the tradition, which incorporated critiques of mainstream religiosity and placed emphasis on achieving the *sahaja* state through the development of Mahāmudrā.[162] These factors link Sahajiyā traditions of Buddhism to the iconoclastic discourses of the Indian Sants, Sikhs, Bāuls, and later Vaiṣṇava traditions that emphasized *nirguṇa-bhakti*.[163]

The Six Dharmas of Nāropa

One of the most influential practice systems associated with the Indo-Tibetan Mahāsiddha tradition is that of the so-called "Six Yogas of Nāropa," more literally the "Six Dharmas" (Tib. *chödruk*, Skt. *ṣaḍdharma*) of Nāropa, a system distinct from the *ṣaḍaṅgayoga* or six-limbed yoga utilized in tantric Buddhism, Kashmir Śaivism, and *haṭhayoga*.[164] Nāropa (Skt. Nāḍapāda, Nāroṭapa), who was the preeminent disciple of Tilopa, taught the Six Dharmas within a framework in which the realization of Mahāmudrā stood as the culmination of all practices at its apogee.[165] The Six Dharmas include the teachings of inner heat (Tib. *tummo*, Skt. *caṇḍālī*), illusory body (*gyulü*, *māyādeha*), dream (*milam*, *svapna*), clear light (*ösal*, *prabhāsvara*), intermediate state (*bardo*, *antarābhava*), and transference (*phowa*, *utkrānti*).[166] The teaching of inner heat (*tummo*, *caṇḍālī*) has strong parallels to *haṭhayoga* and *kuṇḍalinīyoga*, involving the movement of *prāṇa* and *bindu* through the *nāḍī* of the subtle body, and links to a larger set of practices referred to as "channel-wind-instrument" (*tsalung trulkhor*, *nāḍī-vāyu-yantra*).[167] The teachings of the illusory body (*māyādeha*) and of dream (*svapna*) involve the intentional and imaginative construction of an image of oneself as deity (*devatā*) within a *maṇḍala* during both waking and sleeping states. The teachings of the clear light (*prabhāsvara*), the intermediate state (*antarābhava*), and of transference (*utkrānti*) relate to yogic practices of navigating the death-rebirth process. The first of these, the clear light (*prabhāsvara*), is a training in recognizing the foundational clarity and purity of mind at death, the second (*antarābhava*) a training in recognizing the landmarks of the death-rebirth process, and the third (*utkrānti*) a training in the intentional ejection of consciousness from the body at the moment of death. The second of these, *antarābhava*, is translated by the Tibetan term *bardo*, and is the focus of a Tibetan Buddhist text entitled the *Bardo Thödol*, "Liberation in the Intermediate State," the title of which is popularly translated as the "Tibetan Book of the Dead."[168] Through meditative training, a practitioner aims to achieve the ability to navigate the death-rebirth process, recognizing the *prabhāsvara* or the various apparitions of peaceful, wrathful, and elemental appearance in the *antarābhava*, thereby either achieving awakening or deliberately choosing the manner of future birth. These practices, along with long-standing notions regarding the yogic accomplishment (*siddhi*) of possession (*āveśa*) of others' bodies, likely gave rise to Tibetan traditions of the reincarnate teacher, who appears repeatedly in the world as a manifestation body (Tib. *tulku*, Skt. *nirmāṇakāya*). A *tulku* is said to take on repeated physical manifestations, typically in the form of an awakened teacher, out of the compassionate aspiration to free beings from suffering. The Dalai Lama is one of the most prominent examples of a contemporary Tibetan Buddhist *tulku*, being viewed as a human manifestation body (*nirmāṇakāya*) of the Mahāsattva Bodhisattva Avalokiteśvara and serving as a spiritual and political leader within the Gelukpa sect of Tibetan Buddhism.

The Advent of Islam and the Marginalization of Buddhism in India

The early centuries of the second millennium CE in India witnessed the profound transformation of Indian society and culture with the advent of Islam in India and the establishment of a succession of Islamic regimes and empires throughout the region. The Hindu renaissance of the Gupta Empire (4th–6th century CE) and the brief but powerful reign of Harsha (7th century CE) had long faded, and India was ruled by rival principalities that were unable to collectively resist the incursion of the forces of Mahmud of Ghazni from the northwest in the eleventh century.[169] By the twelfth century, the illustrious Buddhist Pāla dynasty in northeastern India had dissolved as well. Small pockets of Hindu resistance to Islamic rule continued to exist, such as those of the Rajputs in northwestern India, the Vijayanagars in southern India, and the Marathas in central India, and the geography of southern India mediated the social and cultural influence of Islamic Persian and Arabic culture in that region, to some degree.[170] Buddhism all but disappeared from India, the great monastic universities of Nālandā and Vikramaśīla being sacked and the larger Buddhist community dwindling in all but remote southern Indian regions. Nonetheless, Buddhism had successfully pollinated much of further South and Southeast Asia (Sri Lanka, Burma, Cambodia, Laos, and parts of Vietnam) and northern Asia (Nepal, Tibet, Mongolia, China, Korea, and Japan), where it continued to meet with considerable success. The *Kālacakratantra*, one of the culminating texts of late Indian Buddhist tantra, recognized and aimed to ritually address the mounting challenge that Islam presented for Buddhism in India during this period.[171]

The first stage of Islamic empire in India, the Delhi Sultanate (13th–16th century CE) gave way to the "golden age" of Islam in India, the reign of the Mughal Empire (16th–18th century CE), which is associated with the Mughal Emperors Babur, Akbar, Jahangir, Shah Jahan (the builder of the iconic Taj Mahal), and Aurangzeb. Akbar, in particular, was renowned for his inclusive, if not ecumenical, attitude toward various religions, and was credited with organizing a meeting akin to a parliament of world religions to facilitate the dissemination of knowledge about various faiths and bring political unity. Muslim rulers and scholars were highly curious about the practice of yoga, resulting in the translation of important texts, such as the *Yogasūtra*, into Arabic and Persian. The development of *fakir* and *dervish* traditions of Sufism in India were marked by a strong mutual influence with the living yoga traditions of the day, especially with regards to their focus on *siddhi* and *mukti*.[172] Later translations of yoga texts in Arabic and Persian document Muslim, especially Sufi, curiosity regarding a range of tantric and *haṭhayoga* practices, notably *mantra*, *prāṇāyāma*, the structure of the subtle body, and postural practice.[173] The Islamic practice of meditative prayer, "remembrance" (*zikr*), in particular, appears to have been viewed as parallel to the use of mantra and *prāṇāyāma* in yoga, creating a point of intersection between Sufi and yoga practice. The Mughal era saw an increasing militarization among Hindu renouncer traditions, and militant traditions of the Daśanāmī and Rāmānandī came to play a highly significant role as mercenaries for the feuding powers of the era, with some Sādhus commanding up to forty thousand foot and horse soldiers.[174] The rise of the Sant traditions and the emergence of Sikhism were, in part, products of the convergence of the streams of Islamic, Hindu, and Buddhist traditions during the Islamic imperial era in India, which reconfigured the religious landscape of India in profound ways.

The Medieval Legacy of Yoga

The medieval era was marked by numerous transformations of the religious landscape of India, including the development of Hindu sectarian and monastic traditions, popular religious devotionalism (*bhakti*), Sant and Sikh traditions, traditions of ritual extension (*tantra*), and Hindu Nāth and Buddhist Mahāsiddha lineages. Traditions of yoga were expanded, systematized, and consolidated, yielding a variety of modes of practice, such as those characterized by the paradigmatic set of *mantrayoga*, *layayoga*, *haṭhayoga* and *rājayoga*. Late medieval and early modern texts of yoga, such as the well-known *Śivasaṃhitā*, *Haṭhapradīpikā*, and *Gheraṇḍasaṃhitā*, document the attempt to integrate the various threads of the classical and medieval traditions of yoga and tantra into a larger, and in some cases, nonsectarian, rubric of *haṭhayoga*, providing a foundation for the development of modern anglophone yoga traditions. The advent of the European colonial era would transform the social, political, cultural, and economic landscape of India, serving as a catalyst for the rapid transformation of the practice of yoga into a modern and global phenomenon. The medieval era stands out as a uniquely fruitful and transformative period in the history of yoga traditions, and continues to offer a range of practical, especially textual, resources for contemporary yoga practitioners and a wealth of historical and literary data for scholars of Indian religion and philosophy.

Chapter 8

Modern Yoga Traditions

The Portuguese explorer Vasco De Gama's discovery of an oversea trade route to India at the end of the fifteenth century opened a new chapter in India's history, one marked by the impact of European colonial powers, including the Portuguese, Dutch, French, and British.[1] Land-based trade dominated by Persian and Arab intermediaries gave way to direct trade between India and Europe, leading to rapid transformation of the Indian subcontinent. The European colonial era culminated in the British "Raj," or "Rulership," in India, a period that began in the mid–eighteenth century and lasted until Indian independence in 1947. During this period, the commercial and corporate influence of the British East India Company gave way to direct imperial rule, with India becoming the "Jewel in the Crown" of the British empire. The shift from Mughal to European colonial rule affected all levels of Indian society, transforming the cultural and religious landscape of India in innumerable ways. Though European missionary efforts to convert the Indian population to Christianity met with minimal success, the pervasive influence of European culture had profound effects on Indian religious life. Colonial rulers amplified existing cultural faultlines, utilizing divide-and-conquer tactics to drive wedges between religious and sectarian traditions and strategically defining the social and legal parameters of Indian caste divisions.[2] The economic and industrial policies of the colonial powers destabilized local economies and exacerbated problems of poverty, hygiene, and health throughout India, in some cases leading to mass disruptions of welfare and livelihood.[3] The British followed the Mughals in using Indian *sādhu* armies as mercenaries, and the popular image of the Indian ascetic and *yogī* was of militant zeal and circus-like showmanship as much as it was of world-renunciation and the pursuit of spiritual liberation.[4] Indian culture was transformed by its encounter with the European empirical sciences and physical cultures of health and the body, novel urban and industrial modes of life, and emergent global nation-state politics. European colonists introduced new religious, spiritual, and occult sensibilities, embodied in movements such as Theosophy, and championed the European academic study of Indian religion and culture, notably the scholastic study of Sanskrit literature referred to as "Orientalism."[5]

Out of this encounter, modern English-based, or anglophone, forms of yoga emerged that would become the basis for widely influential transnational yoga traditions. Practices descended from classical and medieval yoga traditions continued to be taught within the circles of priestly Hindu orthodoxy, the reformed renouncer traditions of the Daśanāmī and Rāmānandī, and in localized *guru-śiṣya* householder lineages. However, distinctively modern yoga traditions emerged that built on these premodern models of yoga, absorbing emergent European and Indian ideologies and physical cultures and softening connections between yoga and Indian sectarian traditions. The success of these modern yoga traditions in Europe and the United States, in turn, had the effect of increasing the valuation of yoga in India, leading to an influx of cultural and economic capital to authoritative figures and institutions across the subcontinent.

Elements of Modern Yoga

Modern yoga traditions exist on a spectrum between secularism and sectarian devotion, often negotiating their rootedness in sectarian lineages through appeal to the notion of yoga as a universal method that transcends religious and cultural identity. One aspect of this universalism is an emphasis on the physical, or *physicalism*, a grounding of the practice of yoga in the physical body, which serves as a *lingua franca* of human experience.[6] The physicalism of modern yoga is, in part, linked to the colonial impact of European physical culture, especially its focus on the disciplining of the body for therapeutic, hygienic, and moral purposes. Physicalism is among a set of factors that characterize modern yoga, of which the following are particularly noteworthy: scientism, medicalism, nationalism and activism, reconstructionism, universalism, orientalism, entrepreneurism and commodification, and body, gender, and sexuality normativism.

Physicalism, Scientism, and Medicalism

The foregrounding of the body in modern yoga practice represents one of the principal elements behind the success of modern postural yoga on a global scale.[7] Emphasis on the physical dimension of yoga, especially yoga posture (*āsana*), places yoga at parity with modern physical culture disciplines such as gymnastics, calisthenics, and the martial arts. This emphasis on physicalism is also associated with the notion of yoga as being "empirical" or "scientific," which is illustrated in expressions such as that of "the science of yoga." Modern proponents of yoga in India, such as Swami Kuvalayananda of the Kaivalyadhama Yoga institute in Lonavla, India, sought to demonstrate the value of yoga in scientific terms through laboratory experiments, deemphasizing its religious metaphysics.[8] The conception of yoga as a first-person empirical enterprise is a pervasive rhetorical component of the discourse of modern yoga, even if such "empiricism" is epistemologically distinct from scientific third-person models.[9] In addition to "Western" or allopathic medicine, modern yoga is also linked with Indian and European non-allopathic medical models such as *āyurveda* and Nature Cure.[10] Modern yoga has also been connected, in some instances, to the pseudo-scientific theories of eugenics and Social Darwinism that postulate a process of "spiritual evolution" through physical and racial purification, ideas associated with early to mid-twentieth-century fascism.[11]

Modern yoga has been similarly associated with a discourse of *medicalism*. Yoga serves as a therapeutic intervention for a range of health issues, including back pain, diabetes, anxiety, trauma, and depression. Yoga is a commonly prescribed intervention within allopathic and osteopathic medicine, and health modalities such as physical therapy have integrated yoga *āsana* into their repertoire. The integration of meditation into psychological and psychiatric practice has also become mainstream, being popularized by a number of Buddhist-meditation-inspired medical interventions, such as mindfulness-based stress reduction (MBSR). It has also been argued that the practice of yoga on a mass public scale may provide a solution to pervasive public mental and physical health problems.[12] However, the widespread use of yoga as a "self-care" health modality has also been critiqued as a reflection of a neoliberal capitalist ethos of individualism that shifts the economic burden of public health away from institutions onto individuals.[13] Additionally, the early twenty-first century saw an increase in public debate regarding the risk of injury, or even death, resulting from the practice of postural yoga traditions, tempering some of the enthusiasm for its application to public health concerns.[14]

Nationalism and Activism

Many early formulators of modern yoga were avid Indian nationalists who viewed yoga as part of a national praxis that would help India overcome its degradation during the colonial period. Swami Vivekananda, perhaps the most famous "Hindu Missionary" of the colonial period, framed yoga as a uniquely Indian gift to the world, a spiritual science of the "East" to be set in contrast to the material science of the "West."[15] Mohandas K. Gandhi, the so-called "Father of the Indian Nation," espoused a political philosophy of "holding to the truth" (*satyāgraha*), which melded yogic-ascetic principles and political activism.[16] Hindu nationalism was also represented in organizations such as the Ārya Samāj, the "Noble Society," which promoted a vision of Hinduism as a socially engaged spirituality. Innovators such as Swami Kuvalayananda of Kaivalyadhama, Shri Yogendra, and Swami Sivananda all viewed yoga as a method for strengthening the nation by strengthening the people of India.[17] The Indian Maharaja Bhavanarao Pant Pratinidhi championed the "Sun Salutation" (Skt. *sūrya-namaskāra*, Hin. *sūrya-namaskār*) exercise as a practice to strengthen and uplift the nation as a whole.[18] Indian yoga gurus of the late twentieth century and early twenty-first century, such as Swami Ramdev, echoed these views, representing yoga as a means for revitalizing India and the world in an era of degeneration.[19] Indian Prime Minister Narendra Modi helped found a United Nations sponsored "International Day of Yoga," which has been celebrated worldwide since 2015, and established a Ministry of Ayurveda, Yoga and Naturopathy, Unani, Siddha and Homeopathy (AYUSH) within the Indian federal government in 2014.[20]

Appeals to yoga and Hindu spirituality have been employed by conservative and nationalist Hindu organizations, such as the RSS and the VHP, in their political efforts in India, and by progressive Hindu environmentalists, such as Vandana Shiva.[21] Swami Ramdev has campaigned for the restoration of the Ganges River and the ending of the Indian "Black Money" economy, while simultaneously championing conservative and nationalist ideals.[22] Buddhists around the globe have embraced an ethos of "Engaged Buddhism" that links Buddhist practice to activism on social, political, and environmental issues.[23] Nonsectarian and anglophone traditions of yoga in Europe and the United States have also embraced social and environmental justice, one prominent example being the "Green Yoga" movement.[24] Modern yoga-inspired activism also includes projects that aim to provide yoga to economically disadvantaged and at-risk groups, such as those in inner cities, drug treatment programs, and correctional institutions.[25]

In India, initiatives to integrate yoga into public education include "Surya Namaskara Day" observances at the state level and the pan-Indian and global "International Day of Yoga." In Madhya Pradesh, the observance of Surya Namaskara Day has been represented as a public health initiative to support healthy minds and bodies. However, in some cases, minority Muslim and Christian communities have viewed such exercises as serving a Hindu nationalist agenda, given that the Sun Salutation (*sūrya-namaskār*) can be interpreted as an act of worship of the Hindu god Sūrya.[26] Advocates of yoga in the United States and Germany have sought to publicize evidence of the physical and psychological benefits of the application of postural yoga and mindfulness meditation within educational contexts.[27] In the United States, some educational yoga programs have been met with legal action that challenges the constitutionality of such practices under the federal establishment clause.[28] In India, a proposal to make yoga a mandatory practice for all primary school children resulted in litigation reaching India's supreme court.[29]

Reconstructionism, Universalism, and Orientalism

A number of formulators of modern yoga traditions, including Vivekananda, Sivananda, and Krishnamacharya, framed their teachings in light of traditional Hindu texts, such as the *Yogasūtra* of Patañjali. Some scholars have questioned the validity of such framing, particularly appeals to Patañjali's *Yogasūtra*, given the limited focus of such texts on the type of postural practice central to modern yoga.[30] However, with respect to the *Yogasūtra*, the appeal to the eight-limbed yoga (*aṣṭāṅgayoga*) model as a framework for understanding yoga practice is consistent with discourses of yoga in the Purāṇa literature and much of the larger *brāhmaṇa* discourse on yoga.[31] In addition to using the *Yogasūtra* and the *aṣṭāṅgayoga* paradigm in framing authority, modern anglophone systems of yoga draw from *haṭhayoga* methodologies, Kashmir Śaiva philosophy, Vaiṣṇava *bhakti* traditions, and Buddhist insight and mindfulness meditation systems, utilizing texts such as the *Haṭhapradīpikā* and *Bhagavadgītā*, among other sources.[32]

Modern yoga traditions, especially their anglophone variations, often frame yoga as accessible to all, regardless of ethnic, religious, or gender identity. The representation of yoga as having a universal application is evident in the modern focus on minimally sectarian Hindu literature, such as practice-oriented *haṭhayoga* texts.[33] It also reflects the impact of Christian Unitarianism and universalizing forms of European spirituality such as Theosophy during the colonial period. As such, yoga is represented as a remedy for the variety of problems of modern life, from individual illness and social disharmony to profound spiritual and metaphysical concerns.[34] It is also adapted to suit various religious contexts, including those of the Abrahamic faiths of Christianity, Judaism, and Islam, as well as modern Indian religions such as Sikhism, often being framed as a "spiritual" practice distinct from the theological or institutional commitments characteristic of "religion."[35]

A primary source for the pervasive universalism found in modern yoga is the Indian philosophical tradition of neo-Vedānta championed by Vivekananda, his teacher Ramakrishna, and other figures associated with the "Hindu Renaissance," such as Swami Sivananda. Neo-Vedānta, which is rooted in modern readings of the *Bhagavadgītā* and Vedānta literature, postulates that though there may be many religious paths, there is ultimately one reality that all of humanity is striving toward, that is, *brahman* or "God." This "many paths, one goal" viewpoint provides a philosophical and ideological basis for asserting that institutional religious affiliation is secondary to the universality of spiritual practice. It may have also served as a counterpoint to colonial missionary efforts in Calcutta (Kolkata) and other intellectual centers of modern Hinduism.[36] Drawing upon the Advaita Vedānta philosophy of Śaṅkara, Vivekananda proposed that different religious paths are like the rungs of a ladder, with early stages being characterized by theistic ritual and devotion and later stages by the development of spiritual insight or wisdom (*jñāna*).[37] Similarly, modern Buddhist traditions also emphasize the universal utility of meditation for people of various religious (or nonreligious) backgrounds, allowing practitioners to retain their non-Buddhist religious or secular identity.[38] Hybrid Jewish-Buddhist identity, for example, comprises a significant part of emergent Buddhist communities in Europe and the United States.[39]

Orientalist scholarship in Europe from the eighteenth to the twentieth century sought to integrate Indian thought into its own universalizing, albeit European, worldview.[40] In turn, Orientalist translations of Indian texts were reappropriated by Hindu modernists such as Vivekananda, creating a recursive cycle of influence and transformation. In the United States, Transcendentalist poets and philosophers, including Ralph Waldo Emerson (1803–1882) and Henry David Thoreau (1817–1862), paved the way for the introduction of Indian philosophy, and specifically yoga, on both elite and popular levels in the United States.[41] Theosophical traditions, based on the teachings of Helena Blavatsky (1831–1891), Henry Steele Olcott (1832–1907), and Annie Besant (1847–1933), provided a cosmopolitan mystical-occult framework for the interpretation of Indian philosophy and facilitated the translation of numerous yoga texts into English, including the *Yogasūtra*.[42] Paul Brunton (Raphael Hurst, 1898–1981), a student of Theosophy, stoked popular interest in yoga and in Indian mysticism with a popular novel, *The Search for Secret India* (1934), in which he described an ecstatic encounter with the Indian saint Ramana Maharishi (1879–1950). The European tradition of "Harmonial Gymnastics," a hybridized tradition that drew upon European gymnastics, occultism, and Indian yoga techniques, provided another important point of intersection with yoga traditions, especially in Europe.[43] On an academic level, Sarvepalli Radhakrishnan (1888–1975) and Aldous Huxley (1894–1963) championed the notion of a "Perennial Philosophy" underlying mystical traditions throughout the world that was deeply indebted to neo-Vedānta.[44] Huxley's philosophical reflections on his experiences with Mescaline in his *The Doors of Perception* (1954) anticipated, if not catalyzed, the intersection of the psychoactive-drug-experimentalism of 1960s counterculture and Hindu and Buddhist spirituality in Europe and the United States.[45]

The universalization of yoga has, in some cases, been met with criticism, a prominent case in point being the "Take Back Yoga" campaign of the United States-based Hindu American Foundation, which sought in the early twenty-first century to publicly delineate the Indian, and especially the Hindu, roots of yoga, shedding light on issues of cultural appropriation and commodification.[46] Some Jewish, Christian, and Muslim leaders in the United States, England, and Australia have argued that yoga is potentially spiritually dangerous or even "demonic," in some cases banning the practice of yoga altogether.[47] A suspicion of a hidden agenda in yoga has led critics to ask the question of whether the practice of yoga leads, on some level, to practitioners "becoming Hindu."[48] The common use of religious icons, the recitation of religious texts, and the existence of various trappings of Indian religiosity provides some basis for the assertion that modern anglophone yoga is proximate to Indian spirituality, if not religion.[49]

Entrepreneurism and Commodification

Swami Vivekananda and Paramahansa Yogananda, among other teachers, became prominent voices for the valorization of yoga in India and the United States through their entrepreneurial, if not evangelical, self-promotion involving public appearances and demonstrations, writing, film, and the deft utilization of media outlets.[50] Printed literature emerged as a major vehicle for the propagation of yoga in the twentieth century, and the use of photography, film, cable television, and digital media vastly expanded popular access to yoga.[51] Modern yoga's association with the wealthy and privileged, especially politicians, heiresses, and celebrity actors and musicians, has also contributed to its longevity and its broad public visibility and appeal.[52] This was illustrated in the lives of prominent North American figures in the early to mid–twentieth century, such as the modern yoga and tantra teacher Pierre Bernard (Perry Baker, 1875–1955), known as the "Omnipotent Oom," his wife Blanche DeVries (1891–1984), and Pierre Bernard's nephew Theos Bernard (1908–1947), who was a popularizer of *haṭhayoga* and Tibetan Buddhism known by the self-proclaimed moniker of the "White Lama."[53]

The configuration of modern yoga, especially in its anglophone postural forms, is deeply tied into its appeal to an emergent Indian middle class and to a larger, economically successful transnational audience that had the capital and leisure to pursue its practice.[54] Over the course of the twentieth century, yoga became the focus of a multibillion dollar industry, a powerful revenue-generating enterprise extending from local communities to transnational institutions and global tourism.[55] Modes of revenue generation in modern yoga include the sale of yoga-themed products, such as yoga apparel, props, books, and electronic media, and fee-based models of payment that quantify the cost of instruction at yoga institutions, studios, retreats, or spas. Yoga products negotiate function and fashion, with yoga apparel being widely adopted in athletics and as everyday attire due to its comfort, versatility, and fashionability, in some cases serving as an indicator of aesthetic value and economic class status. Yoga props, such as mats, blocks, straps, and cushions, perform a range of functions in posture-based yoga practice, with the wide variety of products capitalizing on the consumer market for such goods. The modern yoga studio shares many features with the modern dance studio, such as sprung-wood floors, white walls, and mirrors, and is often decorated with yoga-themed objects, including photographs of teachers and practitioners and religious art and icons.[56] Such items empower and inspire practitioners through association with the spiritual, exotic, and idealized practice of yoga.[57]

In anglophone yoga traditions and, increasingly, in the Indian context, students pay a per-class fee or tuition for yoga course units. In India, it is common for schools to have parallel pay structures for Indian and non-Indian students, reflecting the disparity in wealth between local and international students. Teacher training, workshops, and other programs have various economic thresholds for participation, extending or limiting access. Modern schools such as *Yoga for the People* have sought to challenge the fee-based model, offering yoga courses on a pay-by-choice basis, and many yoga centers hold free or reduced-rate student and community classes.[58] Teacher certification has become increasingly regulated, with the U.S.-based *Yoga Alliance* and *International Association of Yoga Therapists* being the primary institutional authorities for registered teachers of anglophone yoga on an international level, though not without criticism.[59] In India, the Yoga Certification Board at the Morarji Desai National Institute of Yoga of the Indian Ministry of Ayurveda, Yoga and Naturopathy, Unani, Siddha and Homoeopathy (AYUSH) provides and promotes standards for yoga teachers and schools in India.[60] Some contemporary Indian lineages, such as those of K. Pattabhi Jois and B.K.S. Iyengar, have established minimum requirements for teachers but continue to place priority on the judgment of senior teachers with regards to certification.[61]

The branding of styles of yoga, often in association with a particular teacher or lineage, has had both economic and legal implications, creating revenue streams within yoga organizations and precipitating the entry of yoga into the legal spheres of intellectual property and patent law.[62] Yoga chains and franchises, such as *YogaWorks*, have been praised for bringing consistency to the execution of yoga classes and criticized for having a homogenizing influence on yoga practice and an adverse economic impact on smaller yoga studios.[63] Yoga has become a staple in the fitness-club industry in the United States, being common at professional fitness clubs and at YMCA and local community centers. The fluidity of the boundary between "fitness culture" and yoga has led some practitioners to question the distinction between "working out" and practicing yoga.[64] The complexities of differentiating yoga from fitness culture are also evident in debates over whether teaching yoga should be taxable at the state and federal level and whether yoga instructors should be subject to regulation like physical therapists and fitness workers.[65]

Body, Gender, and Sexuality Normativism

The development of modern yoga coincided with the emergence of a worldwide physical culture movement that placed the athletic disciplining and display of the body in a privileged place in global civilization, creating new body, gender, and sexual norms.[66] In concert with this, emergent late and post-Victorian physical ideals provided new paradigms of the aesthetics of beautiful male and female bodies.[67] The emergence of the "modern male physique," patterned after the Greco-Roman ideals of a fit and muscular body, was complemented by the emergence of a physically fit, active, and slender feminine ideal. The promotion of athleticism found worldwide expression in a range of cultural fads, including calisthenics and gymnastics movements, public dancing, circus performance, and contortionism, and coincided with the rise of an ethos of health and morality through physical activity. This era gave birth to "Muscular Christianity," in which the cultivation of the body was equated with the cultivation of the soul, encapsulated in bodybuilding pioneer Eugen Sandow's concept of the "Gospel of Strength" and championed by institutions such as the Young Men's Christian Association (YMCA).[68] In India, engagement with the physical culture movement reflected attempts to combat a colonial discourse that portrayed Indian subjects as feminine, with indigenous body disciplines, yoga among them, being seen as a crucial part of establishing a strong, masculine, and independent India.[69] The Indian bodybuilder K.V. Iyer (1897–1980), an emulator of Sandow, and Iyer's student and collaborator S. Sundaram (1901–1994) played important roles in bridging European bodybuilding, physical culture, and yoga through their teaching, demonstrations, and innovative publications on modern yoga *āsana*.[70]

Though most modern lineages descend from a male *guru*, modern yoga teachers and practitioners have increasingly been female, particularly within the anglophone yoga communities of Europe and the United States.[71] This is partly due to the championing of yoga by middle- and upper-class European and North American women as part of a culture of beautification and as a type of privileged leisure activity. It is also a reflection of countercultural movements in the late nineteenth- to early twentieth-century United States, in which women's liberation and authority was linked with nontraditional spiritualties.[72] The tension between mainstream and countercultural representations of gender and sexuality in yoga is evident in contemporary debates about the "yoga body," in which the idealized youthful, slender, and flexible female body is set in contrast with those of a wider range of ages, body types, gender and sexual identities, and physical abilities.[73] In India, the proliferation of female practitioners of yoga has also been associated with the emergence of a middle-class economy, women's liberation movements, and traditional lineages seeking self-preservation.[74]

Indian yoga modernists have often embraced a householder-yogi paradigm, endorsing traditional heteronormative Hindu parameters regarding sexuality, though in some cases cautioning against the potential dangers of overzealous sexual enjoyment facilitated by yogic mastery.[75] Swami Ramdev, in line with broader conservative modern Hindu views on sexuality, views homosexuality as an aberrant mode of living, one that can be cured by yoga.[76] In contrast, Sri Ravi Shankar has argued that the prohibition of homosexuality is not found in Hindu scriptures.[77] Conservative Hindu views on sexuality in yoga, such as those of Swami Ramdev, stand in contrast to the welcoming attitude toward gay, lesbian, bisexual, transgender, and queer practitioners found in a number of anglophone yoga contexts.[78] Neo-tantra traditions, exemplified by the teachings of Indian, and one-time North American, guru Bhagwan Shree Rajneesh, present sexual expression as means of spiritual transformation, tapping into the "free love" ethos that emerged out of the counterculture of the 1960s in Europe and the United States.[79] The notion that yoga can enhance sexual performance has been explored extensively in anglophone contexts, most notably through print literature and instructional visual media that promises an improved sex life through a regimen of *āsana* and *prāṇāyāma*, augmented, in some cases, with pelvic-floor toning Kegel exercises.[80] Modern yoga has been characterized in its anglophone contexts by the adoption of revealing yoga apparel and the proliferation of visual representations of the idealized female "yoga body" that grace the cover of publications such as *Yoga Journal*.[81] The tension between body-positivity and objectification in anglophone yoga is perhaps most starkly evident in the proliferation of "naked yoga" courses and visual media, which alternately offer the potential for radical self-acceptance and voyeuristic fetishism and titillation.[82] In India, it is common for women to wear a Sari while practicing yoga, as is illustrated by female attendees at mass-attended yoga camps (Hin. *śivir*). However, a bourgeoning market of "yoga workout" videos by Bollywood stars and the emergence of a larger celebrity fitness-yoga culture in India are softening conservative attitudes toward yoga attire.[83]

In the early twentieth century, Hindu yoga gurus and their North American imitators, such as Yogi Ramacharaka, were viewed with considerable suspicion in the United States, particularly with respect to their purported capacity to hypnotize and seduce young and vulnerable women.[84] Though much of this concern, especially in its early manifestations, was a product of media-driven hysteria, paranoia, and xenophobia, the transmission of modern yoga, especially in the anglophone sphere, has been punctuated by numerous high-profile sex scandals and controversies. Accusations, if not well-documented cases, of secret sexual relationships, inappropriate physical contact, and sexual abuse, in some cases involving children, have affected many yoga communities, leading to legal action, negative publicity, and tectonic shifts within the culture of modern yoga.[85] In some contexts, abusive behavior has been connected to a teacher or guru's claims to be providing special or secret teachings to particular disciples, especially women, outside the boundaries of ordinary practice. Access and proximity to the physical presence of the guru, especially when alone, is often highly valued, given the guru's embodiment of power and sacrality, leading to private and intimate contact between student and teacher outside of typical social parameters.[86] Unquestioning faith and loyalty to teachers, gurus, and organizations undoubtedly facilitates abuse and its concealment by the victim and larger community.[87] The *guru* may be conceived of as a perfect embodiment of the practice, inscrutable and therefore beyond moral questioning or reproach, despite clear evidence of abuse.[88] Disciples may also be hesitant to confront such issues given their profound spiritual, moral, and economic investment in a *guru* and their community, particularly when they face potential public embarrassment and ostracism.

Practices of Modern Yoga

Postural styles of yoga that emphasize yoga *āsana* have been highly influential in the modern era, weaving together the physical cultures of India and those of the European and North American worlds. Modern postural yoga systems build on this foundation by incorporating concepts from Hindu and Buddhist tantrism, such as notions of the subtle body (*sūkṣma-śarīra*) with its channels (*nāḍī*) and centers or wheels (*cakra*) in which *prāṇa* and *kuṇḍalinī* are said to move. Meditative forms of modern yoga emphasize practices such as silent *mantra* recitation, mindfulness (*smṛti*) practices of breath and body, and the visualization or cultivation (*bhāvanā*) of mental images. These disciplines of postural and meditative yoga are supplemented with invocatory and devotional chanting of mantras, the musical practice of *kīrtan* (Skt. *kīrtana*, lit. "reciting, repeating"), and the use of ritualized benedictions such as *namaste*.

Āsana, *Prāṇāyāma*, and *Vinyāsa*

Modern postural systems of yoga are marked by the development of a vast vocabulary of both standing and seated yoga postures (*āsana*), building on the framework of premodern traditions such as those of an "eighty-four *āsana*" set that appear in texts of the seventeenth to eighteenth century.[89] Some texts of this era, such as Brajbhasha *Jogapradīpyakā*, "[A] Lamp [on the Practice] of Yoga," use the *aṣṭāṅgayoga* rubric to frame an elaborate practice of yoga *āsana*, anticipating the application of the *aṣṭāṅga* system in modern postural yoga systems.[90] The innovative spirit of twentieth-century modern postural yoga is exemplified by the innovation of a wide range of new standing postures, including the common "triangle pose" (*trikoṇāsana*), "warrior pose" (*vīrabhadrāsana*), and "upright side-angle pose" (*utthitapārśvakoṇāsana*), which are documented visually in modern works such B.K.S. Iyengar's *Light on Yoga.*

The practice of *prāṇāyāma* is largely subsumed into that of yoga *āsana* in modern postural yoga, a configuration exemplified by the practice of *vinyāsa*, in which movement within and between postures is linked to the movement of breath. Typically, exhalation is associated with compressive movements such as forward bending and twisting, and inhalation with decompression movements such as backbending and releasing from twisting movements. In one influential form, *vinyāsa* practice includes a constriction of the throat as an approximation of the *haṭhayoga* practice of "victorious breath control" (*ujjāyī-prāṇāyāma*), supplemented by approximations of the "upward flying" (*uḍḍīyāna*) abdominal and "root" (*mūla*) pelvic lock or binding (*bandha*) and the use of a focused gaze (*dṛṣṭi*) on a point on the body or in space. The principle of *vinyāsa* is exemplified in modern yoga in the "Sun Salutation" (Skt. *sūrya-namaskāra*, Hin. *sūrya-namaskār*), which links inhalation and exhalation with a standardized sequence of prostration-like movements. Contemporary *vinyāsa* is associated with the modern postural rubrics of "Power Yoga" and "Flow Yoga," and is often set apart categorically from static postural approaches to yoga that emphasize remaining in an *āsana* for an extended time.[91] Modern schools referred to with the rubric "Hot Yoga," such as the Bikram Yoga system, augment the practice of dynamic and static *āsana* by heating the yoga practice space to temperatures as high as 105°F (41°C) or more. In many classes, teachers offer hands-on "assists" or "adjustments," which range from attempts to adapt a practice to a student's physical needs to the use of forceful, if not aggressive, pressure, in order to accelerate progress, the latter practice being more common among modern Indian yoga lineages in which liability for injury is assumed by the practitioner.[92]

Kuṇḍalinī, *Śaktipāta*, and *Kriyā*

Though much of modern yoga is focused exclusively on the physical aspect of yoga, especially on health, well-being, and the appearance of the physical body, conceptions of a subtle body (*sūkṣma-śarīra*) are pervasive, especially among yoga traditions with explicit spiritual or religious inclinations. These include the conceptions, rooted in *haṭhayoga* and cognate tantric traditions, that the body contains a system of channels (*nāḍī*) and wheels or centers (*cakra*) in which vital air or energy (*vāyu*, *prāṇa*) and vitality (*bindu*, *bīja*) moves. The notion of the activation or rousing of *kuṇḍalinī* and its ascent from the lowest *cakra* to the highest through the practice of yoga, in particular, has a strong relationship with premodern *haṭhayoga* and tantric forms of yoga. Such ideas, which are often simplified or combined with non-Indian frameworks, serve as a model for conceptualizing how *āsana* and *prāṇāyāma* transforms a person energetically, if not spiritually.[93] In modern yoga traditions such as Kundalini Yoga and Siddha Yoga, the activation of *kuṇḍalinī* is viewed as a central focus of practice, which in some cases is associated with the initiatory practice of the "descent of power" (Hin. *śaktipāt*, Skt. *śaktipāta*), in which a *guru* awakens *kuṇḍalinī* in a disciple through touch, gaze, or other means of physical contact. Modern *kuṇḍalinīyoga* is also associated with the performance of *kriyā*, which are spontaneous vocalizations, physical movements, and inner experiences inspired by *śaktipāta*.[94] Even in traditions that do not explicitly utilize *śaktipāta* and *kriyā*, the touch of the teacher or *guru* is often viewed as uniquely powerful, and spontaneous movement and emotional catharsis in postural practice may be associated with the releasing of trauma from the body.[95]

Satsaṅg, *Sevā*, *Kīrtan*, *Mantra*, and *Namaste*

Many modern yoga traditions embrace practices that are associated either closely or obliquely with traditional, especially Vaiṣṇava, forms of *bhaktiyoga*. This is exemplified by the practice of *satsaṅg* (Skt. *satsaṅga*), literally the "association" with the "good" or the "true," the communal practice of listening to spiritual or *dharma* discourses and the recitation and repetition of devotional mantras and hymns (Skt. *kīrtana*, Hin. *kīrtan*).[96] Similar forms of *dharma* discourse and devotionalism are also found within modern Buddhist and Jain contexts, including didactic teaching and devotional chanting, recitation, and singing. The practice of *satsaṅg* provides a philosophical, moral, and devotional framework for the practice of yoga, which includes a set of goals for practice and insight into how yoga is to be integrated into everyday life. Students may be advised on how to lead a virtuous life, such as how to exercise proper yogic restraint (*yama*), or how to support yoga and address particular health concerns through diet and the use of Indian traditional medicine (*āyurveda*) or other health modalities. Some students may also participate in service (*sevā*), which often takes on the form of volunteer work at an ashram or yoga center and is often rewarded through the reduction or waiver of instructional fees and increased access to the teacher or *guru*.[97]

The performance of *mantra*, or incantation, in modern yoga finds chief expression in the use of the mantra *oṃ* as a ritual signifier in postural forms of yoga, often being recited at the beginning and end of class and as an object of contemplation in meditative contexts. The modern use of *mantra* draws upon Hindu verbal formulas that invoke various deities, such as Śiva, Gaṇeśa, Viṣṇu, or Devī, particularly as representative of various physical, mental, or spiritual qualities, such as strength, compassion, love, and wisdom, either as personal deities or impersonal principles. Modern yoga traditions also commonly use "peace mantras" (*śānti-mantra*) drawn from the Upaniṣads that reference the early Vedic Hindu religious pantheon of deities, such as Indra and Sūrya. *Kīrtan*, the recitation and repetition of the names of Hindu deities with musical accompaniment and participation in ecstatic dance, has deep roots in popular Indian *bhakti* traditions, especially those associated with Viṣṇu and his various incarnations (Skt. *avatāra*, Hin. *avatār*). The widespread practice of *kīrtan* in modern anglophone yoga culture is, in part, due to the influence of the Gauḍīya Vaiṣṇava tradition of the so-called "Hare Krishna" movement popularized in Europe and the United States in the late twentieth century. *Kīrtan*, which is often facilitated by the visual representation of deities in the form of an icon (*mūrti*) or a popular devotional image, serves as a threshold into the more explicitly spiritual or religious aspects of yoga traditions. The performance of *satsaṅg* and *kīrtan* is, in some cases, correlated with life-cycle events, such as birthdays, seasonal changes, and holidays, and occasionally provided during moments of crisis for a community, providing a supportive ritual structure that binds practitioners together.[98]

In modern anglophone contexts, the beginning and end of yoga instruction is commonly marked by the use of the Sanskrit verbal expression *namaste* and the joining of the hands in a prayerful gesture (*mudrā*) of reverence (*namaskāra*) or devotion (*añjali*). The expression *namaste*, along with *namaskār*, is a widespread formal greeting in modern Indian languages, being derived from the Sanskrit *namas* + *te*, literally translating as "[a] bow to you" or "[a] salutation to you." It is sometimes extrapolated to mean "the light in me salutes the light in you" or "the divine in me salutes the divine in you," though it is unclear whether such formulations have any premodern precursors.[99] In addition to the use of *namaste* and *namaskāra-mudrā*, yoga instruction may be followed by some form of closing ritual interaction with the teacher, such as the recitation of *oṃ*, bowing or prostration, gazing (*darśana*), a formal or informal embrace or patting of the head of the student by the teacher, the touching of the feet of the teacher by students, or some combination of such actions.

Dhyāna and *Bhāvanā*

Modern meditative traditions of yoga emphasize the disciplining of the mind for the sake of either mundane or supramundane benefits.[100] Modern meditative yoga traditions are commonly framed in terms of the therapeutic benefits of practice, such as enhanced interoception, and contemporary meditation teachers often appeal to the discourses of the modern psychological and neurobiological sciences in framing its benefits.[101] Among meditative traditions rooted in Hinduism, the most common form of meditation involves the use of a mantra, such as *oṃ*, which is recited verbally or mentally. This is exemplified in the Transcendental Meditation (TM) system of Maharishi Mahesh Yogi, which uses mantra repetition (*japa*) in order to induce states of meditation (*dhyāna*) and contemplation (*samādhi*). Buddhist-derived practices of mindfulness (Skt. *smṛti*, Pāli *sati*), often associated with the practice of insight (Skt. *vipaśyanā*, Pāli *vipassanā*), use meditation on sense experiences, such as awareness of the breath and body, to enhance concentration and facilitate self-reflection. Closely related to Theravāda Buddhist insight meditation practices are Japanese Zen (Chn. *ch'an*, from Skt. *dhyāna*) and Tibetan Mahāmudrā and Dzogchen meditation traditions, which emphasize practices of "open awareness" that aim to cultivate a spacious and receptive, or "sky like," state of mind. Practices such as the meditative cultivation (*bhāvanā*) of loving-kindness (Skt. *maitrī*, Pāli *mettā*) and compassion (*karuṇā*) also continue to be applied widely in modern Theravāda and Mahāyāna Buddhism and in a variety of secular therapeutic contexts. Modern meditative traditions that draw upon Śaiva Hindu, Vajrayāna Buddhist, or Terapanth

Jain *haṭhayoga* and tantric traditions utilize visualization practices on the inner subtle body and on forms of embodied divine and enlightened beings, including Śiva, Devī, Buddhas, Bodhisattvas, and Jinas.[102] Aspects of Śaiva and *haṭhayoga* traditions of breath control (*prāṇāyāma*) and meditation (*dhyāna*) have also been consolidated and reframed under the rubric of "yogic sleep," (*yoga-nidrā*), and serve as a form of therapeutic relaxation or "sleep therapy."[103]

Progenitors, Popularizers, and Schools of Modern Yoga

Modern yoga developed in a period marked by the historical developments of the late- to post-colonial era in South Asia, including the Indian independence movement and the emergence of independent Indian, Pakistani, and Bangladeshi nation-states. Figures such as Paramahansa Yogananda, Swami Sivananda, and B.K.S. Iyengar were instrumental in bringing traditions of modern yoga to a pan-Indian and global audience, ultimately creating a cosmopolitan culture of yoga rooted in Indian soil but looking far beyond it. The transnational and anglophone schools of yoga that emerged in the early twentieth century had varying degrees of connection to Hindu sectarian *sampradāya*-based traditions of renunciation and priestly (*brāhmaṇa*) traditions of householder-yoga. Though Indian teachers were at least initially met with significant suspicion, if not antagonism, in the European and American media, the countercultural appeal of yoga persisted through the twentieth century, with access to teachers enhanced in the United States by the liberalization of its immigration policy in the 1960s. By the early twenty-first century, networks of modern anglophone yoga traditions had been established on virtually every continent, with India serving as a hub for an increasingly global community of practitioners.

Yoga Modernists, Nationalists, and Activists

The Hindu reformer and international guru Swami Vivekananda (Narendranath Datta, 1863–1902), is often hailed as the founder of modern yoga traditions, given his profound impact as a champion of yoga on the world stage in the late nineteenth century. The disciple of a prominent Indian mystic and guru from West Bengal, Swami Ramakrishna (1836–1886),

Vivekananda is often singled out as the embodiment of the globalizing of Hindu spirituality during the late colonial era. Vivekananda's participation at the World Parliament of Religions in Chicago 1893 is often considered a watershed moment in the development of modern yoga.[104] Vivekananda's appearance in Chicago was followed by a tour that paved the way for the establishment of the Vedanta Society, one of the first Hindu missionary organizations in the United States. He championed an Orientalist discourse that imagined India as part of a "mystical East" set apart from the "materialist West," one in which India would offer its spiritual goods to the world in exchange for "Western" scientific knowledge and material wealth. His appeal to Indian and European ideals and his dramatic rhetorical flourishes, which are illustrated in his public discourses and writings, were instrumental in the development of an anglophone discourse of Hindu spirituality and yoga.[105] Vivekananda wrote and published a commentary on the *Yogasūtra* of Patañjali entitled *Rāja Yoga*, in which he integrated neo-Vedāntic thought and European scientific and metaphysical traditions within the umbrella of the *aṣṭāṅgayoga* system.[106] *Rāja Yoga* remains a landmark work in the development of the philosophy of modern yoga and in the formation of an anglophone literature of translation and interpretation of Patañjali's *Yogasūtra*.[107] Vivekananda's role as a spiritual and political leader was later institutionalized in the Vivekananda Kendra, a modern service organization that combines instruction in yoga with service and outreach within an Indian nationalist framework.[108] Among notable Vedanta Society figures in the United States was Swami Prabhavananda (1893–1976), who, along with student and novelist Christopher Isherwood (1904–1986), published a number of popular translations of Hindu texts, including the *Bhagavadgītā* (1944) and the *Yogasūtra* of Patañjali (1953).

Another outstanding figure in the late colonial era in India was Hindu nationalist-turned-guru Aurobindo Ghose (1872–1950), whose publications on "Integral Yoga" sought to link Darwinian evolution with yoga-inspired "spiritual evolution." Like many of his contemporaries, Ghose was also sympathetic to the propagation of modern postural forms of yoga as an indigenous and masculine Indian physical culture.[109] The Sri Aurobindo Ashram in Pondicherry was established in 1926 as a vehicle for the dissemination of Aurobindo's teachings in India, Europe, and North America. Aurobindo's successor in Pondicherry was a European disciple referred to as "The Mother" (Mirra Alfassa, 1878–1973), whom Aurobindo appointed as his successor after recognizing her as an incarnation of the divine mother (*devī-śakti*).[110] The Aurobindo Ashram, in turn, produced a number of influential gurus, including Sri Chinmoy (Kumar Ghose, 1931–2007), who had a considerable impact in the United States through his teachings on yoga and physical fitness and his advocacy for the use of meditative practices at the United Nations.[111]

Another important figure in the Indian independence movement, Mohandas K. Gandhi (1869–1948), known as a "Great Soul" (*mahātma*) and the "Father of the Indian nation," melded spiritual and political life in his concepts of "seizing of the truth" (*satyāgraha*) and "self-rule" (*swarāj*). He established a series of ashrams in India based on the principle of *satyāgraha* and the observance of ascetic-yogic vows (*vrata*), which notably included the *yama* factors of *aṣṭāṅgayoga*.[112] In addition to fasting for health, spiritual purification, and political purposes, Gandhi also conducted controversial tests of his own chastity, purportedly as a means of increasing his *tapas*.[113] Gandhi championed an allegorical interpretation of the *Bhagavadgītā* that framed the practices of *karmayoga* and *bhaktiyoga* as devotional and non-violent service to others, the world, and to God.[114] Gandhi's interpretation of the *Bhagavadgītā* contrasted with those of other Hindu nationalists, such as Bal Gangadhar Tilak and Aurobindo Ghose, who believed that violence, especially retaliatory violence, was morally justified in the spirit of *dharma* advocated by Kṛṣṇa in the *Bhagavadgītā*.[115] Gandhi is said to have at times carried with him a copy of the *Yogasūtra* of Patañjali, and wrote approvingly of the way in which *haṭhayoga* was being used for the purpose of public health and in support of political activism by Indian modernists such as Swami Kuvalayananda.[116]

The founder of the Kaivalyadhama Ashram (1924) in Lonavla, Maharashtra, Kuvalayananda (Jagannath Gune, 1883–1966) was a pioneer in the formulation of modern postural and medicalized forms of yoga. A student of the European-inflected physical culture system of Manick Rao (1878–1954) and the teachings of the Bengali saint Paramahamsa Madhava-dasji (1798–1921), Kuvalayananda championed yoga as both a physical and spiritual culture, the former of which he believed was uniquely suited to scientific study and medical application.[117] Kuvalayananda's experiments played an integral role in the situation of modern yoga within a scientific, as opposed to a metaphysical, context.[118] He was highly influential on many of the modernists that followed him, and the Kaivalyadhama

Ashram continues to be a locus for scholarly and scientific research on yoga, facilitating English-language translations and critical editions of important yoga texts and offering yoga instruction programs that combine technical training and scientific research.[119] Kuvalyananda's work attracted the attention of Jawaharlal Nehru, India's first prime minister, and his daughter and future prime minister, Indira Gandhi, among others.[120] One of Kuvalyananda's most influential students has been O.P. Tiwari (1933–), an advocate and teacher of Kaivalyadhama's therapeutic approach to yoga, especially the modern experimental application of traditional formulations of the practice of *prāṇāyāma*.[121]

Shri Yogendra (Manibhai Haribhai Desai, 1897–1989), was an important innovator and popularizer of the modern yoga class and yoga center, founding the Yoga Institute in Bombay (Mumbai) in 1918.[122] Yogendra's project was marked by the effort to "sanitize, secularize, and rationalize" yoga in such a way as to make it accessible to a modern audience.[123] Like Kuvalayananda, Yogendra was a disciple of Paramahamsa Madhavadasji, and Yogendra adapted his guru's renouncer-focused teachings and practices (including *bhakti, āsana, prāṇāyāma,* and *kriyā*) to fit a modern middle-class householder lifestyle.[124] Madhavadasji was educated at the same school as Vivekananda and Paramahansa Yogananda, the Scottish Church College in Calcutta (Kolkata), in which a vigorous sports regimen was a part of the Muscular Christianity regimen of the day.[125] An avid student of physical culture with a deep affinity for traditional yoga philosophy and practice, Yogendra developed a system of *āsana* and *prāṇāyāma*-focused yoga that resonated with gymnastics, calisthenics, and European physical culture, while also validating traditional representations of yoga in the *Yogasūtra* and other authoritative texts.[126]

Yogananda and Bhishnu Ghosh

Following in the footsteps of Vivekananda, the charismatic Bengali teacher Paramahansa Yogananda (Mukunda Lal Ghosh, 1893–1952) set up the Self Realization Fellowship (SRF) in the United States in 1920, having establishing the Yogoda Satsanga Society in India in 1917.[127] Yogananda's teaching, drawing on that of his teacher Sri Yukteswar, a disciple of Lahiri Mahasaya (1828–1895) and a root-guru referred to simply as "Babaji," incorporated perspectives on Christianity within his practice of Kriya Yoga, which was a combination of physical exercise, progressive relaxation, and *mantra, haṭha*, and *bhaktiyoga* techniques.[128] His *Autobiography of a Yogi* (1946) has been a highly influential English-language publication, playing an important role in the success of the SRF and in the propagation of his teachings on a larger popular scale.[129] Yogananda's more prominent disciples included Swami Kriyananda (James Donald Walters, 1926–2013), who left the SRF in 1962 and formed the Ananda Ashram community, and Swami Daya Mata (Faye Wright, 1914–2010), who led the SRF for over fifty years after the passing of Yogananda.

Yogananda's younger brother, Bhisnu Charan Ghosh (1903–1970), became an avid and popular physical culturist in India, drawing from teachings on "muscle manipulation" from Yogananda and his own research on *haṭhayoga* and bodybuilding.[130] Both brothers found success through bridging *haṭhayoga* techniques with "muscle-control showmanship," and Ghosh's work found resonance with Indian, and especially Bengali, nationalists.[131] Ghosh and Yogananda were both teachers of Buddha Bose (1913–1983), who served as an exemplar of Ghosh's teachings on yoga, such as his "Eighty-Four Postures" sequence, during a world tour in 1938.[132] Bhishnu Ghosh is perhaps best known in the anglophone yoga world as the teacher of Bikram Choudhury (1944–), whose "Hot Yoga" system known as "Bikram Yoga" achieved global commercial success in the late twentieth and early twenty-first centuries, particularly in the United States. Choudhury claimed to have developed this popular mode of practice, in which the temperature in a yoga studio is set to 105°F or higher, while under the guidance of Ghosh, though some scholars believe the method originated in Bikram's studio in Japan.[133] Choudhury's attempts to establish and enforce legal limits on the use of the name "Bikram Yoga" and his sequence of twenty-four yoga postures led to intellectual property litigation in the United States and spurred the establishment of a traditional knowledge database dedicated to protecting yoga as the property of India.[134] Legal actions against Choudhury for sexual misconduct with staff and students brought considerable negative publicity to Bikram Yoga, with Choudhury ultimately leaving the United States to return to India.[135] Bikram's ex-wife, Rajashree Choudhury (1965–), served as the president of the International Yoga Sports Federation, and founded USA Yoga, an organization dedicated to the establishment of yoga as an international sport.[136] Ghosh's granddaughter, Muktamala Mitra (Ghosh), has served as vice principal of the Ghosh Yoga College in contemporary Calcutta (Kolkata), continuing the family tradition and lineage.[137]

Bhavanarao Pant and the Sun Salutation

Bhavanarao Pant Srinivasrao Pratinidhi (1858–1951), the Maharaja of Aundh, a former princely state located in the area of Maharashtra, was instrumental in the development of the modern "Sun Salutation" (Skt. *sūrya-namaskāra*, Hin. *sūrya-namaskār*), which would become a ubiquitous element of modern yoga traditions. In his *Surya Namaskars: Sun Adoration for Health, Efficiency, and Longevity* (1928), he presented the postural practice of the Sun Salutation as an Indian physical culture system aimed at building strength and self-discipline, drawing on his expertise in Indian physical culture and European bodybuilding.[138] Pant's Sun Salutation consists of a "ten point" linking of movement with breath, paralleling the use of *vinyāsa* in later modern yoga systems. Pant's system uses three important proto-yoga postures: the ready position of "even standing" or "mountain pose" (*samasthiti*, *tāḍāsana*) and "upward-" and "downward-facing-dog" postures (*ūrdhva-* and *adhomukhaśvānāsana*), which resemble push-up-like "staff" (Hin. *daṇḍ*, Skt. *daṇḍa*) postures used in Indian wrestling.

The framework of movements in the Sun Salutation are, in part, rooted in a formulaic sequence of prostrations offered by priestly worshippers of the sun-god Sūrya, adapted as a physical exercise routine form.[139] Traditional accounts link the Sun Salutation to the Marathi culture hero Śivaji, who is represented as having learned it from the Maharashtrian saint Samarth Rāmdās (1608–1681).[140] In his *Dāsbodh*, "The Wisdom of the Servant," Rāmdās details the performance of *namaskār* to various deities, including Sūrya, within a larger Hindu religious framework, perhaps lending to this association.[141] Pant argues in *The Ten Point Way to Health: Surya Namaskars* (1938) that the Sun Salutation is a universal offering of respect to the life-giving power of the sun, a power documented in modern science, and that its prostrations only have the appearance of religious ritual.[142] Though encouraging practitioners to recite the Sanskrit names for the sun during practice, he states that those who object on religious grounds can instead use "meaningless" root (*bīja*) mantras.[143] Pant encourages women to take up the practice, presenting it as easing childbearing and postpartum weakness, as a source of strength in child rearing, and as increasing overall physical health, mental health, and beauty.[144] Pant advocates for the use of the Sun Salutation in schools and provides a range of purported health benefits of the practice for individuals and communities.[145]

The Sun Salutation appears to have entered into the popular yoga lexicon around 1940, and played a major role in the transformation of yoga into a practice used and taught by women.[146] An important figure in this process was British journalist Louise Morgan (1883–1964), who interviewed Pant for the London-based *News Chronicle* and wrote a series of popular exposes on the Sun Salutation for the newspaper.[147] The placement of Morgan's series within media coverage of physical culture, and especially that of women's health and beautification, helped set the stage for the reception and adaptation of yoga in the European and American context.[148] Morgan edited and wrote an introduction to Pant's second book, *The Ten Point Way to Health: Surya Namaskars* (1938), cutting significant sections from the original *Surya Namaskar* and modifying the text to highlight the relevance of the practice for women, notably emphasizing beautification and the adaptation of the practice to European life.[149] Morgan appears to have inserted a recommendation of using a rubber mat on linoleum flooring, common in Britain, in order to prevent slippage, providing perhaps one of the earliest references to the use of a "yoga mat."[150]

Swami Ramdev, Sadhguru Jaggi Vasudev, and Sri Ravi Shankar

The Indian yoga guru Swami "Baba" Ramdev (Ramkishan Yadav, 1975–) is likely the most popular and influential guru in the history of yoga traditions in India. Through his cable television series, media appearances, publications, and *āyurveda* products, Ramdev has brought yoga into the mainstream of Indian life at an unprecedented scope. According to his official biography, prior to his fame as a yoga guru, Ramdev lived an ascetic life in the Himalayas and studied in Haridwar, a city synonymous with religious and political revival in India. Ramdev honed his teaching skills through instructing yoga camps (Hin. *śivir*), ultimately being discovered by a cable television magnate in attendance.[151] Following the success of his television program "Om Yog Sadhana," watched daily by millions in the rising middle class of India, Ramdev established the Divya Yoga Trust, headquartered at Patañjali Yogpeeth in Haridwar.[152] Ramdev's "Divine Yoga" (Hin. *divyayog*) combines a focus on the mental and physical health benefits of yoga *āsana* and *prāṇāyāma* with moral and political activism.

In his work *Jeevan Darshan* (2009), Ramdev envisions yoga as a vehicle for bringing unity and morality to the Indian nation, and ultimately the whole world, thereby helping all citizens reach their full potential.[153] Ramdev has received considerable publicity for his environmental activism, for his public protests against government corruption in India, and for his frequent popular media appearances.[154] Ramdev has also been criticized for his conservative Hindu political agenda, for his social views on issues such as homosexuality, and his claims of medical efficacy with respect to his yoga methods and *āyurveda* products.[155] The rise of Narendra Modi and the resurgence of the conservative Bharatiya Janata Party (BJP) in the early twenty-first century, in part due to Ramdev's support, solidified Ramdev's position as a political kingmaker.

Two other popular gurus that have advocated for social, political, and environmental action as a counterpart to the practice of yoga include the southern Indian teachers Sadhguru Jaggi Vasudev (1957–) and Gurudev Sri Ravi Shankar (1956–), who are the developers of the systems of "Isha Yoga" and the "Art of Living," respectively. Both have established a wide following among English and Tamil speaking Indians and among anglophone practitioners of yoga worldwide. Their systems include a focus on yoga *āsana* characteristic of modern yoga but also utilize *mantra* recitation, *prāṇāyāma*, and meditation (*dhyāna*).[156] The Isha Foundation has consultative status with the United Nations Economic and Social Council and supports initiatives for the empowerment of rural society, education, and urban greening and tree planning campaigns.[157] The Art of Living is publicly represented as a vehicle for world peace through stress reduction and as committed to humanitarian efforts including disaster relief, sustainable development, education, and environmental sustainability, among other causes.[158] Much like Swami Ramdev, Vasudeva and Shankar's influence extends well beyond individual practice, helping shape the social and political landscape of India. Both Isha Yoga and the Art of Living have, at times, faced public scrutiny in India, particularly regarding the environmental footprint of their highly popular institutions and festivals.[159]

Tirumalai Krishnamacharya, the "Father of Modern Yoga"

Tirumalai Krishnamacharya (1888–1989) is commonly referred to as the "Father of Modern Yoga," given the impact of his movement- (*vinyāsa*) and sequence- (*krama*) oriented approach to yoga *āsana* propagated by his entrepreneurial students, including B.K.S. Iyengar, K. Pattabhi Jois, Indra Devi, T.K.V. Desikachar, A.G. Mohan, and Srivatsa Ramaswami, among others. Krishnamacharya's life is largely known through biographies written by his disciples, which scholars have argued may be generally considered as hagiography.[160] According to his son, Desikachar, having grown up as a Śrī Vaiṣṇava *brāhmaṇa* in Karnataka in southern India near Mysore, Krishnamacharya traveled widely as a young man to study Sanskrit, Indian philosophy, and yoga, first ending up in Varanasi and then, ultimately, traveling to Lake Mansarovar in Tibet, where he met his guru, Sri Ramamohan Brahmachari.[161] At Mansarovar, according to Desikachar, Krishnamacharya learned several thousand yoga postures, the ability to control his physiological functions, and the recitation of the *Yogasūtra*.[162] Krishnamacharya is said to have returned to Mysore (Mysuru) at the instruction of his guru and established a reputation as an extraordinary practitioner of yoga through public yoga demonstrations. Ultimately, he was invited by the Maharaja, Krishna Wodeyar IV, to establish a *yogaśālā* in the gymnasium at the Mysore Palace. In Mysore, Krishnamacharya systematized an approach to yoga that would prove highly influential in the development of transnational yoga traditions.[163] Krishnamacharya wrote two books, *Yogamakaranda*, "Nectar of Yoga," or *Yogasara*, "Essence of Yoga," and *Yogāsanagaḷu*, "Yoga Āsanas," integrating Pātañjala Yoga (especially *aṣṭāṅgayoga*) and *haṭhayoga* into a modern postural paradigm. Teaching an audience of largely young boys in Mysore, where he was known for his strict demeanor, Krishnamacharya likely drew inspiration from the various physical culture models represented at the Mysore palace, including European gymnastics, Sun Salutation exercises, and Indian wrestling and martial arts techniques.[164] Krishnamacharya's work helped lay the foundation for modern movement-stage (*vinyāsa-krama*) yoga, in which movement and posture is linked to the breath in the manner of the *sūrya-namaskār* and performed as sequences in formation in a manner akin to gymnastic and military exercises.

When the Mysore Palace *yogaśālā* closed after Indian independence, Krishnamacharya moved to Chennai, where his son Desikachar established the Krishnamacharya Yoga Mandiram (1976). In Chennai, Krishnamacharya shifted from his vigorous *vinyāsa* approach to an emphasis on therapeutically focused individual practice, utilizing *āsana*, *prāṇāyāma*, and *mantra* as interventions for various mental and physical conditions. Despite the significant emphasis on the therapeutic aspect of yoga practice, Krishnamacharya continued to frame yoga within a universal Hindu and Vedic framework of authority, emphasizing the primacy of Patañjali's *Yogasūtra* and the authority of the eight-limbed yoga (*aṣṭāṅgayoga*) as a paradigm for yoga practice.[165] The valorization of Patañjali in the Krishnamacharya lineage is evident in the display of icons of Patañjali at the Krishnamacharya Yoga Mandiram in Chennai and the international Iyengar Yoga center in Pune, the Ramamani Iyengar Yoga Institute, among other venues.[166] The Krishnamacharya-based tradition of chanting the *Yogasūtra*, propagated through a range of media developed by Desikachar, his daughter Mekhala, and B.K.S. Iyengar, has played an important role in establishing the recitation of the *Yogasūtra* as an element of modern yoga study, if not as a modern yoga liturgy that is mystical and devotional as well as didactic.[167]

B.K.S. Iyengar and Iyengar Yoga

Two of Krishnamacharya's most influential students were B.K.S. Iyengar (1918–2014) and K. Pattabhi Jois (1915–2009). Both were students of Krishnamacharya at the Mysore Palace *yogaśālā* and founded schools of yoga that had a significant global impact. Iyengar, the brother-in-law of Krishnamacharya and also a Śrī Vaiṣṇava *brāhmaṇa*, claimed to have been, early on, cured of asthma and tuberculosis through Krishnamacharya's yoga. Iyengar was eventually sent by Krishnamacharya to teach in Pune, a city in the western Indian state of Maharashtra. There, Iyengar established a successful yoga institute, completing his yoga training through study of yoga literature and experimentation with *āsana* and *prāṇāyāma*.

Iyengar authored the groundbreaking book *Light on Yoga: Yoga Dipika* (1966), which was hailed early on as the "Bible of *yogāsana*" and later as the "Bible of Modern Yoga."[168] In *Light on Yoga*, Iyengar introduces a range of yoga principles and practices within the *aṣṭāṅgayoga* framework, noting yoga's physical and spiritual benefits.[169] This is followed by images of Iyengar demonstrating numerous yoga postures with brief instructions for performing them, building on the foundational vocabulary of *āsana* found within the Krishnamacharya Mysore-yoga program. Though Iyengar was familiar with Krishnamacharya's *vinyāsa* technique of linking movement and breath and the practice of *sūrya-namaskār*, he deemphasized those elements, instead focusing on the development of bodily "intelligence" within static postural practice.[170] He also wrote at considerable length on the practice of *prāṇāyāma*, most notably in his work *Light on Prāṇāyāma: The Yogic Art of Breathing* (1976). Iyengar developed the extensive use of yoga props, including mats, ropes, blankets, and cushions, in order to assist active yoga practice and to provide support during passive and restorative practice. Iyengar was, in many respects, a pioneer in making yoga accessible to individuals with a range of physical needs, abilities, and disabilities.[171] He was nonetheless known to be quite aggressive in his "hands on" adjustments of students.[172] He was consulted about yoga by prominent Indian gurus (Swami Sivananda), athletes (cricketer Sachin Tendulkar), celebrities (violinist Yehudi Menuhin), and others seeking therapeutic interventions of yoga.[173]

Iyengar, who was known as the "Lion of Pune" for his proud and fierce demeanor, possessed a gift for showmanship, traveling abroad yearly beginning in 1954 and attracting attention through international workshops and television appearances.[174] The success of *Light on Yoga* was complemented by other publications, including *Light on the Yoga Sūtras of Patañjali* (1993), which valorized the study of the philosophical literature of yoga. Iyengar established the Sage Patañjali Temple in his birthplace of Bellur, Karnataka, noting it was the first temple in India to be dedicated to Patañjali as its principal deity.[175] The Ramamani Iyengar Memorial Yoga Institute (RIMYI) was established in Pune in 1975 in honor of Iyengar's late wife, and disciples established affiliated Iyengar Yoga centers worldwide over the following decades. Two of Iyengar's most prominent disciples and teachers of his method were his daughter Geeta Iyengar (1944–2018) and Prashant S. Iyengar (1949–), who served for a number of years as co-directors of the RIMYI. Geeta Iyengar's work included a focus on the application of yoga to women's health issues, a topic outlined in her book *Yoga: A Gem for Women* (1983). Iyengar's influential disciples outside of India have included Patricia Walden (1946–) and Judith Hanson Lasater (1947–), who played an important role in the propagation of Iyengar yoga in the United States and Europe in the late twentieth and early twenty-first century, the latter being a co-founder of *Yoga Journal*.[176]

K. Pattabhi Jois, Ashtanga Vinyasa Yoga, and "Power Yoga"

K. Pattabhi Jois developed the modern Ashtanga Yoga or Ashtanga Vinyasa Yoga system, ostensibly named after the *aṣṭāṅgayoga* of Patañjali, based on the *vinyāsa-krama* system of *āsana* practice developed by Krishnamacharya during his Mysore phase.[177] Jois claimed that his *vinyāsa*-based system was reconstructed by Krishnamacharya from a now-lost text, the *Yoga Korunta* or *Yoga Kurunta* of Vāmanarṣi. As such, the role of the *Yoga Korunta* might be said to parallel the creative reception of the otherwise nonextant *Yoga Rahasya*, or "Secret Yoga," which Krishnamacharya is said to have received in a vision directly from its author, the Vaiṣṇava saint Nāthamuni.[178] One theory is that the titled *Korunta* or *Kurunta* is in fact a transliteration of the Sanskrit *yoga-grantha*, which could mean, generically, a "treatise" or "book" on yoga.[179] Another theory is that Krishnamacharya was referring to Kapālakuraṇṭaka, the author of a text called the *Haṭhābhyāsapaddhati*, "The Pathway of Haṭha Practice," a late *haṭhayoga* text that served as an inspiration for the Mysore Palace tradition of physical culture.[180]

In his work *Yoga Mala* (1999), Jois frames his *āsana* and *prāṇāyāma*-focused system within Hindu philosophical and religious discourse, citing the Upaniṣads, the *aṣṭāṅgayoga* system of Patañjali, and late texts of *haṭha-yoga*. Jois depicts yoga as a means to physical health, especially the curing of disease, which, in turn, serves as a foundation for worldly success and spiritual perfection, with the ultimate goal being the realization of the transcendent self (*ātman*). His system is organized into three successive levels of practice that move from the gross physical body to the subtle energetic body, titled the Primary Series of "curing disease" or "curing through yoga" (*rogacikitsā*, *yogacikitsā*), the Intermediate Series of "purifying the channels" (*nāḍīśodhana*), and the Advanced Series of "imparting stability" (*sthirabhāga*). The *sthirabhāga* series is subdivided into A, B, C, and D sequences, producing a total of six series from the original three. Ashtanga Yoga is also divided into "led" practice, teacher-guided group practice following verbal commands, and "Mysore" practice, self-guided practice often facilitated by forceful or aggressive hands-on adjustments by the teacher. In some cases, Ashtanga teachers, including Jois himself, have been accused of injuring or inappropriately touching students while making such adjustments.[181]

In contrast to the static holding of postures in the Iyengar Yoga system, Jois's system emphasizes the linkage of breath control (*prāṇāyāma*, specifically *ujjāyī prāṇāyāma*), energetic bindings (*bandha*, namely, *mūla*- and *uḍḍīyānabandha*), and the performance of increasingly challenging forms of yoga *āsana*. The vigorous nature of the Ashtanga Vinyasa system is said to cure physical illness and purify the channels (*nāḍī*), or "nerves," in which *prāṇa* moves in the body. Ashtanga Vinyasa integrates the performance of the Sun Salutation as an initial sequence in all three series and as partial *vinyāsa* movements used between yoga *āsana*, and both *vinyāsa* and *āsana* are accompanied by the use of *bandha* and gazing (*dṛṣṭi*) toward a focal point. Though his method is principally associated with arduous routine physical practice, Jois famously stating that "yoga is 99% practice," he and his students have published a number of works that engage yoga philosophy.[182] Ashtanga Vinyasa Yoga practitioners formally venerate Patañjali and the lineage of teachers through recitation of a set of verses (*śloka*) dedicated to them at the beginning of each Led and Mysore practice session.

Jois established the Aṣṭāṅga Yoga Research Institute (AYRI) in Mysore in 1942, eventually building a popular *yogaśālā* to accommodate an increasing number of students from Europe and the United States.[183] After Jois's death in 2009, his grandson Sharath Rangaswami (1971–), now referred to as R. Sharath Jois, took over duties of the *yogaśālā* in Mysore, and the umbrella organization of Ashtanga Yoga was renamed K. Pattabhi Jois Ashtanga Yoga Institute (KPJAYI). Rangaswami is assisted by his mother and fellow teacher Saraswati Rangaswami (1941–), also known as R. Saraswati Jois, who learned the Ashtanga system as a child and had taught women's classes at a Balaji temple in Mysore for a period, in addition to her work at the Mysore *yogaśālā*. Jois's son Manju (1944–), who studied extensively with his father in Mysore, emigrated to the United States in 1975, and has taught the Ashtanga Vinyasa method extensively in yoga centers in the United States and internationally. Other important early students include Lino Miele, an Italian student of Jois's, who is the co-author of a series of books authorized by the AYRI on the Ashtanga method, and Andre Von Lysebeth, a Belgian credited with bringing Jois and his method to the attention of the international yoga community.[184] Miele's school of yoga in Rome took on the rubric of the AYRI when the institute in Mysore was renamed following Jois's death.[185] Jois taught many influential students in the United States, including Norman Allen, David Williams, Nancy Gilgoff, Richard Freeman, Tim Miller, David Swenson, Eddie Stern, Nicky Doane, and Kino Macgregor, among others.

An early variant of Jois's teachings, Power Yoga, was developed by Beryl Bender Birch, a student of Norman Allen, as an adaptation of the Ashtanga Vinyasa system to suit practitioners in the United States, primarily as an accessory to athletic and therapeutic activities.[186] This rubric was expanded and popularized by Rodney Yee, a former dancer and student of B.K.S. Iyengar, who developed both Power Yoga and Flow Yoga sequences as part of a highly successful digital video series produced by the U.S.-based "lifestyle brand" GAIAM.[187] Another popularizer of Power Yoga is Baron Baptiste, a student of Iyengar and Desikachar, whose parents, Walt Baptiste (1918–2001) and Magaña Baptiste (1921–2016), studied with a range of influential teachers, including Indra Devi and Swami Sivananda, and opened one of the first U.S.-based yoga studios in California in 1955.[188] The school of Jivamukti Yoga founded by Sharon Gannon and David Life, established in New York City in 1984, draws upon the *vinyāsa*-style teachings of Jois and other Indian gurus, but also promotes philosophical study, devotion, and lifestyle modification, especially emphasizing a vegan diet.[189] The Prana Vinyasa Yoga, or Vinyasa Flow Yoga, school of Shiva Rea (Bailey), a former student of Jois and Desikachar, is one of the prototypes for various vigorous and dynamic forms of postural yoga that integrate various forms of music into sequence-based *vinyāsa* practice. Rea's system also incorporates Śaiva and Śākta tantric spirituality, dance, diet, and political activism as accessories to postural practice.[190] Another influential teacher of *vinyāsa-krama* styles of yoga is Andrey Lappa, the Ukranian-based formulator of the Universal Yoga system, which promotes a universal theory of yoga *āsana* and *krama* and an integrative approach to yoga philosophy and lifestyle.[191]

T.K.V. Desikachar and Indra Devi

The author of numerous publications, including a biography of Krishnamacharya entitled *Health, Healing, and Beyond* (1998) and an introduction to yoga practice entitled *The Heart of Yoga* (1995), T.K.V. Desikachar (1938–2016) taught extensively based on his father's therapeutic system of *vinyāsa-krama*, at times using the rubric of yogic "application" (*viniyoga*). Under the guidance of Desikachar, KYM established a paradigm of instruction in yoga as a therapeutic intervention for both physical and mental health, utilizing *āsana*, *prāṇāyāma*, *mantra* or "chanting," and meditation (*dhyāna*) as methods. The KYM model, which emphasizes one-on-one relationships between yoga teachers and students, continues to be the primary mode of instruction at KYM, with group-oriented instruction used for some workshops and training courses.[192] The practice of *mantra* and of "chanting" at KYM was drawn from the Vedic *saṃhitā* materials, from the Upaniṣads, and from Patañjali's *Yogasūtra*, though presented as adaptable to suit the needs of practitioners.[193] An emphasis on the authority of Patañjali at KYM is physically represented by icons and images of the philosopher found throughout the institute, as well in the emphasis on the *Yogasūtra* and the *aṣṭāṅgayoga* framework in the center's teachings.[194] In 2006, Desikachar and his son Kausthub (1975–) formed the Krishnamacharya Healing and Yoga Foundation (KHYF) as a separate vehicle for the dissemination of the teachings of Krishnamacharya on a worldwide scale, but its implementation was overshadowed by a controversy over Kausthub's relationships with his students.[195] Desikachar's wife Menaka Desikachar (1947–) also took on a leadership role within the KHYF, having studied personally with Krishnamacharya and Desikachar.[196] Desikachar's daughter Mekhala (1978–) contributed to the development of KYM audiovisual materials promoting Vedic chanting and the oral transmission of the *Yogasūtra*.[197] Desikachar student Gary Kraftsow established the American Viniyoga Institute (1999), which has served as a locus for National Institutes of Health (U.S.)-supported research on yoga as therapy.[198] The American Viniyoga Institute has also developed a widely distributed digital video series on yoga-based interventions for back pain, anxiety, and depression.[199] Another student of Desikachar, Leslie Kaminoff, published a highly popular reference work for yoga practitioners, *Yoga Anatomy* (2007).

Indra Devi (Eugenia Peterson, 1899–2002), also known as Mataji, "Honorable Mother," and the "First Lady of Yoga," played a critical role in advancing women's access to modern yoga practice and forwarding the model of the female yoga teacher in the twentieth century.[200] A displaced pre-Soviet Russian-Latvian aristocrat, Peterson was reluctantly taken up as a student by Krishnamacharya at the request of the Maharaja of Mysore. Peterson, whose stage and (later) teaching name was "Indra Devi," was a socialite and admirer of the Theosophists.[201] She eventually impressed Krishnamacharya with her skill and dedication.[202] She went on to teach in China and the United States, and ultimately counted influential politicians, such as the wife of Chinese nationalist leader Chiang Kaishek, and Hollywood movie stars, such as Gloria Swanson and Greta Garbo, among her students.[203] In 1960, she established the Rancho Cuchuma Ashram in

Tecate, Mexico, which became the primary location for her work during the latter part of her life.[204] Devi played an important role in popularizing yoga in North America, and was an innovator with respect to the development of the fee-based yoga instruction model.[205] Her publications, such as *Forever Young, Forever Healthy* (1953) and *Yoga for Americans: A Complete Six Weeks' Course for Home Practice* (1959), presented an adaptive approach to teaching yoga to an American audience. Later in her life, she became a devotee of the popular but controversial Indian guru Sathya Sai Baba (1926–2011), authoring a book entitled *Sai Baba, Sai Yoga* (1975) that sought to integrate her Krishnamacharya-based postural yoga teachings with the guru-devotion tradition of Sai Baba.[206]

Swami Sivananda Saraswati and the Sivananda Lineage

Swami Sivananda Saraswati of Rishikesh (Kuppuswami Iyer, 1887–1963) established an influential community of yoga practitioners in the foothills of the Himalayas in northwestern India in the early twentieth century. His teachings continue to be propagated through a number of organizations founded by him and by his disciples, including the Divine Life Society (DLS, 1936), Sivananda Yoga Vedanta (1959), and the Bihar School of Yoga (1964). Born into a wealthy *brāhmaṇa* family in Tamil Nadu, Kuppuswami Iyer studied medicine and practiced as a physician in India and Malaysia, publishing an English-language medical newsletter, *The Ambrosia*.[207] Though reportedly successful as a physician, he returned to India to pursue religious interests, in part inspired by the example of Swami Vivekananda.[208] His return to India may have also been catalyzed by the death of his family in Malaysia, though narratives of this rumored scenario have not been confirmed by the DLS.[209] Some DLS accounts imply that he left his family, given that Sivananda's renunciation of worldly life is compared to that of the historical Buddha, who is said to have left his wife and child to pursue awakening.[210] In India, Iyer journeyed to Rishikesh, where he took *saṃnyāsa* and was given the Daśanāmī name Śivānanda Saraswatī.

Sivananda viewed Patañjali's presentation of yoga, especially the concept of *cittavṛttinirodha* and the *aṣṭāṅgayoga* framework, as a benchmark for authoritative yoga, but also recognized the utility of various other systems, writing extensively on various yoga methodologies, including an important early modern treatise on yoga *āsana*.[211] Sivananda cautioned his disciples against the dangers of performing yoga for the achievement of spiritual accomplishments (*siddhi*), due to their potential to impede spiritual progress.[212] Though teaching extensively on the physiological benefits of yoga, his larger body of work frames yoga as a universal spirituality that leads to the realization of union with the "supreme soul."[213] Sivananda utilized his English-language fluency to integrate English-based medical and anatomical language into the yoga lexicon, with many of his publications directed at an English-speaking international audience. He also represented yoga as a panacea for India's ills, framing the welfare of the Indian nation in terms of the first two members of *aṣṭāṅgayoga*, *yama* and *niyama*.[214] Sivananda's prolific writings alternately extol yoga as a universal and scientific enterprise, as the spiritual core of Indian identity, and as a resource for renewal of the Indian nation. The founder of the influential Vishva Hindu Parishad, a right-wing Hindutva organization, was an early disciple of Sivananda.[215]

Swami Chidananda (Sridhar Rao, 1916–2008), served as the head of the DLS in Rishikesh after the death of Sivananda in 1963, playing an important role in its institutional stability.[216] Swami Vishnu Devananda (1927–1993) helped spread Sivananda's teachings outside of India, establishing an influential global network of Sivananda Yoga Vedanta Centers. Devananda also published English-language books popularizing the Sivananda style of yoga, including *The Complete Illustrated Guide to Yoga* (1959) and *Meditation and Mantras* (1978). In India, Swami Satyananda Saraswati (1923–2009) established the Bihar School of Yoga and the Bihar Yoga Bharati, providing an institutional locus for teaching Sivananda-inflected yoga in northeastern India.[217] Satyananda was a prolific author of English-language publications, including the popular *Asana, Pranayama, Mudra, Bandha* (1969). His chief disciples Swami Niranjanananda Saraswati (1960–) and Swami Satyasangananda Saraswati (1953–), took on leadership roles within the Bihar School of Yoga and the Satyananda Yoga tradition after his death, a period marked by the litigation of abuse by Satyananda Yoga teachers in Australia and accusations directed toward others.[218] Sivananda's disciple Swami Satchidananda (1914–2002), established the Yogaville Ashram in the United States, having become widely known in the counterculture for his role in leading the chanting of Sanskrit mantras to open the Woodstock Music Festival in 1969. Satchidananda's *Integral Yoga: The Yoga Sutras of Patanjali* (1978), remains one of the most popular English language publications on yoga philosophy.[219] Satchidananda's student Dean Ornish, a medical doctor, was an early champion for the use of yoga as a therapeutic intervention for heart disease in the United States.[220] Lilias Folan, a student of Vishnu Devananda and Chidananda, was a major influence in bringing Sivananda-inspired yoga to a mainstream audience through her yoga-exercise television program *Lilias, Yoga, and You!*, which aired on public television in the United States from 1972 to 1999.[221] The Sivananda lineage has also been influential in Europe, particularly in Germany, where Boris Sacharow established the first school of yoga after corresponding with Sivananda in the 1940s.[222] Sacharow helped establish a widely-known "Rishikesh Series" of Sivananda Yoga postures that have inspired German practitioners to travel to Rishikesh for generations.[223] Swami Kailashananda (1913–2011), also known as Yogi Gupta, a one-time employee, if not disciple, of Sivananda, established a following in North America, training the influential New York City–based teacher Dharma Mittra, whose "908 Āsanas" chart is a well-known representation of the sequences of modern postural yoga.[224] Another influential New York City guru connected to the Sivananda lineage is Alan Finger, who teaches ISHTA Yoga, an eclectic mix of postural, meditative, and tantra-inflected modern yoga methods.[225]

Mircea Eliade (1907–1986), a central figure in the development of the academic study of religion in the twentieth century, was briefly a student of Sivananda in Rishikesh in the 1930s.[226] Eliade's work *Yoga: Immortality and Freedom* (1958) helped define the academic study of yoga for the latter half of the twentieth century, and continues to be an important scholarly reference work on the topic.[227] Eliade claimed to have had powerful experiences in his study of yoga, which he declined to describe because of the mandate of secrecy between *guru* and *śiṣya*.[228] He ultimately differentiated his academic work from practice, the latter of which he stated was considerably more difficult than amateurs would suggest.[229] Eliade provided glimpses of his Rishikesh experience in his journals and fiction, the latter of which provides perspective on Sivananda as a charismatic religious leader.[230] Sivananda is said to have, in turn, viewed Eliade as the "next Vivekananda," who would spread the teachings of yoga to the "West."[231] Though Eliade rejected this role, his work was instrumental in the development of European and North American popular and academic interest in yoga, with *Yoga: Immortality and Freedom* continuing to be published and circulated extensively well into the twenty-first century.[232]

Popular Gurus and Ashrams of Rishikesh

The popular appeal of Rishikesh was amplified in the 1960s by the celebrity of Maharishi Mahesh Yogi (Mahesh Prasad Varma, 1918–2008), whose Spiritual Regeneration and Transcendental Meditation (TM) systems achieved notoriety in Europe and the United States. Maharishi adapted the teachings of his guru, Swami Brahmananda Saraswati (1868–1953), known as Gurudev, and principles drawn from the Daśanāmī-Śaṅkarācārya tradition into a householder-focused system emphasizing both spiritual and material success.[233] His public image was elevated in 1967 when the popular British rock band The Beatles visited Maharishi in Rishikesh. Though the association was short-lived, in part due to allegations of impropriety on the part of the teacher, it solidified Maharishi's status as a popular transnational guru, and numerous celebrities engaged in TM over the succeeding decades.[234] Maharishi's system, a combination of *mantrayoga* and *dhyānayoga*, particularly utilizing seed (*bīja*) mantras such as *oṃ*, aims to calm and focus the mind through mantra recitation, in some cases evoking ecstatic and visionary experiences in practitioners.[235] Maharishi and his followers claimed that an individual's achievement of peace is a building block for a larger world peace.[236] They have also supported and publicized scientific research that appeared to validate their claims regarding the health benefits of TM, such as the work of Dr. Robert Benson on the "relaxation response," though such efforts have often been controversial.[237] In the 1970s, Maharishi developed a special set of practices referred to as the TM Sidhi (*siddhi*) program, which aimed at the development of extraordinary accomplishments through meditation. The TM-Sidhi program includes contemplation of verses of Patañjali's *Yogasūtra* and the practice of "Yogic Flying," which consists of practitioners making leaps and bounds into the air in lotus posture (*padmāsana*).[238]

In the 1990s, Maharishi moved his headquarters to Vlodrop, the Netherlands.[239] His abandoned ashram in India became a Beatles fan circuit destination, ultimately being renovated by the government of Uttarakhand as "eco-friendly tourist destination" and art exhibition.[240] Leadership of the organization was eventually passed to Tony Nader, a medical doctor with a PhD in Brain and Cognitive Science from the Massachusetts Institute of Technology and an outspoken advocate of bridging the spirituality-science gap in TM.[241] Deepak Chopra (1947–), an Indian-born American author of Neo-Vedānta philosophy and popular alternative-medicine advocate, left medical practice to pursue a life of spiritual reflection and advocacy of mind-body medicine, in part inspired by TM.[242] Along with Andrew Weil (1942–), an influential pioneer of the "holistic" or "integrative" model of medicine in North America, Chopra has been a highly influential figure in promoting yoga and meditation as tools for fighting disease and optimizing health and well-being. Chopra left TM in the early 1990s, and in 1996 joined with another medical doctor, David Simon, to found the Chopra Center for Wellbeing in California, which teaches a variety of subjects, including *āyurveda*-based health and cooking courses, meditation, and *āsana*-based yoga.[243]

Swami Dayananda Saraswati (Natarajan Iyer, 1930–2015), a popular teacher of Vedānta in the Daśanāmī-Śaṅkarācārya tradition, whom the Prime Minister of India, Narendra Modi, once considered his principal guru, established the Dayananda Ashram in Rishikesh in the 1960s.[244] The Dayananda Ashram is a locus for the instruction of a variety of systems of yoga, such as Iyengar yoga and other Krishnamacharya-based traditions, in addition to its primary focus on the study of Vedānta philosophy. Dayananda is described by his followers as having championed interfaith and social-service efforts alongside traditional religious teachings.[245] The nearby Paramarth Niketan Ashram, currently led by H.H. Swami Chidanand Saraswati (1952–), similarly presents itself a hub for social and environmental activism and as a center for instruction in the philosophy and practice of yoga.[246] Paramarth Niketan sponsors a popular annual International Yoga Festival, and in 2017, Prime Minister Modi addressed its attendees, describing yoga as a means of creating harmony and peace within individuals and society.[247] Other notable teachers connected with Rishikesh include Swami Rama (Brij Kishor Kumar, 1925–1996) and his disciple Swami Veda Bharati (Usharbudh Arya, 1933–2015), associated with the Sadhana Mandir and Swami Rama Sadhaka Grama. The Sadhana Mandir and Swami Rama Sadhaka Grama serve as part of the Himalayan International Institute of Yoga Science and Philosophy, or Himalayan Tradition of Yoga.[248] Rama, a charismatic teacher and the author of *Living With the Himalayan Masters* (1978), led the Himalayan Institute in Pennsylvania in the United States from 1971 until the end of his life, though his legacy was shadowed by allegations of misconduct with students toward the end of his life.[249] The Himalayan Institute is currently headed by Rajmani Tigunait (1953–), who was ordained by Rama in 1976, and holds PhD degrees in Sanskrit and in Oriental Studies from the University of Allahabad and the University of Pennsylvania, respectively.[250] A wide variety of other ashrams and centers in contemporary Rishikesh draw an audience of Indian and international students, including the Shree Mahesh Heritage Meditation School, Omkaranda Ganga Sadan and Patanjala Yoga Kendra, Rishikesh Yog Peeth, and Anand Prakash Yoga Ashram. Rishikesh continues to serve as a point of intersection between global, anglophone yoga audiences, formal institutions of renunciation linked to Daśanāmī and Rāmānandī lineages, and itinerant renouncer (*sādhu* and *sādhvī*) communities living in huts along the banks of the Ganges and passing through on pilgrimage.

Modern Tantric, *Haṭhayoga*, and *Bhaktiyoga* Gurus

In the early twentieth century, figures such as Arthur Avalon (Sir John George Woodroffe, 1865–1936) in England and Pierre Bernard and Theos Bernard in the United States brought popular notoriety, and in some cases scandal, to notions of Indian yoga and tantra in the transnational and anglophone contexts.[251] A particularly iconic figure of modern tantra, or "neo-Tantra," is Bhagwan Shree Rajneesh (Rajneesh Chandra Mohan, 1931–1990), also known as "Osho," a Jain-born Indian guru that rose to prominence in the 1970s in India and established a vibrant community of followers across the globe.[252] Rajneesh's teachings linked sexuality, material prosperity, and spiritual life, blending Indian yoga and tantra with pop culture and psychology, spurning both a movement and an industry.[253] In his *Tantra, Spirituality, and Sex* (1983), Rajneesh argues that sexuality has the potential to awaken love and to catalyze mystical experiences, and calls for a radical and global reconfiguration of sexual mores. Rajneesh built a community of "sannyasis," marked by their devotion to Rajneesh, red attire, and unconventional lifestyle, starting in his ashram in Pune, India, and eventually in his community of Rajneeshpuram (1981) in Muddy Creek, Oregon, in the United States. Despite its early success, Rajneeshpuram collapsed in the wake of controversies and conspiracies regarding the legal status and administration of the commune, and Rajneesh was deported to India on immigration charges.[254] Rajneesh's ashram in Pune now functions as the "Osho International Meditation Resort," and Rajneesh is more well-known and popular now than when he was alive.[255] One of Rajneesh's influential disciples is the French-born Margot Anand (1944–), a popular author and speaker, whose work *The Art of Sexual Ecstasy: The Path of Sacred Sexuality for Western Lovers* (1989) brought a Rajneesh-inflected view of sexuality to a broader New Age audience, challenging "sexual myths" and emphasizing the need for body-positivity.[256]

Another influential tantra-based modern tradition is Siddha Yoga, which is associated with the root guru Nityananda or Bade Baba (1897–1961), its founder, Swami Muktananda or Baba Muktananda (Krishna Rau, 1908–1982), and its current guru, Swami Chidvilasananda or Gurumayi (Malti Shetty, 1954–). Chidvilasananda's younger brother, who was dubbed Nityananda (Subhash Shetty, 1962–) by Muktananda, also played an important role in the organization in its early stages, and now leads a separate community.[257] The Siddha Yoga tradition, represented by the Siddha Yoga Dham Associates (SYDA), with centers worldwide, had a strong impact in the United States among popular and academic audiences, in the latter case particularly among North American scholars of Hindu tantra.[258] Important centers for the tradition include the Gurudev Siddha Peeth in Ganeshpuri, India, a site associated with the Siddha-guru Nityananda, and the Shree Muktananda Ashram in upstate New York in the United States. The Siddha Yoga tradition emphasizes the practice of "shaktipat" (*śaktipāta*), the "descending of *śakti*," through the power of a guru's glance and touch. Muktananda drew from his experience of Nityananda, who was said to inspire religious experiences through his mere presence or a glance, serving as the object of intense guru devotion, or *guruyoga*.[259] Disciples, inspired by Muktananda's presence, glances, and touch, would enter into ecstatic states of reverie, often vocalizing and performing spontaneous bodily and hand movements, referred to as *kriyā*.[260] The recitation of the *Guru Gītā*, or "Song to the Guru," plays an important part of the daily liturgy of Siddha Yoga, emphasizing the value of devotion and reverence for the guru. Though Siddha Yoga faced waning numbers in the wake of a series of controversies surrounding Muktananda and Siddha Yoga's New York ashram, it was bolstered by American author Elizabeth Gilbert's popular novel *Eat, Pray, Love* (2006) and subsequent film adaptation, in which the protagonist resides in an ashram in India modeled on the Gurudev Siddha Peeth in Ganeshpuri.[261]

Swami Kripalvananda, also known as Kripalu and Bapuji (Saraswati Chandra Majmudar, 1913–1981), was another important transnational guru who adapted practices of *śaktipāta*, *kuṇḍalinīyoga*, and *haṭhayoga* in teaching to modern and transnational audiences. Kripalvananda, a *saṃnyāsin*, obtained *śaktipāta* from his guru, Swami Pranavananda.[262] For Kripalvananda, the evoking of an initial *kuṇḍalinī* experience was the beginning of the yogic journey perfected through the *haṭhayoga* practices of *khecarī mudrā* and *kevala kumbhaka*, leading to mastery over the subtle body and the preservation of vital fluids.[263] Kripalvananda's disciple Amrit Desai (1932–), known as Gurudev among his followers, established the Kripalu Yoga Ashram, which would eventually become the Kripalu Center for Yoga and Health (1983), one of the most influential and popular hubs for yoga instruction in North America.[264] Desai, who practiced as a householder, developed a system of "meditation-in-motion" that integrated the *śaktipāta* experience with a physically oriented postural system of yoga.[265] Desai left Kripalu following a controversy in 1994, eventually forming the Amrit Yoga Institute in Florida in the early 2000s. The Kripalu Center for Yoga and Health transitioned to a nonsectarian administrative structure and now administers a wide range of courses on topics such as postural yoga, *āyurveda*, holistic healing methods, massage, and diet and cooking, and serves as an important venue for scientific research on the physiological effects of yoga.[266]

The role of devotional yoga (*bhaktiyoga*) in transnational yoga traditions has been significantly influenced by the tradition of ISKCON (International Society for Krishna Consciousness), popularly referred to as the "Hare Krishnas" or "Hare Krishna Movement."[267] An offshoot of the Gauḍīya Vaiṣṇava tradition of Bengal associated with Caitanya (1486–1533), ISKCON is centered on the practice of ecstatic and loving devotion to Kṛṣṇa as the supreme godhead, emphasizing the accessibility of such practice to people of all social levels and backgrounds. The founder of ISKCON, A.C. Bhaktivedanta Prabhupada (Charan De, 1896–1977), established a series of centers in the United States in the late 1960s and early 1970s, sparking a popular but controversial movement, attracting a young and largely countercultural audience. The success of ISKCON in the United States led to the establishment of centers in India and integration with South Asian immigrant populations in Europe and North America, fueled by Prabhupada's missionary activity and ISKCON publications. Association with celebrities such as The Beatles' George Harrison brought additional visibility, momentum, and resources to the movement in the late 1960s and 1970s.[268] Controversies over its missionary activities, internal conflicts, and a series of scandals marked a period of instability leading up to and following the founder's death in 1977. In the early 2000s, ISKCON moved toward a "family-friendly" model that emphasized the academic study of religion and the propagation of mainstream Hindu values and practices over impassioned missionary service.[269] This was complemented by the emergence of Kṛṣṇa-devotion infused postural yoga traditions, in which *bhakti* was integrated into mainstream *āsana* practice, without reference to its sectarian roots.[270] The broader impact of ISKCON-inspired spirituality on modern yoga is illustrated in the work of Wai Lana (Huilan Zhang, 1955–), a daughter of Chinese immigrants born in Hong Kong, who attained celebrity through the success of her popular Hawai'ian-inspired North American public television yoga series "Wai Lana Yoga" (1998–).[271] Wai Lana credits her "spiritual master" and husband, Jagad Guru Siddhaswarupananda Paramahamsa (Chris Butler, 1948–), a former disciple of Prabhupada and the founder of the Science of Identity Foundation (1977), for her success.[272] In 2016, she was awarded the prestigious Padma Shree Award for her work popularizing yoga by the Government of India.[273] Her song "Namaste" was broadcast at the United Nations and in Times Square in New York City at the inauguration of the first International Day of Yoga.[274]

Another influential *bhakti*-oriented teacher on the world stage in the late twentieth century was spiritual "father" (Hin. *bābā*) Neem Karoli Baba (Lakshmi Narayan Sharma, 1900–1973). Neem Karoli Baba's teachings of unconditional devotion were forwarded by Baba Ram Dass (Richard Alpert, 1931–), a former Harvard-based psychologist who had been a co-investigator with Timothy Leary in the therapeutic use of psychoactive substances.[275] Alpert's work with Leary included a Tibetan Buddhism-informed guide to LSD experimentation, which was published as *The Psychedelic Experience: A Manual Based on the Tibetan Book of the Dead* (1964). Later, in the wake of his experiences with Neem Karoli Baba, Ram Dass wrote *Be Here Now* (1973), a widely popular introduction to Hindu-based spirituality. The impact of Neem Karoli Baba as an international guru is paralleled by that of another teacher, Meher Baba (Merwan Sheriar Irani, 1894–1969), who similarly attracted a worldwide following of devotees, including celebrities, to his guru-focused and *bhakti*-centered spiritual path.[276]

A thread of contemporary Indian *bhakti*-focused tradition that has cross-pollinated with modern yoga traditions is devotion to female Hindu gurus who are, in some cases, viewed as incarnations of the Goddess (*devī* or *śakti*), especially in the form of a spiritual "mother" (Hin. *mā, mātā*, Tamil *ammā*). These guru figures inspire deep emotive, and often ecstatic, sentiments in their followers through gazing (*darśana*), teaching, and, often, touch. Notable "mothers" include Gauri Ma (Mridani Chattopadhyaya, 1857–1938), Anandamayi Ma (Nirmala Sundari, 1896–1982), Amma, Ammachi, or Mata Amritanandamayi Devi (Sudhamani Idamannel, 1953–), who is also known as the "Hugging Saint," and Mother Meera (Kamala Reddy, 1960–).[277] These female gurus often head their own renunciation orders, which offer a heightened organizational status to women and promote women's education and social liberation. In some cases, their authority is inflected through wider connections with spiritual figures and institutions, such as Gauri Ma's association with Sarada Devi, Ramakrishna's wife and spiritual partner, and Mother Meera's connection to the Sri Aurobindo Ashram in Pondicherry.[278]

Modern Buddhist and Buddhist-Inspired Traditions

As with Hinduism, modern Buddhist traditions have been transformed through the transition from the colonial to the post-colonial era in South Asia. Parallels can be drawn between the Sri Lankan lay-monastic Buddhist practitioner Anagarika Dharmapala (Don David Hewavitarne, 1864–1933), an influential advocate of a lay-oriented modern and nationalist Buddhism, and Vivekananda, with whom Dharmapala shared the stage at the 1893 Parliament of the World's Religions in Chicago.[279] Dharmapala, who had connections with the Theosophical Society, founded the Maha Bodhi Society in 1891, dedicated to preserving Buddhist traditions and archeological sites, and championed the teaching of meditation to laypeople.[280] Dharmapala's work helped prepare the ground for the global success of lay-oriented Theravāda *vipassanā* traditions and for the broader popular dissemination of Buddhism, including Mahāyāna traditions such as Tibetan Buddhism and Zen Buddhism. Traditions referred to under the broad rubric of "mindfulness meditation" have been particularly popular and successful, informing both Buddhist and non-Buddhist practice and being widely adapted for use in popular therapeutic and self-help discourse.[281]

In the late nineteenth and early twentieth century, the Theravāda Buddhist Burmese monk Ledi Sayadaw (U Nyanadaza, 1846–1923) helped forward an agenda of reviving the practice of *vipassanā* or "insight" meditation, especially in bringing its practice to a lay audience.[282] Another Burmese teacher, Mahasi Sayadaw (U Thobana, 1904–1982), a monk closely identified with the "forest tradition" of Buddhist meditation, was instrumental in adapting *vipassanā* in its modern form, developing a method widely adopted throughout the Theravāda Buddhist world.[283] Other influential *vipassanā* teachers and innovators in Burma included U Ba Khin (1899–1971) and his Indian-Burmese student S.N. Goenka (1924–2013), and in Thailand, teachers such as Ajahn Chah (Chah Subhaddo, 1918–1992) and Buddhadasa (Ngeuam Panich, 1906–1993) taught to an increasingly international audience.[284] Buddhadasa presented *vipassanā* as at parity with modernism and nationalism, arguing for a universalist vision of Buddhism that minimized supernatural elements and appeals to sectarian identity.[285] Lay *vipassanā* practice was popularized on an international level by European and North American students of Sri Lankan and Burmese teachers, including Jack Kornfield, Joseph Goldstein, and Sharon Salzberg, who together founded the Insight Meditation Society (1975) in the United States.[286] The *vipassanā* method served as a building block in the development of the Mindfulness Based Stress Reduction program of Jon Kabat-Zinn, a widely utilized meditation-based health intervention that also incorporates postural yoga practice.[287] The *vipassanā* method also informs the Insight Yoga method of Sarah Powers, a system of contemplative mind-body practice that builds on the Daoism- and Chinese martial arts-informed Yin Yoga tradition developed by Paulie Zink and Paul Grilley.[288]

Modern *vipassanā* practice is characterized by the cultivation of mindfulness (*sati*) in the form of a dispassionate moment-to-moment awareness of physical sensations and mental activity. One of the most popular contemporary vehicles for the teaching of *vipassanā* is the ten-day retreat model developed by S.N. Goenka and administered by the Vipassana International organization at their main center at Igatpuri, India, the Dhamma Giri, or "Hill of Dharma," and at over one hundred other retreat locations worldwide.[289] *Vipassanā* is often distinguished from serenity-oriented *samatha* (Skt. *śamatha*) meditation, a concentration-oriented form of meditation that is, in some cases, critiqued as either an inferior or an extinct mode of Buddhist practice. However, basic *samatha* forms of breath-awareness (*ānāpānasati*) and loving-kindness (*mettā*) meditation are typically taught as a precursor to *vipassanā* practice, and some contemporary Theravāda lineages, such as those of Pa Auk Sayadaw and Ajahn Chah, teach the *samatha* practice of meditation (*jhāna*) as a living tradition.[290]

With respect to Mahāyāna Buddhism, a central figure in the global spread of Tibetan Buddhism in the twentieth and twenty-first centuries has been the fourteenth Dalai Lama, Tenzin Gyatso (1935–), a Gelukpa-sect Buddhist monk and teacher (*lama*) who has served as a political and spiritual leader of Tibetan Buddhism and the Tibetan refugee community in exile. The Dalai Lama is viewed by Tibetan Buddhists as a reincarnate teacher (*tulku-lama*) and manifestation of the Bodhisattva of compassion, Avalokiteśvara. The Dalai Lama fled Tibet following the 1959 invasion of Tibet by China, establishing an exile government in India, and in 1989 won the Nobel Peace Prize for his commitment to nonviolent political action. His worldwide efforts to preserve Tibetan culture and to promote Tibetan Buddhism, along with his charismatic persona and popular publications, elevated him to international celebrity status. He also played an important role in the growth of the academic study of Tibetan Buddhism and of Buddhism and Neuroscience in Europe and the United States, the latter evident in his role in the formation of the Mind and Life Institute (1987) in cooperation with neuroscientist Francisco Varela (1946–2001) and entrepreneur R. Adam Engle (1942–).[291] A close associate of the Dalai Lama, Geshe Lhundub Sopa (1923–2014), was instrumental in the development of the academic study of Buddhism and the establishment of institutional Gelukpa practice in the United States. Robert Thurman (1941–), a professor of religion at Columbia University, a close friend and supporter of the Dalai Lama, and a well-known author and public speaker on Tibetan Buddhism, helped bring greater visibility to the political and humanitarian situation in Tibet and has continued to be an important figure in the popular dissemination of Buddhist contemplative practice in the United States.

The establishment of the Nyingma Institute in Berkeley, California, in 1972 by Tarthang Tulku (1934–), the founder of Dharma Publishing, marked an important moment in study and practice of Tibetan Nyingma Buddhism in the United States.[292] Chögyam Trungpa Rinpoche (1940–1987) drew upon the Kagyü and Nyingma lineages of Tibetan Buddhism in founding the Naropa Institute (1974), now Naropa University, in Boulder, Colorado.[293] Trungpa, a prolific author known for an eccentric lifestyle and antinomian approach to teaching Buddhism, found resonance with the 1960s countercultural movement, attracting celebrity students such as the poet Allen Ginsberg. His international organization, Vajradhatu (1973), was the foundation for the later development of a worldwide network of Shambhala Meditation Centers, headed by Sakyong Mipham Rinpoche (1962–), Trungpa's son. Both Sakyong Mipham and Trungpa have been the subject of investigations and controversy over their personal behavior and relationships with students.[294] Another important figure in the Shambhala tradition is the Buddhist nun Pema Chödrön (Deirdre Blomfield-Brown, 1936–), a student of Trungpa whose popular writings and audio programs have established her as an authoritative and influential voice in the reception of Buddhist meditation practice in the anglophone context.

Meditative yoga practices in modern Tibetan Buddhism include the development of breath-focused *shinay* (Skt. *śamatha*) meditation and deity yoga (Tib. *lha-naljor*, Skt. *devatā-yoga*), the latter being practices focused on the visualization of Buddhas and Bodhisattvas. Advanced practitioners have access to tantric initiations into deity yoga involving wrathful deities, advanced *maṇḍala* visualizations, and practices such as Nāropa's Six Dharmas, Dzogchen, and *ṣaḍaṅgayoga*. As with Theravāda *vipassanā* practice, popular modern Tibetan Buddhist forms of meditation emphasize the cultivation of mindfulness (Tib. *drenpa*, Skt. *smṛti*) and insight (Tib. *lhagthong*, Skt. *vipaśyanā*) as a basis for the development of skillful mental states conducive to psychological well-being. The cultivation of loving-kindness (*maitrī*) and compassion (*karuṇā*) are also utilized as foundational meditative practices, or mind training (Tib. *lojong*), including extending love to others through "sending and receiving" (Tib. *tonglen*), visualizing all beings as having been one's mother in previous lives, and contemplation of the Bodhisattva Avalokiteśvara (Tib. *chenrezig*) as an exemplar of compassion.

The system of Yantra Yoga developed by Chögyal Namkhai Norbu (1938–), based on the Tibetan practices of *tsalung trulkhor* (Skt. *nāḍī-vāyu-yantra*), demonstrates parity with other modern postural forms of yoga, being adapted to suit practitioners at a variety of levels of commitment and physical ability. Norbu, a respected Nyingma-Bön Tibetan *lama* and *rinpoche* and a scholar and practitioner of Dzogchen, was invited by the influential Italian Orientalist Giuseppe Tucci (1894–1984) in 1960 to work in Rome at the Istituto Italiano per il Medio ed Estremo Oriente.[295] Norbu was appointed as Professor of Tibetan and Mongol Linguistics at the University of Naples L'Orientale, subsequently founding the International Dzogchen Community in the 1970s and the Shang Shung Institute in 1989.[296] Yantra Yoga, which links breath and posture in a mode similar to *vinyāsa* styles of yoga, is represented by Norbu as a *trulkhor*-based practice descended from the Indian Mahāsiddhas and related genealogically to *haṭhayoga*, being taught to him by his uncle Togden Ugyen Tendzin (1888–1962).[297] Yantra Yoga's *prāṇāyāma* and *āsana* exercises are intended to relax body, voice, and mind into a "natural condition" that serves to restore health and create optimum conditions for contemplative practice, especially Dzogchen.[298] Another proponent and modern adaptor of the Tibetan *trulkhor* system is Geshe Tenzin Wangyal Rinpoche (1961–), a Bön teacher and founder of the Ligmincha Institute in the United States (1992).[299] Wangyal presents the principles of *āsana*, *prāṇāyāma*, and linked movement in yoga as instrumental to physical and psychological health and a foundation for spiritual practice.[300] Another movement-oriented modern Tibetan system is Kum Nye Relaxation, or Kum Nye Tibetan Yoga, developed by the Nyingma teacher Tarthang Tulku. Much like Norbu and Wangyal's systems, the postures and movements of Kum Nye Tibetan Yoga are presented as a vehicle for physical and psychological health and as a foundation for more sophisticated modes of Buddhist practice.[301]

Zen Buddhist meditation, and especially *zazen*, or seated meditation, is an iconic form of modern Japanese contemplative practice popularized in the United States and Europe in the mid–twentieth century by writers such as D.T. Suzuki (1870–1966) and Alan Watts (1915–1973).[302] The Japanese term *zen* is derived from the Chinese *ch'an*, which is, in turn, a translation of the Sanskrit term for meditation (*dhyāna*) in its form as a spiritual perfection (*pāramitā*) in the Mahāyāna Buddhist tradition. As in modern Theravāda traditions, modern Zen traditions emphasize the importance of mindfulness, and seated meditation and walking meditation are commonly presented as complementary practices.[303] An important figure in the propagation of Zen practice in North America was Shinryu

Suzuki (1904–1971), the founder of the San Francisco Zen Center (1962) and the author of a popular introduction to Zen Buddhism, *Zen Mind, Beginner's Mind* (1970). The Vietnamese Buddhist Zen (Viet. Thiền) monk Thich Nhat Hanh (Nguyen Xaun Bao, 1926–) was another instrumental figure in the global success of Zen Buddhism and the establishment of a worldwide popular discourse on mindfulness. Nhat Hanh was nominated for the Nobel Peace Prize by American civil rights activist Martin Luther King Jr. for his work on reconciliation in Vietnam and is an advocate of "Engaged Buddhism." Despite being exiled from Vietnam due to his activism, he propagated a worldwide Buddhist monastic community called the Order of Interbeing starting in Saigon in 1966, establishing its principal headquarters in Plum Village near Bordeaux in southern France in 1982.[304] His numerous publications, including *The Miracle of Mindfulness* (1975), and his many public appearances around the world established him as a central figure in the discourse of mindfulness meditation in the late twentieth and early twenty-first century.

Jain and Sikh Yoga Systems

The Jain (Skt. *jaina*) Preksha Meditation system, developed by Acharya Shri Mahapragya (Nathmal Choradia, 1920–2010), a monk in the Śvetāmbara Terāpanth tradition, is presented as a means to this-worldly health and success and as a support for the path to liberation in a manner akin to other modern yoga systems.[305] Mahapragya's Preksha Foundation (1972) provides instruction on Preksha Meditation at centers around the world, with a concentration in western India where it has close ties to the local Śvetāmbara Jain population. Preksha Meditation integrates monastic, lay, and non-Jain practice, and the Terāpanth tradition frames the practice and its goals in both soteriological and therapeutic language.[306] Preksha Meditation includes regimens of linked *āsana* and *prāṇāyāma* similar to modern *vinyāsa*-type yoga, the practice of *sūrya-namaskār*, and *vipassanā*-like contemplation of the body.[307] Aspects of Preksha Meditation resemble *haṭhayoga*, *layayoga*, and *kuṇḍalinīyoga*, including a practice of inner journeying (*antaryātrā*) that approximates the ascension of *kuṇḍalinī* through the subtle body. The use of *āsana* and *prāṇāyāma*, gesture (*mudrā*), and sound (*dhvani*) together aim to facilitate deep relaxation (*kāyotsarg*), spiritual ascension through inner journeying (*antaryātrā*), contemplation of the breath, body, and the subtle body centers (*cakra*), and concentration on *mantra*.[308]

One of the most visible forms of transnational and anglophone modern Sikh yoga is the Kundalini Yoga system developed by Yogi Bhajan (Haribhajan Singh Puri, 1929–2004), the founder of the Happy, Healthy, Holy Organization (3HO, 1969) and the Sikh Dharma Brotherhood (1973).[309] Yogi Bhajan's teachers included Swami Dhirendra Brahmachari (1924–1994) and Maharaj Virsa Singh (1934–2007), who taught him *haṭhayoga*-based techniques of *āsana*, *prāṇāyāma*, and *bandha*, and Sikh mantra-based contemplation on the name of the divine, or *nām*, respectively.[310] Brahmachari had a high-profile clientele, counting Jawaharlal Nehru and Indira Gandhi among his students.[311] The 3HO tradition emphasizes Yogi Bhajan's linkage to another teacher, Sant Hazara Singh, whom they credit as Bhajan's original teacher of *kuṇḍalinī yoga kriyā*.[312] The core group of Yogi Bhajan's early followers were American converts to Sikhism who observed the ritual dress-code of the Punjabi Sikh Khalsa, though opting for white colored robes and turbans over the variety of colors worn by Sikh practitioners in India.[313] Yogi Bhajan received considerable criticism from Indian Sikh communities, in part due to a perceived overemphasis on yoga in his teachings.[314] At the end of his life and after his death, a number of disciples sued Bhajan and his estate regarding his business practices and claims of abusive relationships.[315]

Practice in 3HO, referred to as *sādhana*, includes a combination of prayer (the Sikh *jāpji sāhib*), *kuṇḍalinī yoga kriyā*, a set of mantra-based and utopian-themed "Aquarian Sadhana Mantra Meditations," and readings from the principal Sikh scripture, the *Gurū Granth Sāhib*, or "Honorable Guru Book."[316] The wider teaching of Kundalini Yoga to non-3HO practitioners is administered through the International Kundalini Yoga Teachers Association (1994), which certifies teachers in the system, advocates for unity, and pursues the broader dissemination of Yogi Bhajan's teachings.[317] Kundalini Yoga practice, *kuṇḍalinī yoga kriyā*, utilizes dynamic movement in association with *āsana*, *prāṇāyāma*, *bandha*, and *mudrā* to engage and manipulate *prāṇa* in the subtle body, with the goal of effecting health, stabilizing emotions, and providing insight into the nature of the universe and the self.[318] The 3HO organization has also promoted "White Tantra," a couples-based Kundalini Yoga presented as a vehicle for rapidly evoking *kuṇḍalinī* energy through the intersection of personal "magnetic fields."[319]

Women have played an important role in the development and success of Kundalini Yoga, one important leader being Gurmukh Kaur Khalsa (Mary Mae Gibson, 1943–), a direct disciple of Yogi Bhajan who helped popularize the tradition in Europe and the United States through her books, multimedia presentations, and association with celebrities.[320] The countercultural nature of the 3HO organization and the Kundalini Yoga community has, in some cases, allowed women to often assume positions of power and influence uncharacteristic of other yoga communities.[321] More broadly, the emotive, ecstatic, and communal nature of the Kundalini Yoga system, including *kuṇḍalinī yoga kriyā* and the devotional practice of *kīrtan*, distinguishes it from physicalist systems of yoga and has contributed to its appeal among more spirituality-minded yoga practitioners.

Abrahamic Yoga and Hybrid Yoga Systems

Despite negative attitudes toward yoga among a number of contemporary Christian groups, Indian contemplative traditions, and yoga specifically, have made significant contributions to modern Christian spirituality. This is particularly evident in the work of twentieth-century figures in Christian spirituality such as Bede Griffiths (1906–1993), Thomas Merton (1915–1968), and Jean-Marie Déchanet (1906–1992), who drew extensively on Indian traditions.[322] The question of whether yoga is compatible with Abrahamic faith has been a topic of considerable debate within Jewish and Muslim, as well as Christian, communities in the modern era.[323] The Christian system of "Praise Moves" and the Jewish system of "Torah Yoga," developed by American teachers Laurette Willis (1957–) and Diane Bloomfield (1959–), respectively, incorporate recitation and contemplation of Biblical scripture into postural practice, adapting yoga to fit Abrahamic-style religious devotion.[324] The Jewish Yoga Network presents yoga as a means to recapture Jewish wisdom, and Christian groups have championed "Christian Yoga" or "Yoga Prayer" as a way of revitalizing Abrahamic faith.[325] The latter are among a range of Christian forms of yoga that include "Christoga," "Yahweh Yoga," "Christ Centered Yoga," and "Christian Meditation."[326] In some cases, contemporary Islamic practitioners of yoga have compared the Sun Salutation (*sūrya-namaskār*) to the Islamic practice of daily prayer (Urdu-Hindi *namāz*, etymologically related to *namaste*) as a set of movements beneficial for mind and body.[327]

Hybridized forms of yoga include a range of verbal conjunctions, such as "Acroyoga," "Cycling Yoga," "Boxing Yoga," "Yogalates," "Laughter Yoga," "Doga," "Goat Yoga," and many others.[328] In addition to illustrating the power of the rubric of "yoga" as a branding or marketing device, such appellations often indicate the notion of a spirituality or "whole life" practice that brings self-discipline together with a focal point of topical interest or commitment. Yoga may also be viewed as providing a competitive edge in an activity, such as in contemporary athletic competition, and the practice of yoga, both postural and meditative, has found a place within training regimens of elite professional athletes in various sports.[329] Beyond this secondary application of yoga in support of athletic training, the government of India recognizes yoga as itself being a "sports discipline" and USA Yoga and the International Yoga Sports Federation have sought inclusion of yoga as a sport in Olympic competition.[330] The Yoga Federation of India currently conducts a National Yoga Sports Championship competition, a tradition that dates back to the mid-twentieth century, if not earlier.[331] Though it might seem intuitive to view the athletic or sport-centered model of yoga as inherently physicalist or secular, it should be noted that various forms of athletics, including Olympic competition, have roots in sectarian traditions, and the relationship between sport and religion is complex and multifaceted.[332]

Transformations of Yoga in a New Millennium

The formulation of modern and anglophone forms of yoga in late nineteenth to early twentieth-century India was deeply informed by the vast influx of European physical culture, medicine, philosophy, and spirituality during the colonial era in South Asia. However, the foundation for the development of modern yoga can be found in premodern practices and principles, especially in medieval *haṭhayoga* and tantric yoga traditions and in widely disseminated philosophical and practical formulations of yoga such as the *aṣṭāṅgayoga* framework. The success of yoga in Europe and in the Americas, in turn, transformed yoga in India, helping bring about a "yoga renaissance," one that culminated in yoga's status as an iconic representation of India itself. While yoga was increasingly taken up as a householder practice by an emerging middle class, Indian renouncer traditions such as the Nāths and Rāmānandīs sought to claim, or perhaps reclaim, authority over its heritage.[333] The success of postural and meditative householder-yoga systems formulated by Hindu teachers was paralleled by the success of similar systems among lay practitioners in Buddhism, Jainism, and Sikhism, with transnational enthusiasm linking together spirituality, health, and tourism.[334] The nonsectarian and universalizing nature of yoga, particularly its physicalism, allowed for the adaptation of yoga to suit a plurality of religious identities, including Jewish, Christian, and Muslim, and for its hybridization with a wide range of other secular activities, including fitness and athletics. Modern yoga served as the foundation for the emergence of a global industry and a set of novel professions that saw extraordinary economic growth in the late twentieth and early twenty-first centuries. Modern yoga has touched every part of the globe, and its impact as a driving cultural force remains unabated well into the twenty-first century as it continues to be adapted to suit changing religious, political, economic, and technological contexts and conditions.

Conclusion

Tracing the Path of Yoga

Yoga has a long and complex history, and any large-scale study such as this cannot be complete in its coverage. However, as has been demonstrated, the larger arc of yoga's history and philosophy is largely a coherent one, with threads of continuity and points of divergence shedding light on its theory and practice from its premodern manifestations to its contemporary practice. Yoga can be principally defined as an Indian mode of mind-body discipline, a "yoking" of mental and physical capacities, in which a practitioner masters what would be otherwise autonomous aspects of embodied life, resulting in heightened capacities of knowledge and action. By extension, as the goal of the practice of such a discipline, the term "yoga" can refer to a union or conjoining of the personal self with a personal or impersonal deity (such as Śiva or *brahman*) or a state of liberation (*mokṣa*) from the processes of embodied existence, especially the cycle (*saṃsāra*) of birth and rebirth. The impulse toward liberation (*mokṣa*) or cessation (*nirodha*) in yoga has a counterpart in the conception of yoga as leading to various accomplishments (*siddhi*) or powers (*vibhūti*), especially the attainment of extraordinary capacities of action and perception that blur the boundaries between the human and the divine. The dynamic tension between numinous and cessative dimensions of yoga extends into modern forms of yoga practice, in which the practice of yoga is just as often viewed as a gateway to health, beautification, and worldly success as it is viewed a means of obtaining the goals of insight, peace, unification, or liberation.

Yoga is commonly represented in "limbed" forms, such as the eight-limbed yoga (*aṣṭāṅgayoga*) and six-limbed yoga (*ṣaḍaṅgayoga*), and the suffix *-yoga* and prefix *yoga-* are also used extensively to represent a range of different yoga methodologies. The *aṣṭāṅgayoga* system is the most pervasive of all of the paradigms of yoga practice, having its roots deep in yoga's prehistory and extending its influence throughout the classical, medieval, and modern eras into the present. Among other well-established conceptions of yoga forms or paths (*mārga*) are those of the "yoga of action" (*karmayoga*), the "yoga of devotion" (*bhaktiyoga*), and the "yoga of knowledge" (*jñānayoga*), as well as the designations of "incantation yoga" (*mantrayoga*), "yoga of dissolution" (*layayoga*), "yoga of force" (*haṭhayoga*), and "royal yoga" (*rājayoga*). The medieval development of forms of tantra, which aim to accelerate spiritual transformation through the use of extraordinary ritual means, yielded various modes of tantric practice that pervasively influenced the development of yoga systems in Hinduism, Buddhism, and Jainism.

Practitioners of yoga, the *yogin* and *yoginī*, or simply "yogis," represent the embodiment of the practice of yoga as it is typically passed from preceptor (*guru*) to disciple (*śiṣya*), serving in narrative and philosophical literature as embodiments of spiritual wisdom and as masters of occult powers. The figure of the yogi extends through the worlds of the householder and renouncer traditions and navigates the elite orthodoxy of priestly (*brāhmaṇa*) traditions and the popular grassroots practice associated with "folk heroes" such as the Nāths and Mahāsiddhas. Though many, if not most, of the texts that delineate the practice of yoga privilege male voices, images and conceptions of female ascetic and *yoginī* figures appear at critical points to offer testimony to the virtuosity of female practitioners of asceticism and yoga in the Indian tradition. Though the figures of the *yogin* and *yoginī* are often represented as outside of conventional society, practitioners of yoga have, at times, also had considerable political influence and power, a point amply demonstrated by the considerable political influence and economic success of yoga gurus in contemporary India and in the global sphere.

Though the ongoing question of whether yoga has its origins in the Indus Valley civilization or in a non-*brāhmaṇa* culture that existed outside of the Vedic tradition continues to be an interesting one, it is not necessary to appeal to extra-Vedic traditions to find many of the building blocks of later yoga traditions. The Vedic tradition, with its conceptions and practices of *mantra, tapas, prāṇāyāma*, and *brahmacarya*, and its valorizing the proto-yogi figures of the Ṛṣi, Muni, and the *viṣa*-imbibing ecstatic Keśin, provides numerous examples of parallels to the full-fledged yoga disciplines and exemplars of yogic virtuosity evident in later literature. The emergence of *brāhmaṇa* asceticism and the *śramaṇa* traditions consolidated and extended this Vedic legacy, bringing coherence to ascetic practices of renunciation, conceptions of cyclic existence (*saṃsāra*) and liberation (*mokṣa*), and modes of spiritual discipline (*yoga*), including meditation (*dhyāna*). These elements found systematic expression in the classical and scholastic literature of Hinduism, Buddhism, and Jainism in the early centuries of the Common Era. This literature included the *Yogasūtra*, which forwarded the influential eight-limbed yoga (*aṣṭāṅgayoga*) rubric, Buddhist and Jain path (*mārga*) literature, and the Hindu epic and Purāṇic (*itihāsa-purāṇa*) and Law (*dharma*) texts of that era. Late classical forms of yoga emphasized the concept of liberation-in-life (*jīvanmukti*) and the perfection of compassion (*karuṇā*), idealized in figures such as the Mahāyāna Bodhisattvas and Buddhas, whose liberation is viewed as only the beginning of their story of self- and world-transformation.

Medieval traditions of yoga in Hinduism, Buddhism, and Jainism extended classical modes of practice through the integration of *bhakti* and *tantra*, which were exemplified and embodied in the Sant, Nātha, and Mahāsiddha traditions. In some cases, this represented a shift toward yoga as "union" with the divine object of meditative practice, such as Śiva, Viṣṇu, or a formless (*nirguṇa*) supreme being. Other traditions sought the integration of ascetic and tantric conceptions of the subtle body (*sūkṣma-śarīra*), with its channels (*nāḍī*), wheels (*cakra*), and latent power (*śakti*), such as *kuṇḍalinīyoga*. Medieval traditions were also the locus for the development of a larger range of *haṭhayoga* practices, from body-cleansing *kriyā* practices, to the somatic and energetic practices of *āsana*, *bandha*, *mudra*, and *prāṇāyāma*, seeking to preserve and transform the essence (*bindu*) of life within the body. Hindu, Buddhist, and Jain tantric practices aimed to accelerate the attainment of spiritual knowledge or wisdom (*jñāna, prajñā*) and accomplishment (*siddhi*) through ritual worship (*pūjā*) and meditative visualization (*bhāvanā*) of deities. In some cases, these tantric disciplines incorporated transgressive practices and substances to catalyze religious experience, as well as disciplines such as *ṣaḍaṅgayoga* and subtle-body practices cognate with *kuṇḍalinīyoga*. The medieval traditions of *bhaktiyoga* and *haṭhayoga* each contributed elements to the modern practice of yoga in its sectarian and nonsectarian contexts.

The modern and anglophone era of yoga has been characterized by the elevation of yoga to a pan-Indian and global phenomenon, with yoga being practiced on a scale not seen before in its historical development. Modern yoga is marked by the profound transformation of Indian culture over centuries of colonial impact, by the ascendancy of Indian nationalism, and by its formulation within an emergent transnational physical and spiritual culture in the nineteenth, twentieth, and twenty-first centuries. It has, at times, been adapted and presented as a secular physical culture and framed as a scientific and therapeutic health intervention. It has also taken the form of a competitive sport in which human virtuosity in terms of strength, flexibility, and beauty are displayed through the medium of yoga *āsana*. Yoga has become a sort of "philosopher's stone" that, when appended to any activity, raises that activity to the level of a spiritual discipline, giving it the luster of something exotic or extraordinary. The spiritual, political, and economic impact of modern yoga only appears to be growing as the twenty-first century unfolds. In many respects, the history and philosophy of yoga anticipates the extraordinary technological transformations of the human organism that appear on the horizon of human civilization today. It brings to mind and to light the considerable moral, if not spiritual and religious, issues associated with the augmentation of human capacities of human action and perception. It also evokes reflection on the perennial human quest for a lasting peace, happiness, and success in this life and the attainment of serenity in the face of death—if not liberation from it altogether.

Notes

Introduction

1. The significant variability within the umbrella terms of "Hinduism," "Buddhism," and "Jainism" will be explored at length over the course of the text. On the complexities of the definition of the rubric of "tradition," see Paul Valliere, "Tradition," in *Encyclopedia of Religion*, ed. Lindsay Jones, 2nd ed., vol. 13 (Detroit, MI: Macmillan Reference USA, 2005), 9267–9281.

Chapter 1

1. Gerald James Larson and Ram Shankar Bhattacharya, *Encyclopedia of Indian Philosophies: India's Philosophy of Meditation. Yoga. Volume XII* (Motilal Banarsidass Publishers, 2008), 30–33. As might be anticipated, the truth of the matter is likely to be found somewhere between such extreme positions, where there is recognition of the impact of yoga as an iconic modern Indian and cosmopolitan tradition and acknowledgment that it is one facet of a vast Indian heritage of religion and philosophy.

2. The scholarly impulse to construct a coherent and comprehensive understanding of yoga might have been part of the motivation for the development of various *yogaśāstra*, or scholastic discourses on yoga, and of formulaic representations of yoga such as the eight-limbed (*aṣṭāṅga*) and six-limbed (*ṣaḍaṅga*) forms.

3. However, this is not intended to isolate an "ideal" or "pure" yoga, a *yoga pur*, that exists outside of, or that can be abstracted from, particular traditional and contextual parameters. On this topic, see Louis de La Vallée Poussin and others, "Le Bouddhisme et Le Yoga de Patañjali," *Mélanges Chinois et Bouddhiques* 5 (1937): 223–241.

4. Mircea Eliade, *Yoga: Immortality and Freedom*, trans. Willard Ropes Trask (Princeton, NJ: Princeton University Press, 2009).

5. A discussion of this issue can be found in David Gordon White, *Sinister Yogis* (Chicago & London: University of Chicago Press, 2009). See also Asko Parpola, *The Roots of Hinduism: The Early Aryans and the Indus Civilization* (New York: Oxford University Press, 2015), 306. Parpola proposes that the seated figures are derived from a "Proto-Elamite sitting bull" figure. Further reflection, including a discussion of Parpola's work, can be found in Geoffrey Samuel, *The Origins of Yoga and Tantra: Indic Religions to the Thirteenth Century* (Cambridge: Cambridge University Press, 2008), 2–8.

6. However, as an exception to this rule, Parpola has theorized conceptual and linguistic linkages between later Vedic ascetic-yogic concepts linking the subtle body and cosmology and the Indus civilization. See Parpola, *The Roots of Hinduism*, 310–311.

7. Stuart Ray Sarbacker, "The Numinous and Cessative in Modern Yoga," in *Yoga in the Modern World: Contemporary Perspectives*, ed. Mark Singleton and Jean Byrne (New York: Routledge, 2008), 161–183. A brief survey of yoga in the Upaniṣads can be found in Dermot Killingley, "The Upaniṣads and Yoga," in *The Upaniṣads: A Complete Guide*, ed. Signe Cohen (New York: Routledge, 2018), 174–185.

8. *Yogasūtra* 1.2.

9. *Yogabhāṣya* 1.1.

10. Larson and Bhattacharya, *Encyclopedia of Indian Philosophies*, 28.

11. These are two "types" of modern yoga identified in Elizabeth De Michelis, *A History of Modern Yoga: Patañjali and Western Esotericism* (London & New York: Continuum, 2005), 187–189; two others De Michelis identifies are "Modern Psychosomatic Yoga" and "Modern Denominational Yoga."

12. Somadeva Vasudeva, *The Yoga of the Mālinīvijayottaratantra*, chapters 1–4, 7, 11–17 (Pondichery: Institut français de Pondichéry: École française d'Extrême-Orient, 2004), 367; Alexis Sanderson, "Yoga in Śaivism" (Unpublished Draft), 1999, 31–32; James Mallinson and Mark Singleton, *Roots of Yoga* (London: Penguin Books, 2017), 11. It is, however, also common in modern pedagogy to use the term "limb," given its wide conventional usage as an anatomical and/or botanical metaphor for the components of yoga practice.

13. Hemacandra and Olle Qvarnström, *The Yogaśāstra of Hemacandra: A Twelfth Century Handbook of Śvetāmbara Jainism* (Cambridge, MA: Harvard University Press, 2002), 9; Vesna A Wallace, *The Inner Kālacakratantra: A Buddhist Tantric View of the Individual* (Oxford: Oxford University Press, 2001), 2–30.

14. In some variations of *haṭhayoga*, the performance of *āsana*, *prāṇāyāma*, and other body-focused techniques is seen as efficacious with respect to the goals of the religious or spiritual life. Some traditions of *haṭhayoga*, for example, subsume *rājayoga*, the "royal" or meditative yoga, within physical and energetic practices that

aim to bring the mind into a meditative state through control of the body and the vital air (*vāyu*) or breath (*prāṇa*) within it, rather than through a formal meditative praxis that involves mental training. *Āsana* and *prāṇāyāma* can be linked more broadly to conceptions of Indian asceticism, especially with respect to the idea that disciplining the body by means of strenuous physical activity or breath retention yields spiritual purity, power, and insight, and preserves physical vitality in the body.

15. But, as will be discussed below, both *aṣṭāṅgayoga* and *ṣaḍaṅgayoga* (or *ṣaḍaṅga*) *ṣaḍaṅga* have variant forms and are interpreted and explained differently depending on their philosophical and sectarian context.

16. *Bhāgavata Purāṇa* 11.20.6–8.

17. The designation *rājayoga* is not modern in origin, but Vivekananda's use of the term to refer specifically to Patañjali's yoga system represents a distinct contextual application of the term. A larger examination of the term and its history can be found in Jason Birch, "Rājayoga: The Reincarnations of the King of All Yogas," *International Journal of Hindu Studies* 17, no. 3 (December 2013): 399–442. The rubric of *rājayoga* has historically referred to the meditative aspect of yoga or a mental state achieved through yogic practice (such as *samādhi*), linking it conceptually to the meditatively oriented Pātañjala Yoga system, but suggesting a broader semantic field of application. Nicholson argues that Vivekananda may have developed the "four yoga" scheme out of the division of yoga into *dhyāna-*, *jñāna-*, *bhakti-*, and *karmayoga* found in *Īśvaragītā* of the *Kūrma Purāṇa*, a text Vivekananda utilized extensively. Andrew J. Nicholson, ed., *Lord Śiva's Song: The Īśvara Gītā* (Albany, NY: SUNY Press, 2014), 167 n.4.24.

18. This is the compound form of the Sanskrit stem *karman*, used for clarity given its common conventional usage.

19. As in the case of the five spiritual faculties (*pañca-indriya*) common to the Buddhist and Hindu yoga traditions, namely faith (*śraddhā*), vigor (*vīrya*), mindfulness (*smṛti*), contemplation (*samādhi*), and wisdom (*prajñā*). See Stuart Ray Sarbacker, *Samādhi: The Numinous and Cessative in Indo-Tibetan Yoga* (Albany, NY: SUNY Press, 2005), 78–79.

20. This dynamic is exemplified in the *bhakti* dimension of modern *viniyoga* practices developed from the teachings of Tirumalai Krishnamacharya, one of the key figures in the development of modern yoga. See Klas Nevrin, "Krishnamacharya's Viniyoga: On Modern Yoga and Sri Vaisnavism," *Journal of Vaishnava Studies* 14, no. 1 (2005): 65–94. The role of *bhakti* in yoga practice often signifies the existence, emergence, or re-emergence of sectarian identity and religious sentiment within a yoga community.

21. See, for example, *Yogatattva Upaniṣad* 1.19. This classification is discussed briefly in Jason Birch, "The Meaning of *Haṭha* in Early *Haṭhayoga*," *Journal of the American Oriental Society* 131, no. 4 (2011): 527–554.

22. White, *Sinister Yogis*, 2009, 59–71; John Brockington, "Sūrya Ivāparaḥ: Exemplary Deaths in the Mahābhārata," in *Release from Life–Release in Life*, ed. Andreas Bigger and Peter Schreiner (New York: P. Lang, 2010), 21–35.

23. Vasudeva, *The Yoga of the Mālinīvijayottaratantra*, 235–246.

24. A discussion of yoga as both method and goal can be found in Knut Jacobsen's Introduction to Gerald James Larson and Knut A. Jacobsen, *Theory and Practice of Yoga: Essays in Honour of Gerald James Larson* (Leiden & Boston: Brill, 2005), 3–5.

25. Iyengar points to both spiritual and mundane possibilities with respect to yoga: "By definition, yoga means union. On a spiritual plane it is the union of the Universal Soul with the individual self. Yoga is also the union of the senses, body and mind. The union of these three significantly impacts and enhances a player's game." B.K.S Iyengar, *Yoga for Sports: A Journey towards Health and Healing* (Chennai: Westland, 2015), 25.

26. Discussed briefly in White, *Sinister Yogis*, 38.

27. Christopher Key Chapple, "Introduction," in *Yoga in Jainism*, ed. Christopher Key Chapple (New York: Routledge, 2016), 1–2.

28. The practice of yoga is often framed in terms of an understanding of the nature of the "true" spiritual self (*ātman*) as separate from the non-self (*anātman*). This view is encapsulated by the Yoga Philosophy's dynamic between the soul or person (*puruṣa*) and nature (*prakṛti*) and the Jain contrast between the soul (*jīva*) and the non-soul (*ajīva*). Advaita Vedānta philosophy, drawn from the Upaniṣad literature, postulates an inner self (*ātman*) that is recognized as the ultimate reality (*brahman*), set apart from material existence or nature (*prakṛti*) and the illusion (*māyā*) that nature creates about the world and human embodiment. Likewise, ultimate identity of the *ātman* might be framed in terms of either unity or relationship with a supreme personal deity or "lord" (*īśvara*). Buddhist traditions typically emphasize the characteristic of non-self (*anātman*) found in the mental and physical processes (*nāma-rūpa*) that compose the phenomenal person, postulating that embodiment is the result of processes that dependently co-arise (*pratītya-samutpāda*) and are empty (*śūnya*) of any abiding essence. These traditions share the view that due to ignorance (*avidyā*), human beings habitually, if not instinctively, cling to erroneous conceptions of self-identity that drive a process of bondage and misery in *saṃsāra*. Given this, spiritual discipline (*yoga*) can facilitate liberation (*mokṣa*) through supporting renunciation and the cultivation of knowledge or wisdom (*jñāna*, *prajñā*). As such, nature (*prakṛti*) is of a particular order, and mastery of its elements (*bhūta*) and their principles (*tattva*) in their concrete and subtle forms is viewed as a gateway to power and freedom.

29. Sarbacker, *Samādhi*, 27–51.

30. Sarbacker, *Samādhi*, 104–109.

31. A discussion of these can be found in David Gordon White, *Kiss of the Yoginī: "Tantric Sex" in Its South Asian Contexts* (Chicago & London: University

of Chicago Press, 2003), 199. The list of eight types of *siddhi* is referred to in YS 3.45, *tato'ṇimādiprādurbhāvaḥ kāyasampat taddharmānabhighātaś ca*, as *aṇimādi*, "beginning with *aṇimā* (smallness)." On the *siddhi* in Pātañjala Yoga, see Hariharananda Aranya's commentary in Patañjali et al., *Yoga Philosophy of Patañjali: Containing His Yoga Aphorisms with Vyasa's Commentary in Sanskrit and a Translation with Annotations Including Many Suggestions for the Practice of Yoga* (Albany, NY: SUNY Press, 1983), 325–327.

32. The six types of *abhijñā* are a uniquely Buddhist presentation of such powers, but most of the *abhijñā* powers, especially the *ṛddhi* (Pāli *iddhi*), are coextensive with larger Indian traditions regarding the *vibhūti* and *siddhi*. For their philological context, see Franklin Edgerton, *Buddhist Hybrid Sanskrit Grammar and Dictionary* (New Haven, CT: Yale University Press, 1953), 50, 151. A larger examination of the role that *abhijñā* and *ṛddhi* play within Buddhist meditation theory, cosmology, and metaphysics can be found in Louis de La Vallée Poussin, *Abhidharmakośabhāṣyam* (Berkeley: University of California Press, 1988), 1157–1181. The final Buddhist *abhijñā* is represented as resulting in liberation from the cycle of rebirth (*saṃsāra*), and said to be a uniquely Buddhist attainment..

33. Padmanabh S. Jaini, *The Jaina Path of Purification* (Delhi: M. Banarsidass, 2001), 21–25; Hajime Nakamura and Gaynor Sekimori, *Gotama Buddha: A Biography Based on the Most Reliable Texts* (Tokyo: Kosei Publishing Co., 2000), 292–308.

34. For a range of sectarian perspectives on liberation in the Hindu tradition, see Andrew O. Fort and Patricia Y. Mumme, *Living Libertaion in Hindu Thought* (Albany, NY: SUNY Press, 1996). With respect to the Buddhist tradition, similar discussions are presented in John J. Makransky, ed., *Buddhahood Embodied: Sources of Controversy in India and Tibet* (Albany, NY: SUNY Press, 1997). In these contexts, the disciplining of the body is a means of obtaining power over embodiment and the world, with liberation itself being referred to, in some cases, as the supreme accomplishment or perfection (*siddhi*). In *haṭhayoga*, bodily practices such as *āsana*, *prāṇāyāma*, *mudrā*, and *bandha* may be understood as a means of rapidly attaining to the transcendent practices of *rājayoga*, especially the accomplishment of deep contemplation (*samādhi*). In *layayoga*, manipulating the body and its *prāṇa* links together the numinous and cessative paradigms of worldly and otherworldly perfection, as spiritual liberation and bodily perfection are accomplished simultaneously. The state of Buddhahood as articulated in Mahāyāna and Vajrayāna Buddhism is characterized as simultaneously being dispassion toward worldly objects and as a state of higher knowledge and manifestation (*abhijñā*, *nirmāṇa*), the latter capacities being utilized for the sake of assisting beings caught up in *saṃsāra*.

35. Śiva is often characterized as a capricious god whose powers and roles demonstrate a profound tension within Indian society between world-affirming and world-denying tendencies, embodying the ambiguity of yogic mastery. Wendy

Doniger, *Śiva, the Erotic Ascetic* (New York: Oxford University Press, 1981), 255–313. Doniger's theory might be said to diverge in significant ways from that of Eliade with respect to the nature and role of *tapas* in the theory and practice of yoga. In contrast to Eliade, who appears to see an emphasis on *kaivalya* as the litmus test of authentic yoga, Doniger situates *tapas* and yoga within the scope of narrative and its rich range of complexities and contradictions, emphasizing the "unorthodox" elements of the iconography of Śiva, and thus yoga.

36. Stuart Ray Sarbacker, "The Icon of Yoga: Patañjali as Nāgarāja in Modern Yoga," in *Sacred Matters: Material Religion in South Asian Traditions*, ed. Tracy Pintchman (Albany, NY: SUNY Press, 2015), 24–25.

37. White, *Sinister Yogis*, 1–37. Stuart Sarbacker, "Rudolf Otto and the Concept of the Numinous," *Oxford Research Encyclopedia of Religion*, August 31, 2016.

38. Stuart Ray Sarbacker, "Power and Meaning in the Yogasūtra of Patañjali," in *Yoga Powers: Extraordinary Capacities Attained through Meditation and Concentration*, ed. Knut A Jacobsen (Leiden: Brill, 2011), 195–222.

39. Sarbacker, *Samādhi*, 63–74.

40. Aranya, *Yoga Philosophy of Patañjali*, 249–345.

41. *Haṭhapradīpikā* of Svātmārāma, 1:1, 10, 17.

42. Patrick Olivelle, *The Āśrama System: The History and Hermeneutics of a Religious Institution* (New York: Oxford University Press, 1993), 73–82; Patrick Olivelle, *Upaniṣads* (Oxford: Oxford University Press, 2008), xxiii–lx; Johannes Bronkhorst, *The Two Traditions of Meditation in Ancient India* (Delhi: Motilal Banarsidass, 1993), 54–77; Johannes Bronkhorst, *The Two Sources of Indian Asceticism* (New Delhi: Motilal Banarsidass, 1998), 43–66.

43. See, for example, the "orthogenetic" theory in Johannes C. Heesterman, *The Inner Conflict of Tradition: Essays in Indian Ritual, Kingship, and Society* (Chicago: University of Chicago, 1985), 39–41; a "heterogenetic" argument can be found in Johannes Bronkhorst, *Greater Magadha: Studies in the Culture of Early India* (Leiden & Boston: Brill, 2007), 75–136. Questions regarding the emergence of larger rubrics of Hindu, Buddhist, and Jain identity, especially with respect to *brāhmaṇa* traditions, are investigated in Nathan McGovern, *The Snake and the Mongoose: The Emergence of Identity in Early Indian Religion* (New York: Oxford University Press, 2018).

44. One particularly important example is that of Rāvaṇa, the villain of the *Rāmāyaṇa* epic, who obtains the boon of invulnerability to the attacks of the gods as a reward from the great god Brahmā for his austerities, thus prompting the human incarnation of Viṣṇu as Rāma. See John L Brockington, *The Sanskrit Epics* (Leiden: Brill, 1998), 444. The trope of the use of yogic powers appears in a

range of literary contexts in India. With respect to conceptions that the abuse of such power is a degradation of yoga, see Eliade, Trask, and White, *Yoga*, 38–142 *et passim*. Eliade places emphasis on the cessative dimension of yoga, and therefore sees the "magical" dimension of yoga as an aberration from ideal forms of practice. For a discussion of the ambiguity of *tapas* in the broader context of Indian religious literature, see Brockington, *The Sanskrit Epics*, 237–240.

45. Bronkhorst, *The Two Sources of Indian Asceticism*, 13, 29–36.

46. Walter O. Kaelber, *Tapta Mārga: Ascetism and Initiation in Vedic India* (Albany, NY: SUNY Press, 1989), 2–4.

47. The systems of Bikram Choudhury and K. Pattabhi Jois offer two cases in point in this regard.

48. Stuart Ray Sarbacker, "The Numinous and Cessative in Modern Yoga," in *Yoga in the Modern World: Contemporary Perspectives*, ed. Mark Singleton and Jean Byrne (New York: Routledge, 2008), 175.

49. This would include the adoption of ascetic discipline generally and *tapas* specifically as a component of *niyama* in variations of *aṣṭāṅgayoga* as represented in Hindu and Jain traditions. Likewise, this notion of subsuming asceticism into a larger frame is an important part of the "Middle Way" thought of Buddhism, which Gavin Flood has correctly noted does not eschew asceticism *in toto* but only the most extreme forms of it. See Christopher Key Chapple, Haribhadra Sūri, and John Thomas Casey, *Reconciling Yogas: Haribhadra's Collection of Views on Yoga* (Albany, NY: SUNY Press, 2003), 15–38; Hemacandra and Qvarnström, *The Yogaśāstra of Hemacandra*, 27–30; Gavin Flood, *The Ascetic Self: Subjectivity, Memory and Tradition* (Cambridge: Cambridge University Press, 2005), 120–122.

50. Richard Gombrich and Gananath Obeyesekere, *Buddhism Transformed: Religious Change in Sri Lanka* (Delhi: Motilal Banarsidass, 1990), 21.

51. Karen Pechilis, ed., *The Graceful Guru: Hindu Female Gurus in India and the United States* (New York: Oxford University Press, 2004), 26.

52. A discussion of some of the complexities of viewing the *guru* as a god in a contemporary yoga tradition can be found in John Paul Healy, *Yearning to Belong: Discovering a New Religious Movement* (Farnham: Ashgate Publishing, 2013), 20–21.

53. Sarbacker, "Power and Meaning in the Yogasūtra of Patañjali," 214–218.

54. Paul Williams, *Mahāyāna Buddhism: The Doctrinal Foundations* (New York: Routledge, 1989), 49–54. Williams discusses *upāya-kauśalya* in connection with the Mahāyāna Buddhist conception of the Bodhisattva, the embodiment of the Mahāyāna virtue of compassion (*karuṇā*), and thus the goal of leading beings out of *saṃsāra*.

55. One case mentioned briefly in Williams, *Mahāyāna Buddhism*, 26.

56. See, for example, the discussions of economic, political, and sexual abuse in Lise McKean, *Divine Enterprise: Gurus and the Hindu Nationalist Movement* (Chicago: University of Chicago Press, 1996), 305–313.

57. Important in this respect is the *pativrata*, devotion to the husband and ascetic *tapas* aimed at the welfare and protection of the husband and the family. Sītā, the heroine of the epic *Rāmāyaṇa*, is often seen as paradigmatic model of such devotion. On these issues, see David R. Kinsley, *Hindu Goddesses: Visions of the Divine Feminine in the Hindu Religious Tradition* (Berkeley: University of California Press, 1997), 70–78.

58. Sarah Strauss and Laura Mandelbaum, "Consuming Yoga, Conserving the Environment: Transcultural Discourses on Sustainable Living," in *Yoga Traveling: Bodily Practice in Transcultural Perspective*, ed. Beatrix Hauser (Heidelberg: Springer, 2013), 175–200.

59. Sarah Strauss, *Positioning Yoga: Balancing Acts across Cultures* (Oxford: Berg, 2005), 87–114.

60. Following the usage of "anglophone yoga" developed in Mark Singleton, *Yoga Body: The Origins of Modern Posture Practice* (Oxford & New York: Oxford University Press, 2010), 7.

61. See, for example, *Muṇḍaka Upaniṣad* 1.2.12.

62. James L. Fitzgerald, "A Prescription for Yoga and Power in the Mahābhārata," in *Yoga in Practice*, ed. David Gordon White (Princeton, NJ: Princeton University Press, 2012), 43–50; John Brockington, "Yoga in the Mahābhārata," in *Yoga: The Indian Tradition*, ed. Ian Whicher and David Carpenter (London & New York: RoutledgeCurzon, 2003), 13–24.

63. Jonathan A. Silk, "The Yogācāra Bhikṣu," in *Wisdom, Compassion, and the Search for Understanding: The Buddhist Studies Legacy of Gadjin M. Nagao*, ed. Jonathan A. Silk (Honolulu: University of Hawai'i Press, 2000), 265–314.

64. The female gendered Sanskrit counterparts to *sādhaka* and *vīra* being *sādhakā* and *vīrā*.

65. Liz Wilson, *Charming Cadavers: Horrific Figurations of the Feminine in Indian Buddhist Hagiographic Literature* (Chicago: University of Chicago Press, 1996), 48–57; Arti Dhand, *Woman as Fire, Woman as Sage: Sexual Ideology in the Mahābhārata* (Albany, NY: SUNY Press, 2008), 127–149.

66. Wilson, *Charming Cadavers*, 141–179.

67. Dhand, *Woman as Fire, Woman as Sage*, 55–93.

68. Sarbacker, "The Numinous and Cessative in Modern Yoga," 2008, 169–170.

69. See, for example, the discussion of Mīrābāī's life and work in John Stratton Hawley and Mark Juergensmeyer, *Songs of the Saints of India* (New York: Oxford University Press, 2004).

70. T.W. Rhys Davids and William Stede, *The Pali Text Society's Pali-English Dictionary* (Chipstead, 1921), 559.

71. István Keul, *"Yoginī" in South Asia: Interdisciplinary Approaches* (London & New York: Routledge, Taylor & Francis Group, 2013), 7–14.

72. See, for example, the work of Lal Dēd (Lalla), explored in detail in Ranjit Hoskote, *I, Lalla: The Poems of Lal Dēd* (New Delhi: Penguin Books, 2013), as well as the role of women among the Buddhist Mahāsiddha traditions, such as Niguma and Lakṣmīṅkarā, discussed below.

73. On defining the term *yoginī*, see Shaman Hatley, "What Is a Yoginī? Towards a Polythetic Definition," in *"Yoginī" in South Asia: Interdisciplinary Approaches*, ed. István Keul (London & New York: Routledge, Taylor & Francis Group, 2013), 21–31. A sexual aspect of *yoginī* practice is alluded to in the *Haṭhapradīpikā* 3.99–102, notably discussed as resulting in flight (*khecarī*), a signature power of a *yoginī*. The development of *yoginī* traditions is discussed at length in White, *Kiss of the Yoginī*.

74. Frederick M. Smith, *The Self Possessed: Deity and Spirit Possession in South Asian Literature and Civilization* (New York: Columbia University Press, 2006).

75. A ritual distinction developed by de Heutsch and utilized in I.M. Lewis and Athlone Press, *Arguments with Ethnography: Comparative Approaches to History, Politics & Religion* (London & New Brunswick: Athlone Press, 1999), 106–114.

76. This thesis, which has been the subject of considerable controversy, is examined in Miranda Shaw, *Passionate Enlightenment: Women in Tantric Buddhism* (Princeton, NJ: Princeton University Press, 2011).

77. Richard F. Gombrich, *Theravada Buddhism: A Social History from Ancient Benares to Modern Colombo* (NY: Routledge, 2006), 56–60. The perceived virtues of the *kṣatriya* class for Jains are discussed in Jaini, *The Jaina Path of Purification*, 7–8. An important later narrative regarding the foundation of the Jain community centers upon *brāhmaṇa* converts referred to as *gaṇadhara*. See Paul Dundas, *The Jains* (London & New York: Routledge, 2002), 37–39. Both Mahāvīra and the Buddha are represented as attempting to redefine the status of *brāhmaṇa* into a term for moral and spiritual attainment as opposed to a class or caste designation. A broader discussion of *śramaṇa* traditions in the context of caste and class discussions can be found in Greg Bailey and Ian Mabbett, *The Sociology of Early Buddhism* (Cambridge: Cambridge University Press, 2006).

78. Olivelle, *Upaniṣads*, xxxiv–xxxvi.

79. *Yogabhāṣya* 2.30, for example.

80. Patrick Olivelle, *Saṃnyāsa Upaniṣads: Hindu Scriptures on Asceticism and Renunciation* (Oxford: Oxford University Press, 1992), 11–18.

81. James Mallinson, "Yoga: Haṭha Yoga," in *Brill's Encyclopedia of Hinduism*, ed. Knut Jacobsen et al. (Leiden & Boston: Brill, 2011), 770–781; James Mallinson, "Śāktism and Haṭhayoga," in *Goddess Traditions in Tantric Hinduism: History, Practice, and Doctrine*, ed. Bjarne Wernicke-Oleson (London: Routledge, 2016), 109–140.

82. Keith Dowman, *Masters of Mahāmudrā: Songs and Histories of the Eighty-Four Buddhist Siddhas* (Albany, NY: SUNY Press, 2010), 2–5.

83. Dowman, *Masters of Mahāmudrā*. The social transformation brought on by Buddhist tantrism is discussed in Ron Davidson, *Indian Esoteric Buddhism: A Social History of the Tantric Movement* (New York & Chichester: Columbia University Press, 2005).

84. K. Pattabhi Jois, another important formulator of modern yoga from the *brāhmaṇa*-class, having quoted *Haṭhapradīpikā* 1.64 on yoga's applicability, states: "Indeed, only lazy people find the practice of the yogic limbs useless. Otherwise, yoga is very important for anyone eight years or older, regardless of sex." K. Pattabhi Jois, *Yoga Mala* (New York: North Point Press, 2002), 27.

85. Sarbacker, *Samādhi*, 169–170.

86. Sondra L. Hausner, "The Category of the Yoginī as a Gendered Practitioner," in *"Yoginī" in South Asia: Interdisciplinary Approaches*, ed. István Keul (London & New York: Routledge, Taylor & Francis Group, 2013), 32–43.

87. It can be noted, however, that women in positions of power in the anglophone yoga community tend to be white and of relatively high economic class, with some exceptions. Enoch H. Page, "The Gender, Race, and Class Barriers: Enclosing Yoga as White Public Space," in *Yoga, the Body, and Embodied Social Change: An Intersectional Feminist Analysis*, ed. Beth Berila, Melanie Klein, and Chelsea Jackson Roberts (Lanham, MD: Lexington Books, 2016), 49–52.

88. The attempt to discern the origins of any phenomenon may contain an implicit valuation of its earlier manifestations, implying that what is prior or ancient is more true or authentic. It may have the opposite effect as well, to the degree to which is implied that what is chronologically prior is less significant than a later or contemporaneous, and thus more complete, version of the phenomenon. Instead, adaptation should be understood a critical part of living tradition, and so it makes sense to consider each permutation as complete in its own terms. A brief but lucid discussion of issues of "origin" and "completeness" can be found in Gavin D. Flood, *An Introduction to Hinduism* (Cambridge: Cambridge University Press, 2011), 23–24.

89. One theory regarding the origin of the term "shaman" links it to the Tungus word *saman* and in turn to the Sanskrit term *śramaṇa*, or spiritual "striver." Andrei A. Znamenski, *Shamanism: Critical Concepts in Sociology* (London: RoutledgeCurzon, 2008), 64–65.

90. Thematic connections between yoga and shamanism are explored at length in Eliade, *Yoga*, 318ff.

91. Dominik Wujastyk, "The Path to Liberation through Yogic Mindfulness in Early Āyurveda," in *Yoga in Practice*, ed. David Gordon White (Princeton, NJ: Princeton University Press, 2012), 31–42.

92. Bailey and Mabbett, *The Sociology of Early Buddhism*, 13–36.

93. Hans Penner, "The Mystical Illusion," in *Mysticism and Religious Traditions*, ed. Steven T. Katz (New York: Oxford University Press, 1983), 89–116. Penner argues that this dynamic model continues in the present. The liminoid, or parallel, communities of renouncers, in this theory, simultaneously rejects and affirms the mainstream society that it sets itself apart from. The parallelism between householder and renouncer communities evokes a distinction between economic and cultural capital in which the world-affirming sphere places primary value on material welfare and the renouncer sphere on spiritual welfare, with many points of intersection between the two in which exchange can take place. In the modern context, yoga has a number of links to issues such as urban commerce and individualism, the relationship between capitalism and spirituality, and the power and economic capital associated with yoga teaching and products. Over the past century, yoga has also had an intimate relationship with Indian identity, especially with respect to Indian nationalism, as connected to its formulation as a universal system of physical culture comparable to European and American physical fitness, gymnastic, and calisthenic traditions.

94. On the connections between the development of this ideology and Hindu Nationalism, see Joseph S. Alter, *Yoga in Modern India: The Body between Science and Philosophy* (Princeton, NJ: Princeton University Press, 2004), 142–177.

95. This is sometimes referred to as the "pizza effect" and has played an extremely important role in the formation of contemporary yoga and meditation movements in Hinduism and Buddhism. See Agehananda Bharati, "Indian Expatriates in North America and Neo-Hindu Movements," in *The Communication of Ideas,* ed. J.S. Yadava and Vinayshil Gautam (New Delhi: Concept Publishing, 1980), 245–255. See also Strauss, *Positioning Yoga*, 8–11; Stuart Ray Sarbacker, "Reclaiming the Spirit through the Body: The Nascent Spirituality of Modern Postural Yoga," *Entangled Religions*, no. 1 (2014): 99–100. This has led to a mushrooming of yoga practices in the popular sphere in India and in the global context, often paired with a downplaying in popular and academic discourse of the elements of ritualism and devotion in yoga. This might be referred to as "Protestant Yoga" in a manner akin to the rubric of "Protestant Buddhism" developed in Gombrich and Obeyesekere, *Buddhism Transformed*, 202–240.

96. Alter, *Yoga in Modern India*, 73–108.

97. Another important aspect of living yoga traditions is the process of hybridization that occurs due to the encounter of different traditions within yoga with each other and with other systems of physical and mental discipline. An example of the complexity of this process is the influence of yoga on the development of the physical discipline of Pilates, and the counter-influence that Pilates has exerted on the practice of yoga. Penelope Latey, "The Pilates Method: History and Philosophy," *Journal of Bodywork and Movement Therapies* 5, no. 4 (October 2001): 275–282.

The Pilates system is itself a highly hybridized system. Likewise, the confluence of the practice of yoga with Chinese, Japanese, and Korean variations of martial arts and Daoist practices, which in turn may have roots in or have been influenced by Indian traditions cognate to yoga, demonstrates the complex relationship between such disciplines in an era of globalization and encounter. The possible historical connections, or lack thereof, between yoga and Chinese systems are discussed in Harold David Roth, *Original Tao: Inward Training (nei-yeh) and the Foundations of Taoist Mysticism* (New York & Chichester: Columbia University Press, 1999), 135–138. See also Livia Kohn, *Chinese Healing Exercises: The Tradition of Daoyin* (Honolulu: University of Hawai'i Press, 2008); Livia Kohn, *Daoist Body Cultivation: Traditional Models and Contemporary Practices* (Magdalena, NM: Three Pines Press, 2006). Thematic connections are discussed in Eliade, *Yoga*, 284–290, 412–413, 417–418. On the connections between Chinese gymnastics, European gymnastics, and yoga, see Mark Singleton, "Transnational Exchange and the Genesis of Modern Postural Yoga," in *Yoga Traveling: Bodily Practice in Transcultural Perspective*, ed. Beatrix Hauser, Transcultural Research—Heidelberg Studies on Asia and Europe in a Global Context (Cham & New York: Springer, 2013), 35–56.

98. De Michelis, *A History of Modern Yoga*, 187–193.

99. Sarbacker, "Reclaiming the Spirit through the Body: The Nascent Spirituality of Modern Postural Yoga," 97–99.

100. Sarbacker, "Reclaiming the Spirit." In late *haṭhayoga* texts, such as the *Haṭhapradīpikā* (see 1.1, for example), *haṭhayoga* is framed as a preliminary to *rājayoga*, a state of deep contemplation (*samādhi*), which arises spontaneously upon the perfection of the techniques of *haṭhayoga*, especially *prāṇāyāma*. This paradigm, in which physical and energetic practices are viewed as productive in and of themselves, producing a transformation of mind and emotion without recourse to philosophical reflection or metaphysical ideals, parallels the physicalism of many modern traditions of yoga.

101. De Michelis, *A History of Modern Yoga*, 2005. This is a simplification of De Michelis's fourfold schema, but captures the dynamic between physical and cognitive emphases that is a major division between modern yoga forms.

102. One representative example from this emerging field of literature is Eugene G. D'Aquili and Andrew B. Newberg, *The Mystical Mind: Probing the Biology of Religious Experience* (Minneapolis: Fortress Press, 1999).

103. Alter, *Yoga in Modern India*, 14–31; Mark G. Williams and Jon Kabat-Zinn, *Mindfulness: Diverse Perspectives on Its Meaning, Origins and Applications* (NY: Routledge, 2013). As such, modern meditative traditions of yoga often distance their presentation of meditative practice from explicit sectarian trappings and commitments, at least in their initial stages of practice, appealing instead to

a shared universal human psychology and benefits of practice that can be studied and documented. Sarbacker, *Samādhi*, 3–6.

104. Mallinson and Singleton argue, on the other hand, that the primary definition of *yoga* is as a goal, though they recognize a variability of usage within the larger literature of yoga. Mallinson and Singleton, *Roots of Yoga*, 4–6. Commentators that establish technical definitions of *yoga* and *aṅga* based on the *Yogasūtra*, such as Vyāsa, Vācaspati Miśra, and Bhoja Rāja, may have conflated "method" and "goal" in their attempts to bring etymological coherence to the terms *yoga* and *samādhi*. Additionally, the relationship of the *aṣṭāṅgayoga* system of Patañjali to the Buddhist *aṣṭāṅgamārga*, discussed below, also suggests a close relationship between *yoga* and *mārga*, that is, between "discipline" and "path," that suggests its character as a method as opposed to a goal.

105. More technical discussions of the parameters of tantra can be found in André Padoux, "What Do We Mean by Tantrism?," in *The Roots of Tantra*, ed. Katherine Anne Harper and Robert L Brown (Albany, NY: SUNY Press, 2002), 17–24; David Gordon White, "Tantra in Practice: Mapping a Tradition," in *Tantra in Practice*, ed. David Gordon White (Princeton, NJ: Princeton University Press, 2000), 3–38.

106. Ándre Padoux, *The Heart of the Yoginī: The Yoginīhṛdaya, a Sanskrit Tantric Treatise* (New York: Oxford University Press, 2013), 1–2; Navjivan Rastogi, "The Yogic Disciplines of the Monistic Śaiva Tantric Traditions of Kashmir: Threefold, Fourfold, and Six-Limbed," in *Ritual and Speculation in Early Tantrism: Studies in Honour of André Padoux*, ed. André Padoux and Teun Goudriaan (Albany, NY: SUNY Press, 1992), 247. Tantra can also refer, more generically, to a spiritual discipline or to a topical discourse.

107. On the "mainstreaming" of tantric ritual and ideology, see White, *Kiss of the Yogini*, 2–7.

108. Hugh B. Urban, "The Cult of Ecstasy: Tantrism, the New Age, and the Spiritual Logic of Late Capitalism," *History of Religions* 39, no. 3 (February 2000): 268–304.

109. Sudhir Kakar, *Shamans, Mystics, and Doctors: A Psychological Inquiry into India and Its Healing Traditions* (New Delhi: Oxford, 2012), 151–190; June McDaniel, *Offering Flowers, Feeding Skulls: Popular Goddess Worship in West Benagal* (New York: Oxford University Press, 2004), 9–10. McDaniel postulates a distinction between folk/popular and classical modes of tantra.

110. Olivelle, *Upaniṣads*, xxiv–xxix.

111. See, for example, Thomas R Trautmann, ed., *The Aryan Debate* (New Delhi: Oxford University, 2007); Edwin F. Bryant and Laurie L. Patton, *The Indo-Aryan Controversy: Evidence and Inference in Indian History* (London &

New York: Routledge, 2005); Edwin F. Bryant, *In Quest of the Origins of Vedic Culture: The Indo-Aryan Migration Debate* (New York: Oxford University Press, 2000).

Chapter 2

1. For a discussion of the meaning of the term "Dravidian" and theories regarding its genesis as a cultural-linguistic group, see Bhadriraju Krishnamurti, "Introduction," in *The Dravidian Languages*, ed. Bhadriraju Krishnamurti (Cambridge: Cambridge University Press, 2003), 1–47.

2. One contemporary scholarly attempt to translate the Indus "script" can be found in Asko Parpola, *Deciphering the Indus Script* (Cambridge: Cambridge University Press, 2010). Parpola suggests linkages between the Indus script and the Dravidian language family, but postulates that proto-Vedic ideas are represented in the Indus seals as well. An argument against the "script" interpretation can be found in Steve Farmer, Richard Sproat, and Michael Witzel, "The Collapse of the Indus-Script Thesis: The Myth of a Literate Harappan Civilization," *Electronic Journal of Vedic Studies* 11, no. 2 (2016): 19–57.

3. Flood, *An Introduction to Hinduism*, 30–35. Discussions of the AMT, and the critiques of the CTT and OIT can be found in Michael Witzel, "Indocentrism: Autochthonous Visions of Ancient India," in *The Indo-Aryan Controversy: Evidence and Inference in Indian History*, ed. Edwin F. Bryant and Laurie L. Patton (New York: Routledge, 2005), 341–404. CTT suggests a link between Indus and Vedic traditions in India, whereas OIT suggests that Aryan traditions originated in India and spread to Central Asia and Europe.

4. Susan L. Huntington, *The Art of Ancient India: Buddhist, Hindu, Jain* (Boston: Weatherhill, 1985). Huntington suggests that the headdress of seal 420, which resembles the horns of a bull, might suggest a link between Indus and Mesopotamian art and culture. Variants of this seal appear to represent a "vegetative" headdress or crown.

5. *Mūlabandhāsana* is suggested in Jonathan M. Kenoyer, *Ancient Cities of the Indus Valley Civilization* (Karachi & Islamabad: Oxford University Press; American Institute of Pakistan Studies, 2011), 111–112.

6. Huntington, *Art of Ancient India*. The Indus archeologist Sir John Marshall was a strong proponent of this theory; his work is discussed in Eliade, *Yoga*, 353–358.

7. Christopher Chapple, *Nonviolence to Animals, Earth, and Self in Asian Traditions* (Albany, NY: SUNY Press, 1993), 5–7.

8. Huntington, *Art of Ancient India*, 22.

9. Huntington, *Art of Ancient India*, 21; Eliade, *Yoga*, 355.

10. Huntington, *Art of Ancient India*.

11. White, *Sinister Yogis*, 2009, 48–59; Doris Srinivasan, "Unhinging Śiva from the Indus Civilization," *Journal of the Royal Asiatic Society of Great Britain and Ireland*, no. 1 (1984): 77–89; Geoffrey Samuel, *The Origins of Yoga and Tantra: Indic Religions to the Thirteenth Century* (Cambridge: Cambridge University Press, 2008), 2–8. For example, the forms of yoga *āsana* that the Indus figure is said to approximate appear in texts only thousands of years later during the medieval era. Similarly, attempts to connect the Indus civilization to medieval practices related to *kuṇḍalinī* draw connections from vastly distant cultural eras. See, for example, Thomas McEvilley, "An Archaeology of Yoga," *Res: Anthropology and Aesthetics* 1 (March 1981): 44–77.

12. A number of examples are given in White, *Sinister Yogis*, 2009.

13. David M. Knipe, *Vedic Voices: Intimate Narratives of a Living Andhra Tradition*, 2015, 40–41.

14. See, for example, the *Ṛgveda* on the goddess Pṛthivī at 1.160.6, and on the god Indra at 8.1.2.

15. On the larger discussion of the place of the cow in Hindu traditions and the development of vegetarianism, see D.N. Jha, *The Myth of the Holy Cow* (London: Verso, 2004).

16. Witzel, "Indocentrism: Autochthonous Visions of Ancient India."

17. *Kaṭha Upaniṣad* 3:3–17; *Milindapañha* 2.1.1.

18. David M. Knipe, "Becoming a Veda in the Godavari Delta," in *India and Beyond: Aspects of Literature, Meaning, Ritual, and Thought. Essays in Honor of Frits Staal*, ed. Dick van der Meij (Leiden: International Institute for Asian Studies, 1997), 306–322.

19. Knipe, *Vedic Voices*, 47–49. Knipe points to the relative artificiality of the association of the *brahman* with the *Artharvaveda*. The term *atharvan* refers to a type of priest that may have contributed to the composition of the *Artharvaveda*.

20. Stuart Ray Sarbacker, *Samādhi: The Numinous and Cessative in Indo-Tibetan Yoga*, 17–18. This is drawing on a larger discussion of the concept found in J. Gonda, *The Vision of Vedic Poets* (Berlin & New York: De Gruyter Mouton, 2011). Gonda argues that the concept of *dhī* in the Vedic literature is the conceptual and linguistic precursor of the term *dhyāna*.

21. Arthur Anthony Macdonell, *Vedic Mythology* (New Delhi: Munshiram Manoharlal, 2000), 8–11.

22. Macdonell, 19.

23. Macdonell, 15–114.

24. As will be discussed below (see chapter 3), in the *śramaṇa* tradition of Buddhism, the realms of the *deva* and *asura* represent different modes of rebirth

resulting from distinct admixtures of meritorious (*puṇya*) and unmeritorious (*apuṇya*) action (*karma*) in a human life.

25. A five-fire system was developed as well. See David M. Knipe, "One Fire, Three Fires, Five Fires: Vedic Symbols in Transition," *History of Religions* 12, no. 1 (August 1972): 28–41.

26. Stephanie W. Jamison and Joel P. Brereton, *The Rigveda: The Earliest Religious Poetry of India* (New York: Oxford University Press, 2014), 30–32; Harri Nyberg, "The Problem of the Aryans and the Soma: The Botanical Evidence," in *The Indo-Aryans of Ancient South Asia: Language, Material Culture, and Ethnicity*, ed. George Erdosy, n.d., 382–406; Harry Falk, "Soma I and II," *Bulletin of the School of Oriental and African Studies, University of London* 52, no. 1 (1989): 77–90. See also Matthew James Clark, *The Tawny One: Soma, Haoma, and Ayahuasca* (New York: Muswell Hill Press, 2017).

27. Liz Wilson, *The Living and the Dead: Social Dimensions of Death in South Asian Religions* (Albany, NY: SUNY Press, 2014), 37–38.

28. The wife as co-sacrificer in modern *vaidika* ritual is discussed in Knipe, *Vedic Voices*, 160–161.

29. Laurie L. Patton, *Bringing the Gods to Mind: Mantra and Ritual in Early Indian Sacrifice* (Berkeley: University of California Press, 2006), 142–51.

30. On the reconstitution of the world in Vedic ritual, see Johannes C. Heesterman, *The Broken World of Sacrifice: An Essay in Ancient Indian Ritual* (Chicago: University of Chicago Press, 1993).

31. Jonathan Z. Smith, "Religion, Religions, Religious," in *Critical Terms for Religious Studies*, ed. Mark C. Taylor (Chicago: University of Chicago Press, 1998), 269–284.

32. *Ṛgveda* 10.90.

33. Anand Teltumbde, *Dalits: Past, Present and Future* (New York: Routledge, 2017), 2–3.

34. A more common rendering of *viṣa* is as "poison," rendered here as "agent" to highlight the psychoactive properties that are the basis for consuming it.

35. Martin G. Wiltshire, *Ascetic Figures before and in Early Buddhism: The Emergence of Gautama as the Buddha* (Berlin: Mouton de Gruyter, 1990), 245–247.

36. Finnian M.M. Gerety, "This Whole World Is OM: Song, Soteriology, and the Emergence of the Sacred Syllable" (Harvard University: Graduate School of Arts & Sciences, 2015), 400.

37. Kaelber, *Tapta Mārga*, 45–60.

38. Kaelber, *Tapta Mārga*, 19, 46, 111, 61–62.

39. Eliade, *Yoga*, 111–114.

40. Eliade, *Yoga*, 111–114; Kaelber, *Tapta Mārga*, 102, 106.

41. Kaelber, *Tapta Mārga*, 114–124.

42. Samuel, *Origins of Yoga and Tantra*, 131–133.

43. Samuel, *Origins*, 131–133.

44. Stephen Hillyer Levitt, "New Considerations Regarding the Identity of the Vedic Sóma as the Mushroom Fly-Agaric," in *Studia Orientalia, Volume 111*, ed. Lotta Aunio (Helsinki: Finnish Oriental Society, 2011), 105–118; Kevin Feeney, "Revisiting Wasson's Soma: Exploring the Effects of Preparation on the Chemistry of Amanita Muscaria," *Journal of Psychoactive Drugs* 42, no. 4 (December 2010): 499–506.

45. Falk, "Soma I and II."

46. Discussed at length in David Gordon White, *The Alchemical Body: Siddha Traditions in Medieval India* (Chicago & London: University of Chicago Press, 2007).

47. Stuart Ray Sarbacker, "Herbs (Auṣadhi) as a Means to Spiritual Accomplishments (Siddhi) in Patañjali's 'Yogasūtra,'" *International Journal of Hindu Studies* 17, no. 1 (2013): 37–56.

48. Barbara A. Holdrege, *Veda and Torah: Transcending the Textuality of Scripture* (Albany, NY: SUNY Press, 1996).

49. Holdrege, *Veda and Torah.*

50. Wendy Doniger O'Flaherty, *The Rig Veda: An Anthology: One Hundred and Eight Hymns* (Harmondsworth: Penguin Books, 2007), 137–138; Jamison and Brereton, *The Rigveda*, 1621–1622.

51. The later Purāṇic narratives portray Śiva (who is genealogically related to Rudra) as drinking a poison (*hālahala*) that emerges from the gods churning the cosmic ocean in pursuit of the nectar of immortality (*amṛta*), presumably to protect the others.

52. Olivelle, *The Āśrama System*, 78–79. Olivelle discusses one permutation in which a student takes up permanent residence in a teacher's house (pp. 108–109).

53. *Atharvaveda* 11.5–7.

54. Sarbacker, "The Numinous and Cessative in Modern Yoga," 169.

55. Samuel, *Origins of Yoga and Tantra*, 183–185.

56. Eliade, *Yoga*, 103–105.

Chapter 3

1. Following the distinction in Samuel, *The Origins of Yoga and Tantra*, 153–172.

2. Bronkhorst, *Greater Magadha.*

3. Bronkhorst, *Greater Magadha.*

4. The question of "agency" in the Ājīvika tradition is a matter of dispute, with respect to whether it presented a strict form of fatalism or not. See Jeffery D. Long, *Jainism: An Introduction* (London & New York: I.B. Tauris, 2009), 43–44.

5. Stanley Tambiah, "The Reflexive and Institutional Achievements of Early Buddhism," in *The Origins and Diversity of Axial Age Civilizations*, ed. S.N. Eisenstadt (Albany, NY: SUNY Press, 1986), 453–471.

6. Patrick Olivelle, *The Early Upanisads: Annotated Text and Translation* (New York: Oxford University Press, 1998), 29–30, 145–149.

7. The template for understanding the diversity of modes of being in *saṃsāra* may have been, in part, the broader spectrum of urban life experience, from that of the wealthy and powerful to the impoverished and disenfranchised.

8. Olivelle, *The Early Upanisads*, 29.

9. A brief survey of their contents can be found in Signe Cohen, "The Yoga Upaniṣads," in *The Upaniṣads: A Complete Guide*, ed. Signe Cohen (New York: Routledge, 2018), 405–411. Mallinson and Singleton, following Bouy, argue that the Yoga Upaniṣads were a late product of the consolidation of earlier *haṭhayoga* texts. Mallinson and Singleton, *Roots of Yoga*, xxi; Christian Bouy, *Les Nātha-yogin et les Upaniṣads: étude d'histoire de la littérature hindoue* (Paris: Diffusion De Boccard, 1994).

10. *Muṇḍaka Upaniṣad* 1.1.3–5.

11. *Muṇḍaka Upaniṣad* 1.1.3–5.

12. *Muṇḍaka Upaniṣad*, 1.2.5–10. Hume notes the parallelism between this passage and *Kaṭha Upaniṣad* 2.5 and *Maitrī Upaniṣad* 7.9. Robert Ernest Hume and George C.O. Haas, *The Thirteen Principal Upanishads* (London: Oxford University Press, 1968), 368 n.4. See also, below, the discussion of this trope in the *Bhagavadgītā*.

13. *Muṇḍaka Upaniṣad*, 1.2.11

14. *Muṇḍaka Upaniṣad*, 1.2.12–13

15. *Muṇḍaka Upaniṣad*, 2.1.1

16. *Muṇḍaka Upaniṣad*, 2.2.3–4

17. *Muṇḍaka Upaniṣad*, 3.2.6

18. Eliade, *Yoga*, 117–118. A larger discussion of the term "yoga" in the Upaniṣads under the rubric of "self-discipline," including in the *Taittirīya Upaniṣad,* can be found in Stephen H. Phillips, *Yoga, Karma, and Rebirth: A Brief History and Philosophy* (New York: Columbia University Press, 2009), 163–175. Olivelle translates yoga in the passage (2.4) as "performance." Olivelle, *The Early Upaniṣads*, 303.

19. *Taittirīya Upaniṣad*, 2.1–5. Mallinson and Singleton have theorized that this framework, which is found extensively in modern yoga pedagogy, was later grafted on to *haṭhayoga* practices by Vedānta interpreters, having found little application in yoga texts prior to the seventeenth century. Mallinson and Singleton, *Roots of Yoga*, 184.

20. *Chāndogya Upaniṣad*, 8.6

21. *Bṛhadāraṇyaka Upaniṣad*, 5.15.

22. *Chāndogya Upaniṣad*, 1.1.
23. *Kaṭha Upaniṣad*, 2.12, 11.11.
24. *Kaṭha Upaniṣad*, 1.1–25.
25. In Buddhism this is represented in the connection between the god of desire (*kāma*) and the god of death (*māra*), who become interchangeable. This is most famously evident in the narrative of the Buddha's "temptation" by Māra on the eve of his enlightenment. Catherine Benton, *God of Desire: Tales of Kāmadeva in Sanskrit Story Literature* (Albany, NY: SUNY Press, 2006), 161–164.
26. *Kaṭha Upaniṣad*, 2.15–17.
27. *Kaṭha Upaniṣad*, 3.3–6.
28. *Kaṭha Upaniṣad*, 6.16–17.
29. *Kaṭha Upaniṣad*, 6.18.
30. *Śvetāśvatara Upaniṣad*, 1.3.
31. *Śvetāśvatara Upaniṣad*, 1.7.
32. *Śvetāśvatara Upaniṣad*, 2.1–4.
33. *Śvetāśvatara Upaniṣad*, 2.8–9.
34. *Śvetāśvatara Upaniṣad*, 2.10–11.
35. *Śvetāśvatara Upaniṣad*, 2.12–15.
36. *Śvetāśvatara Upaniṣad*, 4.11–20.
37. *Śvetāśvatara Upaniṣad*, 4.1.
38. *Śvetāśvatara Upaniṣad*, 6.13, 1.14.
39. *Śvetāśvatara Upaniṣad*, 6.22–23. Following the translation in Olivelle, *Early Upaniṣads*, 433. However, Olivelle translates *bhakti* as "love."
40. *Maitrāyaṇīya Upaniṣad*, 2.6. Utilizing the vulgate edition in J.A.B. van Buitenen, *The Maitrāyaṇīya Upanisad: A Critical Essay with Text, Translation and Commentary* (Boston: De Gruyter Mouton, 2017).
41. *Maitrāyaṇīya Upaniṣad*, 6.21.
42. *Maitrāyaṇīya Upaniṣad*, 6.19.
43. *Maitrāyaṇīya Upaniṣad*, 6.10.
44. Olivelle, *Early Upaniṣads*, 1998, 27.
45. *Bṛhadāraṇyaka Upaniṣad*, 6.3–4.
46. *Kauṣītaki Upaniṣad*, 2.3–9.
47. Edward Fitzpatrick Crangle, *The Origin and Development of Early Indian Contemplative Practices* (Wiesbaden: Harrassowitz Verlag, 1994), 59–89.
48. Discussed by Plutarch, among other sources. See Plutarch, Robin Waterfield, and Andrew Erskine, *Hellenistic Lives* (Oxford: Oxford University Press, 2016), 66–68. The story is retold in other versions, including one in which Alexander encounters a group of Rabbis. See Luitpold Wallach, "Alexander the Great and the Indian Gymnosophists in Hebrew Tradition," *Proceedings of the American Academy for Jewish Research* 11 (1941): 47–83.
49. Jaini, *The Jaina Path of Purification*, 7.

50. Signe Cohen, "The Upaniṣads and Early Buddhism," in *The Upaniṣads: A Complete Guide*, ed. Signe Cohen (New York: Routledge, 2018), 73–80. Cohen notes the shared usage of *brāhmaṇa* names and tropes within Buddhist narrative and philosophical literature.

51. Chapter 25 of the *Dhammapada*, for example, defines the *brāhmaṇa* in terms of Buddhist virtue and meditative accomplishment. Jaini, *Jaina Path*, 7.

52. Jaini, *Jaina Path*, 15–21.

53. Jaini, *Jaina Path*, 15–21

54. Jaini, *Jaina Path*, 11.

55. Jaini, *Jaina Path*, 25–27; Dundas, *The Jains*, 26–28.

56. Dundas, *The Jains*, 33–34.

57. *Kalpasūtra*, 121.

58. *Kalpasūtra*, 122.

59. John E. Cort, *Jains in the World: Religious Values and Ideology in India* (Oxford & New York: Oxford University Press, 2001), 22–23.

60. Jaini, *Jaina Path*, 37.

61. Jaini, *Jaina Path*, 220.

62. Cort, *Jains in the World*, 93–99.

63. Olle Qvarnström, "Hemacandra on Yoga," in *Yoga in Jainism*, ed. Christopher Key Chapple (London & New York: Routledge, Taylor & Francis Group, 2016), 142.

64. Chapple, Haribhadra Sūri, and Casey, *Reconciling Yogas*, 26–38.

65. Jaini, *Jaina Path*, 167.

66. Jaini, *Jaina Path*, 168.

67. *Yogasūtra* 2.30–31.

68. Dundas, *The Jains*, 15.

69. Jaini, *Jaina Path*, 21.

70. Dundas, *The Jains*, 155.

71. Long, *Jainism*, 43.

72. Paul Dundas, "A Digambara Jain Prescription of the Yogic Path to Deliverance," in *Yoga in Practice*, ed. David Gordon White (Princeton, NJ: Princeton University Press, 2012), 144.

73. Jaini, *Jaina Path*, 252–253.

74. Dundas, "Digambara Jain Prescription," 144.

75. An event paralleled in Jain narratives of Vardhamāna's conception. See Jaini, *Jaina Path*, 6.

76. His human life and ultimate enlightenment is viewed as such as the culmination of many lifetimes of spiritual striving, with stories of those previous lifetimes developed in a literature of its own, the *Jātaka*, which parallels the fable-literature of India, such as the *Pañcatantra*, and other parts of the ancient world as a medium for moral instruction.

77. John S. Strong, *The Buddha: A Short Biography* (Oxford: Oneworld, 2006), 59–60. However, this might be contrasted with a passage in which Aśvaghoṣa likens Siddhārtha's life of blissful ignorance in the palace to that of the gods in heaven, who, caught up in heavenly sport and enjoyment, are unaware of the pain and misery in other realms of *saṃsāra*. *Buddhacarita*, 2.30–34.

78. Discussed in detail in Bronkhorst, *The Two Traditions of Meditation in Ancient India*, 1–25. It also represents a tension between two traditions of asceticism and meditation, one that aimed at suppression of physical and mental activity, and another that aimed at contemplative insight, the latter being central to Buddhism, the former peripheral. On this point, see Bronkhorst, *Two Traditions*, 128.

79. A tenfold (*daśāṅgamārga*), lit. "ten-limbed path," adds correct knowledge (Skt. *jñāna*, Pāli *ñāṇa*) and release (Skt. *vimukti*, Pāli *vimutti*). See Roderick S. Bucknell, "The Buddhist Path to Liberation: An Analysis of the Listing of Stages," *Journal of the International Association of Buddhist Studies* 7, no. 2 (1984): 7–40.

80. White, *Sinister Yogis*, 2009, 42–45.

81. G.P. Malalasekera et al., *Encyclopaedia of Buddhism* (Colombo: Govt. of Ceylon, 1961), 799.

82. *Dhammapada*, 282, 209.

83. Jois, *Yoga Mala*, 799.

84. Aśvaghoṣa and Patrick Olivelle, *Life of the Buddha* (New York: New York University Press, 2009), 53.

85. Discussed in Eliade, *Yoga*, 179. See also Keren Arbel, *Early Buddhist Meditation: The Four Jhānas as the Actualization of Insight*, 2017, 180–190; L.S. Cousins, "Scholar Monks and Meditator Monks Revisited," in *Destroying Mara Forever: Buddhist Ethics Essays in Honor of Damien Keown*, ed. Damien Keown, John Powers, and Charles S. Prebish (Ithaca, NY: Snow Lion Publications, 2010), 31–46.

86. Johannes Bronkhorst, "Yoga and Seśvara Sāṃkhya," *Journal of Indian Philosophy* 9, no. 3 (1981): 309–320. Also discussed in White, *Sinister Yogis*, 2009, 123–124.

87. *Dhammapada* 14.8 (183).

88. *Vinaya Piṭaka* 5.131, 193. Also discussed in Wilson, *Charming Cadavers*, 42–43; Flood, *The Ascetic Self: Subjectivity, Memory and Tradition*, 124–125.

89. Kate Crosby, *Theravada Buddhism: Continuity, Diversity, and Identity* (Chichester, West Sussex & Malden, MA: Wiley Blackwell, 2014), 125–129.

90. Crosby, *Theravada Buddhism*, 125–129.

91. Crosby, *Theravada Buddhism*, 125–129.

92. Peter Harvey, "The Dynamics of Paritta Chanting in Southern Buddhism," in *Love Divine: Studies in Bhakti and Devotional Mysticism*, ed. Karel Werner (London & New York: Routledge, Taylor & Francis Group, 1993), 53–84. *Paritta* chanting, as such, may be viewed as an aspect of the numinous dimension of yoga,

in which the human-divine boundary becomes fluid, the practitioner of *mettā*, in this case, obtaining a state of "divine abiding" (*brahmavihāra*).

93. Sarah Shaw, *Buddhist Meditation: An Anthology of Texts from the Pali Canon* (London; New York: Routledge, 2006), 8–10; Henepola Gunaratana, *The Path of Serenity and Insight: An Explanation of the Buddhist Jhanas* (Delhi: Motilal Banarsidass, 1985), 22–26.

94. See, for example, *Yogasūtra* 1.33; *Tattvārthasūtra* 7.11.

95. Shaw, *Buddhist Meditation*, 48–49; Leah Zahler, Lati Rinpoche, and Denma Lochö Rinbochay, *Meditative States in Tibetan Buddhism* (Boston: Wisdom Publications, 1998), 69–72.

96. Bronkhorst, *Two Traditions*, 78–95.

97. Sarbacker, *Samādhi*, 104–108.

98. Sarbacker, "The Numinous and Cessative in Modern Yoga," 167–168. The use of *abhijñā* in conversion "miracles" (*prātihāra*), lit. "carrying away," is listed in the *Abhidharmakośa* as being linked to *ṛddhi*, mind reading (*ādeśanā*), and admonition (*anuśāsanī*).

99. Gunaratana, *The Path of Serenity and Insight*, 136–137.

100. Some scholars have argued that the focus on *vipaśyanā* (Pāli *vipassanā*) is a later superimposition on an original *jhāna*-focused spiritual discipline in early Buddhism. See, for example, Tilmann Vetter, *The Ideas and Meditative Practices of Early Buddhism* (Leiden & New York: E.J. Brill, 1988). *Śamatha* meditation is viewed in some contexts as the foundation for the practice of *vipaśyanā*, due to the need for stability and serenity in contemplating the nature of mental (*nāma*) and physical (*rūpa*) aspects of embodiment. However, some Buddhist traditions suggest the possibility of a practice of "dry insight" that uses momentary concentration instead of the sustained concentration characteristic of *śamatha*. Shaw, *Buddhist Meditation*, 18–20.

101. There is some scholarly disagreement as to how much the practice of mindfulness (*smṛti*) represents a projection of a Buddhist framework of ideas onto experience versus establishing an "open awareness" of the field of experience that sees things as they are. The practice aims, either way, to yield a state of peace and detachment in the face of the flux of moment to moment of awareness.

102. Hajime Nakamura, *Indian Buddhism: A Survey with Bibliographical Notes*, Intercultural Research Institute Monograph, no. 9 (Hirakata, Japan: KUFS Publication, 1980), 84–85.

103. Kauṭalya and L.N. Rangarajan, *The Arthashastra* (New Delhi & London: Penguin Books, 1992), 3–8. It is notable that in his discussion of statecraft in the *Arthaśāstra*, Kauṭilya advises kings to have spies pose as ascetics to gather information, having spread rumors about such purported ascetics powers to create a receptive audience. Patrick Olivelle, "King and Ascetic: State Control of Asceticism in the Ārthaśāstra," in *Festschrift Ludo Rocher*, ed. Richard Lariviere and Richard

Salomon (Madras: Adyar Library and Research Centre, 1987), 39–59. The ability of the ascetic or renouncer to cross social boundaries is viewed as a virtue in the gathering of intelligence from various sources, and the political power of ascetic communities is implicit in many such discussions.

104. Hermann Kulke and Dietmar Rothermund, *A History of India* (London & New York: Routledge, 2016), 36–39; Helmuth von Glasenapp and Shridhar B. Shrotri, *Jainism: An Indian Religion of Salvation* (Delhi: Motilal Banarsidass Publishers, 1999), 40–44.

105. Kulke and Rothermund, *A History*, 39–45.

Chapter 4

1. The rubric of "classical" utilized here indicates the manner in which the consolidation and systematization of Vedic and *śramaṇa* thought and practice during this era established a formative model of Hinduism that served as a foundation for later developments. The term "classical" will also be applied in chapter 5 to similar developments in Buddhist and Jain traditions. For a discussion of the rubric of "classical" within the context of the study of religion, see Valliere, "Tradition," 9275–9277.

2. Samuel, *The Origins of Yoga and Tantra*, 197–198.

3. Samuel, *Origins*, 199.

4. Nicholson argues that referring to Patañjali as "Hindu" may obscure the complexity of the situation on the ground, given that Sāṃkhya-Yoga systems, in some respects, bear more similarity to Jain and Buddhist traditions than to Vedānta and other "Hindu" systems, and were criticized as such by some Hindu sects. Nicholson also notes that in spite of these historical issues, modern Hindu organizations invoke Patañjali and the *Yogasūtra* as a way of claiming yoga as being uniquely "Hindu." Andrew J. Nicholson, "Is Yoga Hindu? On the Fuzziness of Religious Boundaries," *Common Knowledge* 19, no. 3 (2013): 492–498. The use of "Hindu" here is in reference to, among other factors, the rootedness of Pātañjala Yoga in the use of Vedic and Upaniṣadic terminology and the Brāhmaṇical context of its commentarial literature, as well as its later formal consolidation as an *āstika* viewpoint (*darśana*) and its use within sectarian Hindu traditions, as exemplified by the role of *aṣṭāṅgayoga* in the Purāṇa literature.

5. Flood, *An Introduction to Hinduism*, 225.

6. Flood, *Introduction*, 231.

7. Knut A. Jacobsen, "Introduction: Yoga Traditions," in *Theory and Practice of Yoga: Essays in Honor of Gerald James Larson*, ed. Knut A. Jacobsen (Leiden & Boston: Brill, 2005), 14.

8. Jacobsen, "Yoga Traditions," 14.

9. The latter link occurring in the commentary of Vācaspati Miśra. *Yogasūtra* 1.23–26; *Yogabhāṣya* 1.25. Ram Shankar Bhattacharya and Gerald James Larson, *Samkhya: A Dualist Tradition in Indian Philosophy* (Princeton, NJ: Princeton University Press, 1987), 112, 119.

10. Larson and Bhattacharya, *Encyclopedia of Indian Philosophies*, 37–42.

11. Ian Whicher, *The Integrity of the Yoga Darsana: A Reconsideration of Classical Yoga* (Albany, NY: SUNY Press, 1998), 42–45; Johannes Bronkhorst, "The Reliability of Tradition," in *Boundaries, Dynamics and Construction of Traditions in South Asia*, ed. Federico Squarcini (Firenze, Italy: Firenze University Press, 2005), 74. One possible linkage to living yoga traditions is through the Pāśupata Śaiva traditions, in which *aṣṭāṅgayoga* and Pātañjala Yoga figure in important ways. See Andrew J. Nicholson, *Lord Śiva's Song: The Īśvara Gītā* (Albany, NY: SUNY Press, 2014); Stuart Ray Sarbacker, "The Yoga of the Śiva Purāṇa" (17th World Sanskrit Conference, Vancouver, 2018). Modern monastic practice associated with Sāṃkhya-Yoga and Patañjali is documented in Knut A. Jacobsen, *Yoga in Modern Hinduism: Hariharānanda Āraṇya and Sāṃkhyayoga* (Abingdon: Routledge, 2018).

12. Larson and Bhattacharya, *Encyclopedia*.

13. Larson and Bhattacharya, *Encyclopedia*.

14. Larson and Bhattacharya, *Encyclopedia*.

15. One theory is that this is a conflation of the terms for a premier (*ādiśiṣta*) grammarian and the name Ādiśeṣa. This thesis, forwarded by Deshpande, is discussed in Stuart Sarbacker, "The Icon of Yoga: Patañjali as Serpent-King in Modern Yoga," in *Sacred Matters: Material Religion in South Asian Traditions*, ed. Tracy Pintchman and Corinne Dempsey (Albany, NY: SUNY Press, 2015), 27.

16. *Patañjalicarita* 2.1–11. This is typically considered a "folk etymology." Sarbacker, "Icon of Yoga," 28. See also Larson and Bhattacharya, *Encyclopedia*, 59.

17. Sarbacker, "The Icon of Yoga: Patañjali as Nāgarāja in Modern Yoga," 27–31. On the iconography of Patañjali, see also Gudrun Bühnemann, "Nāga, Siddha, and Sage: Visions of Patañjali as an Authority on Yoga," in *Yoga in Transformation*, ed. Phillip A. Maas and Karin Preisendanz (Göttingen: Vienna University Press, 2018), 575–622.

18. Sarbacker, "Icon of Yoga," 23–25.

19. Larson and Bhattacharya, *Encyclopedia*, 61–65.

20. The use of *Pātañjalayogaśāstra* serves, in part, to distinguish it from other texts referred to as *Yogaśāstra*, such as that of the Jain author Hemacandra. David Gordon White argues that the rubric of *Yogasūtra* may be a relatively recent invention, with its widespread use being evidence of the impact of modernist reconstructions of the tradition. David Gordon White, *The Yoga Sutra of Patanjali: A Biography* (Princeton, NJ: Princeton University Press, 2014). See also Mark

Singleton, "The Classical Reveries of Modern Yoga," in *Yoga in the Modern World: Contemporary Perspectives*, ed. Mark Singleton and Jean Byrne (London and New York: Routledge, Taylor & Francis Group, 2008), 77–99.

21. Bronkhorst, "Reliability," 71; Philipp A. Maas, *Samādhipāda: Das erste Kapitel des Pātañjalayogaśātra zum ersten Mal kritisch ediert* (Aachen: Shaker Verlag, 2006), xii–xix. Larson also notes that this view is found among later commentators, including Abhinavagupta. Larson and Bhattacharya, *Encyclopedia*, 39–40. Chapple, however, has noted inconsistencies between the *sūtra* and *bhāṣya* texts that suggest Patañjali and Vyāsa were not necessarily in full agreement conceptually, a point seemingly at odds with the "auto-commentary" thesis. Christopher Chapple, *Yoga and the Luminous: Patanjali's Spiritual Path to Freedom* (Albany, NY: SUNY Press, 2008), 219–236. Other possible inconsistencies are discussed in Stuart Ray Sarbacker, "Svādhyāya and Bhakti: Saguṇa Devatā and Nirguṇa Īśvara in Aṣṭāṅgayoga" (Dharma Association of North America, Boston, 2017).

22. Larson and Bhattacharya, *Encyclopedia*, 39–40; Bronkhorst, "Reliability," 71.

23. Sarbacker, "Power and Meaning in the Yogasūtra of Patañjali," 200 n.11. See also Carl W. Ernst, "Situating Sufism and Yoga," *Journal of the Royal Asiatic Society* 15, no. 1 (2005): 15–43; Carl W. Ernst, "Accounts of Yogis in Arabic and Persian Historical and Travel Texts," *Jerusalem Studies in Arabic and Islam* 33 (2007): 409–426; Andrea Acri, "Dharma Pātañjala: A Śaiva Scripture from Ancient Java; Studied in the Light of Related Old Javanese and Sanskrit Texts" (Forsten, 2011).

24. John Brockington, "Yoga in the Mahābhārata," in *Yoga: The Indian Tradition*, ed. Ian Whicher and David Carpenter (London & New York: RoutledgeCurzon, 2003), 13–24.

25. Jacobsen, "Yoga Traditions," 12 n.15.

26. Sarbacker, *Samādhi*, 75–109.

27. Brockington, "Yoga in the Mahābhārata."

28. Whicher, *Integrity*, 65–70.

29. *Yogasūtra* 1.3.

30. *Yogasūtra* 2.1–2.

31. *Yogasūtra* 2.29.

32. Some scholars have argued that the inclusion of the two yogic disciplines of *kriyāyoga* and *aṣṭāṅgayoga* is evidence that the *Yogasūtra* is a composite text, though others have viewed the two systems as complementary in nature, moving from more general to specific instructions for practice. Larson and Bhattacharya, *Encyclopedia*, 62–65.

33. Āraṇya suggests they act, respectively, on "natural afflictive actions," "speech," and "mind." Patañjali et al., *Yoga Philosophy of Patañjali: Containing His Yoga Aphorisms with Vyasa's Commentary in Sanskrit and a Translation with*

Annotations Including Many Suggestions for the Practice of Yoga (Albany, NY: SUNY Press, 1983), 114.

34. *Yogabhāṣya* 2.32.

35. *Yogabhāṣya* 2.32.

36. *Yogasūtra*, 2.33. This "paralleling" is, arguably, bidirectional, in that Pātañjala Yoga likely draws from Vedic, epic, and Purāṇic materials and contributes to the consolidation and systematization of the principles and practices that it draws upon. Sarbacker, "Svādhyāya and Bhakti."

37. *Yogabhāṣya* 1.32. However, this may be a conflation of *svādhyāya* and *īśvarapraṇidhāna*.

38. *Yogasūtra* 1.23–28.

39. Bronkhorst, "Yoga and Seśvara Sāṃkhya."

40. A thesis particularly associated with Hermann Jacobi. See Hermann Jacobi, "Uber Das Ursprüngliche Yoga-System," *Sitzungsberichte Der Preusischen Akademie Der Wissenschaften* (Berlin: Academic Verlag, 1929), 581–624.

41. Eliade, *Yoga*, 73–76.

42. Andrew J. Nicholson, *Unifying Hinduism: Philosophy and Identity in Indian Intellectual History* (New York: Columbia University Press, 2014), 69–74; Andrew Nicholson, "Hindu Disproofs of God: Refuting Vedāntic Theism in the Sāṃkhya-Sūtra," in *The Oxford Handbook of Indian Philosophy*, ed. Jonardon Ganeri (New York: Oxford University Press, 2017), 598–619.

43. Brockington, "Yoga in the Mahābhārata," 22. Additionally, later texts use the term *aṣṭaguṇa* to refer to the eight forms of perfection or accomplishment (*siddhi*).

44. Wujastyk, "The Path to Liberation through Yogic Mindfulness in Early Āyurveda."

45. Jacobsen, "Yoga Traditions," 12 n15.

46. A useful chart of various "limbed" systems can be found in Mallinson and Singleton, *Roots of Yoga*, 9–10.

47. *Yogasūtra* 2.28.

48. *Yogasūtra* 2.30–31.

49. See, for example, *Liṅga Purāṇa* 1.8.17–20

50. *Yogasūtra* 2.35–39.

51. *Yogasūtra* 2.40–45.

52. *Yogasūtra* 2.46–55. For a more detailed examination of the role of *āsana* in Pātañjala Yoga, see Phillip A. Maas, "Sthirasukham Āsanam: Posture and Performance in Classical Yoga and Beyond," in *Yoga in Transformation*, ed. Phillip A. Maas and Karin Preisendanz (Göttingen: Vienna University Press, 2018), 49–100.

53. *Yogasūtra* 3.1–8.

54. *Yogasūtra* 1.16–17. *Saṃprajñāta* is mentioned in the *sūtrapāṭha*; *asaṃprajñāta* is not.

55. Larson and Bhattacharya, *Encyclopedia*, 125–132; Sarbacker, "Power and Meaning," 203–205. These parallel, to some degree, the Buddhist conception of the meditative attainments of *abhijñā* and *nirmāṇa*, "higher knowledge" and "manifestation."

56. *Yogabhāṣya* 3.45.

57. *Yogasūtra* 3.29–34, 39–40.

58. Sarbacker, *Samādhi*, 107–108.

59. *Yogasūtra* 3.50. On the complexity of conceptions of omniscience in Indian Philosophy, see Padmanabh S. Jaini, "On the Sarvajñatva (Omniscience) of Mahāvīra and the Buddha," in *Buddhist Studies in Honour of I.B. Horner*, ed. L. Cousins, Arnold Kunst, and K.R. Norman (Dordrecht: Springer Netherlands, 1974), 71–90.

60. *Yogabhāṣya* 3.51.

61. *Yogasūtra* 3.37.

62. *Yogasūtra* 4.1–6.

63. Vasubandhu and Louis de La Vallée Poussin, *Abhidharmakośabhāṣyam* (Berkeley, CA: Asian Humanities Press, 1988), 1161–1176. Patañjali is theorized to have drawn heavily from Buddhist Abhidharma material, and this may be one example.

64. Sarbacker, "Herbs (Auṣadhi) as a Means to Spiritual Accomplishments (Siddhi) in Patañjali's 'Yogasūtra.' "

65. Sarbacker, "Power and Meaning."

66. *Yogasūtra* 2.25, 3.55, 4.29–34. It is possible that *kaivalya* as represented at the end of the third *pāda* of the *Yogasūtra* represents a preliminary liberation and that of the fourth *pāda* a final liberation in which the *guṇa* factors return to their source. This would be consistent with Purāṇic accounts of *kaivalya* that suggest some yogis may continue to exist in the world for a time before entering into a final state. See, for example, *Śiva Purāṇa* 7.2.38.44–45. This might be considered in some respects analogous to the Buddhist distinction between an initial *nirvāṇa* in life and a final *nirvāṇa* (*parinirvāṇa*) at death.

67. *Yogabhāṣya* 3.55, 4.34.

68. *Yogasūtra* 3.32.

69. Whicher, *Integrity*, 301–308. Or, alternately, one might read 4.34 to indicate an option to either enter a final state of liberation or to exist as a *jīvanmukta*.

70. *Yogasūtra* 4.4–7.

71. Singleton, "The Classical Reveries of Modern Yoga." A larger discussion can be found in White, *Yoga Sutra of Patanjali*. Birch notes, however, that the

utilization of the *Yogasūtra* and *aṣṭāṅgayoga* paradigm as a syncretic framework for understanding yoga is evident in late medieval works such as the *Yogacintāmaṇi* of Śivānandasarasvatī and the *Yuktabhavadeva* of Bhavadeva, anticipating Vivekananda's efforts in that respect. Birch, "Rājayoga," 401–402.

72. White, *Sinister Yogis*, 2009, 47.

Chapter 5

1. Samuel, *The Origins of Yoga and Tantra*, 193.

2. With respect to the Purāṇas, the date of 500 CE correlates with an "early recension" period, in which a formative nexus of Purāṇic concepts and narratives had been developed, with much of the Purāṇic corpus compiled much later. On the complexity and difficulty of dating the *The Purāṇas*, see Ludo Rocher, *The Puranas* (Wiesbaden: Otto Harrassowitz, 1986), 100–103.

3. The *itihāsa-purāṇa* literature is mentioned as an extension of Vedic literature in *Bṛhadāraṇyaka Upaniṣad* 2.4.10; it is explicitly mentioned as the fifth Veda in *Chāndogya Upaniṣad* 7.1.4.

4. Brockington, *The Sanskrit Epics*, 2.

5. The term *sūta* may have also referred to a son produced by a *kṣatriya* father and a *brāhmaṇa* mother, but it is unclear whether the term for bard (*sūta*) is the same. Rocher, *The Purāṇas*, 53–59.

6. James L. Fitzgerald, Sushil Mittal, and Gene Thursby, "Mahābhārata," in *The Hindu World*, ed. Sushil Mittal and Gene Thursby (New York: Routledge, 2004), 52–54.

7. Brockington, "Yoga in the *Mahābhārata*," 17.

8. Brockington, "Yoga," 17.

9. Fitzgerald, Mittal, and Thursby, "Mahābhārata," 58.

10. With respect to the concept of Kṛṣṇa as a manifestation (*avatāra*) of Viṣṇu, *Bhagavadgītā* 4.7 is often cited, though the term *avatāra* does not appear in the verse, being considered implicit. David Kinsley, "Avatāra," in *Encyclopedia of Religion*, ed. Lindsay Jones, 2nd ed., vol. 2 (Detroit, MI: Macmillan Reference USA, 2005), 707–708.

11. Brockington, "Yoga," 19–20.

12. Fitzgerald, Mittal, and Thursby, "Mahābhārata," 68.

13. V.M. Bedekar, "Dhyānayoga in the Mahābhārata," *Bharatiya Vidya Bhavan* 20–21 (1960–1961): 116–125; Brockington, "Yoga," 20.

14. Brockington, "Yoga," 19.

15. Brockington, "Yoga," 17.

16. Brockington, "Yoga," 20; White, *Sinister Yogis*, 141–145.

17. Dhand, *Woman as Fire, Woman as Sage*, 68.

18. Brockington, "Yoga in the Mahābhārata," 22.

19. *Bhagavadgītā* 2.48, 2.50, 14.26, 8.12–16.

20. *Bhagavadgītā* 9.20–23, *Muṇḍaka Upaniṣad* 2.7–11.

21. Ithamar Theodor, *Exploring the* Bhagavad Gitā*: Philosophy, Structure, and Meaning* (Burlington, VT: Ashgate, 2010), 61–63.

22. Angelika Malinar, The Bhagavadgītā*: Doctrines and Contexts* (Cambridge: Cambridge University Press, 2009), 126–127.

23. *Bhagavadgītā* 4.1.

24. Jacobsen, "Introduction: Yoga Traditions," 14.

25. *Bhagavadgītā* 10.26. Malinar, The Bhagavadgītā*: Doctrines and Contexts*, 2009, 162–163.

26. *Bhagavadgītā* 33.5–35. Malinar argues, however, that this does not mean Kṛṣṇa is subsumed to Viṣṇu in the manner of the *avatāra* doctrine. Angelika Malinar, The Bhagavadgītā, 172–173. Explicit references by Arjuna to Kṛṣṇa as being *brahman* are found earlier in the text (pp. 157–158).

27. Following the excellent summary of the story in R.P. Goldman and S.J. Sutherland Goldman, "Rāmāyaṇa," in *The Hindu World*, 75–96.

28. Sally J. Sutherland Goldman, "The Voice of Sītā in Vālmīki's Sundarakāṇḍa," in *Questioning Ramayanas: A South Asian Narrative Tradition*, ed. Paula Richman (Berkeley: University of California Press, 2001), 223–238.

29. On the genealogy of the *Yogavāsiṣṭha*, see John Brockington and Mary Brockington, eds., "Re-Creation, Refashioning, Rejection, Response . . . How the Narrative Developed," in *The Other Ramayana Women: Regional Rejection and Response* (New York: Taylor & Francis, 2016), 10.

30. Christopher Key Chapple, "The Sevenfold Yoga of the Yogavāsiṣṭha," in *Yoga in Practice*, ed. David Gordon White (Princeton, NJ: Princeton University Press, 2012), 117–139.

31. Chapple, "Sevenfold Yoga," 122.

32. *Yogavāsiṣṭha* 6.1.77–82. This is an inversion of a common trope of the guru-śiṣya dynamic between a male renouncer and his female spouse. Wilson, *Charming Cadavers*, 224 n.57. Further discussion can be found in Ana Laura Funes Maderey, "Kuṇḍalinī Rising and Liberation in the Yogavāsiṣṭha: The Story of Cūḍālā and Śikhidhvaja," *Religions* 8, no. 11 (November 2017): 248–263.

33. Rocher, *The Purāṇas*, 67–80.

34. Freda Matchett, "The Purāṇas," in *The Blackwell Companion to Hinduism*, ed. Gavin D. Flood (Malden, MA: Blackwell, 2007), 134–135.

35. Rocher, *The Purāṇas*, 30–33.

36. Velcheru Narayana Rao, "Purāṇa," in *The Hindu World*, 101.

37. *Viṣṇu Purāṇa* 3.6.20–24. Matchett, "The Purāṇas," 133.

38. *Śiva Purāṇa* 7.2.37.41–44; 7.2.38.7–45.

39. Ramachandra Dīkshitar, "Yoga," in *The Purāṇas Index* (Madras: University of Madras, 55 1951–55).

40. Nicholson, *Lord Śiva's Song*, 2. The *Īśvaragītā* is a section of the *Kūrma Purāṇa* comparable in some respects to the *Bhagavadgītā* and *Yogavāsiṣṭha*, exemplifying the syncretic nature of yoga discourse in the Purāṇa literature, as it blends together Śaiva theism, Sāṃkhya-Yoga, and Vedānta (see Nicholson, pp. 35–153).

41. Matchett, "The Purāṇas," 139.

42. Antonio Rigopoulos, Dattatreya: *The Immortal Guru, Yogin, and Avatara: A Study of the Transformative and Inclusive Character of a Multi-Faceted Hindu Deity* (Albany, NY: SUNY Press, 1998), xi–xii, 26–37, 228–229.

43. The Buddhist critique is discussed in Nathan McGovern, "Brahmā: An Early and Ultimately Doomed Attempt at a Brahmanical Synthesis," *Journal of Indian Philosophy* 40, no. 1 (2012): 1–23.

44. Thomas J. Hopkins, "Saura Hinduism," in *Encyclopedia of Religion* (Detroit: Macmillan Reference USA, 2005).

45. See, for example, *Agni Purāṇa* 372–379; *Vāyu Purāṇa* 1.10–14; *Kūrma Purāṇa* 2.11; *Garuḍa Purāṇa* 2.226–237; *Śiva Purāṇa* 7.2.37–39; *Liṅga Purāṇa* 1.8–9; *Bhāgavata Purāṇa* 3.27–28; *Viṣṇu Purāṇa* 6.7.

46. Edwin F. Bryant, "Patañjali's Theistic Preference, or, Was the Author of the Yoga Sūtras a Vaishnava?," *Journal of Vaishnava Studies 14*, no. 1 (Fall 2005): 7–28. In addition to the possibility of Patañjali being a Vaiṣṇava or a Śaiva, it might be considered that he was *smārta* (or, perhaps, proto-*smārta*) in orientation, which would align with the priestly framework of the text and its apparent lack of sectarian commitment. Sarbacker, "Svādhyāya and Bhakti: Saguṇa Devatā and Nirguṇa Īśvara in Aṣṭāṅgayoga."

47. The *Śiva Purāṇa*, for example, contrasts the inner processes of meditation and the reality of the inner *ātman* over the outer, concrete worship of sacrifice (*yajña*), following the thread of critique of the sacrificial model. *Śiva Purāṇa* 7.2.39.28–30.

48. *Liṅga Purāṇa* 1.8.20.

49. *Śiva Purāṇa* 7.2.37.19.

50. *Śiva Purāṇa* 7.2.38.44–45.

51. *Liṅga Purāṇa* 1.9.56–61.

52. *Liṅga Purāṇa* 1.8.16–20; *Bhāgavata Purāṇa* 2.27–28.

53. Arvind Sharma, *Classical Hindu Thought: An Introduction* (New Delhi & New York: Oxford University Press, 2003), 40.

54. Eliade, *Yoga*, 144–145.

55. Eliade, *Yoga*, 144–145

56. Eliade, *Yoga*, 138–142.

57. Eliade, *Yoga*, 138–142.

58. R.N. Dandekar, "Vedānta," in *Encyclopedia of Religion*, ed. Lindsay Jones, 2nd ed., vol. 14 (Detroit, MI: Macmillan Reference USA, 2005), 9543–9549.

59. In this analysis, the multiplicity of individual bodies and souls make up, as a totality, the body of God or *brahman*. John B. Carman, "Rāmānuja," in *Encyclopedia of Religion*, ed. Lindsay Jones, 2nd ed., vol. 11 (Detroit, MI: Macmillan Reference USA, 2005), 7615.

60. T.S. Rukmani, "The 'Yogasūtrabhāṣyavivaraṇa' Is Not the Work of Śaṅkarācārya the Author of the 'Brahmasūtrabhāṣya,'" *Journal of Indian Philosophy* 26, no. 3 (1998): 263–274. Rukmani rejects the association of the two Śaṅkara figures, though other scholars are more willing to consider them the same person. A discussion of scholarship on this issue can be found in Kengo Harimoto and Śaṅkara, *God, Reason and Yoga: A Critical Edition and Translation of the Commentary Ascribed to Śaṅkara on Pātañjalayogaśāstra 1.23–28* (Hamburg: Department of Indian and Tibetan Studies, Universität Hamburg, 2014), 225–251. One clear ground to reject this association is to note that in *Brahmasūtrabhāṣya* 2.1.3, Śaṅkara quotes a Yogaśāstra that opens *atha tattvadarśanopāyo yogaḥ*, likely referring to a Nyāya text, rather than the first *Pātañjalayogaśāstra* verse, *atha yoganuśāsanam*. If Śaṅkara were the author of the *Pātañjalayogaśāstravivaraṇa*, it would seem much more likely that Śaṅkara would have quoted the opening verse of the *Pātañjalayogaśāstra, atha yogānuśāsanam,* instead.

61. T.S. Rukmani, "Śaṅkara's Views on 'Yoga' in the 'Brahmasūtrabhāṣya' in the Light of the Authorship of the 'Yogasūtrabhāṣyavivaraṇa,'" *Journal of Indian Philosophy* 21, no. 4 (1993): 395–404.

62. Smith, *The Self Possessed*, 294–297.

63. Rukmani, "Śaṅkara's Views on 'Yoga' in the 'Brahmasūtrabhāṣya' in the Light of the Authorship of the 'Yogasūtrabhāṣyavivaraṇa,'" 397–398. Another significant critique is the emphasis on action (*karma*) and the "goal orientation" of the practice of yoga, which contrast with Śaṅkara's views on the centrality of *jñāna* in the achievement of liberation. Wilhelm Halbfass, *Tradition and Reflection: Explorations in Indian Thought* (Albany, NY: SUNY Press, 1991), 224–228; Andrew O. Fort, *Jivanmukti in Transformation: Embodied Liberation in Advaita and Neo-Vedanta* (Albany, NY: SUNY Press, 1998), 45–46.

64. Surendranath Dasgupta, *A History of Indian Philosophy* (Cambridge: Cambridge University Press, 1961), 96–99.

65. Andrew O. Fort, "On Destroying the Mind: The Yogasūtras in Vidyāranya's Jīvanmuktiviveka," *Journal of Indian Philosophy* 27, no. 4 (1999): 377–395. Fort notes how the *Yogasūtra* text is quoted selectively, omitting portions that utilize Sāṃkhya philosophical principles.

66. Nicholson, *Unifying Hinduism*, 7, 32–34.

67. Nicholson, *Unifying Hinduism*, 108–123.

Chapter 6

1. Silk, "The Yogācāra Bhikṣu." On the development of *yogācāra* rubric, see also Daniel M. Stuart, "Yogācāra Substrata? Precedent Frames for Yogācāra Thought among Third-Century Yoga Practitioners in Greater Gandhāra," *Journal of Indian Philosophy* 46, no. 2 (April 2018): 193–240.

2. Jaini, *The Jaina Path of Purification*, 4–5.

3. Jaini, *Jaina Path*, 5–6.

4. Dundas, *The Jains*, 86.

5. Dundas, *The Jains*, 87.

6. *Tattvārthasūtra* 1.1.

7. Dundas, *The Jains*, 87; Jaini, *Jaina Path*, 81.

8. Jaini, *Jaina Path*, 81–82.

9. Jaini, *Jaina Path*, 82.

10. *Tattvārthasūtra* 7.6.

11. Umāsvāti, *That Which Is: Tattvārtha Sūtra*, trans. Nathmal Tatia (New Haven, CT: Yale University Press, 2011), 232–233.

12. Umāsvāti, *That Which Is*, 236–237.

13. *Tattvārthasūtra* 9.43–46.

14. Umāsvāti, *That Which Is*, 243, 279.

15. *Tattvārthasūtra* 10.1–6.

16. Umāsvāti, *That Which Is*, 257–264; Kenneth Roy Norman, "The Pratyeka-Buddha in Buddhism and Jainism," in *Collected Papers* 2 (Oxford: Pali Text Society, 1991), 210–223; Wiltshire, *Ascetic Figures before and in Early Buddhism*; Ria Kloppenborg, *The Paccekabuddha: A Buddhist Ascetic: A Study of the Concept of the Paccekabuddha in Pali Canonical and Commentarial Literature* (Leiden: Brill, 1974).

17. Chapple, Haribhadra Sūri, and Casey, *Reconciling Yogas*, 1.

18. Chapple, Haribhadra Sūri, and Casey, *Reconciling*, 18.

19. Chapple, Haribhadra Sūri, and Casey, *Reconciling*, 20.

20. Chapple, Haribhadra Sūri, and Casey, *Reconciling*, 19.

21. Qvarnström, "Hemacandra on Yoga," 141.

22. Hemacandra and Qvarnström, *The Yogaśāstra of Hemacandra*, 7–8; Olle Qvarnström, "Jain Tantra: Divinatory and Meditative Practices in the Twelfth-Century Yogaśāstra of Hemacandra," in *Tantra in Practice*, ed. David Gordon White (Princeton, NJ: Princeton University Press, 2000), 596–597.

23. Hemacandra and Qvarnström, *Yogaśāstra*, 9.

24. Hemacandra and Qvarnström, *Yogaśāstra*, 96–98.

25. Qvarnström, "Jain Tantra: Divinatory and Meditative Practices in the Twelfth-Century Yogaśāstra of Hemacandra," 168–197.

26. Vasubandhu and La Vallée Poussin, *Abhidharmakośabhāṣyam*, xxx–xxxvii.

27. Charles S. Prebish, "Buddhist Councils and Divisions of the Order," in *Buddhism: A Modern Perspective*, ed. Charles S. Prebish (University Park: Pennsylvania State University Press, 1989), 25.

28. Hajime Nakamura, *Indian Buddhism: A Survey with Bibliographical Notes*, Intercultural Research Institute Monograph, no. 9 (Hirakata, Japan: KUFS Publication, 1980), 116.

29. Upatissa, *The Path of Freedom: Vimuttimagga*, trans. N.R.M Ehara, Soma Thera, and Kheminda Thera (Kandy; Sri Lanka: Buddhist Publication Society, 1995), xxxvi–xlii.

30. Upatissa, *Path*, 4.

31. Upatissa, *Path*, 27.

32. The *Vimuttimagga* is not currently extant in Pāli, and translators vary on their interpretation of the existing Chinese versions, utilizing the terms *yogin* and *yogāvacara* alternately. See, for example, the variants in Upatissa, *The Path of Freedom: Vimuttimagga*; P.V. Bapat, *Vimuttimagga and Visuddhimagga: A Comparative Study* (Calcutta: Calcutta Oriental Press, Ltd., 1937).

33. Gombrich, *Theravada Buddhism*, 153.

34. Gunaratana, *The Path of Serenity and Insight*, 24–25.

35. Buddhaghosa and Ñāṇamoli, *The Path of Purification: Visuddhimagga* (Seattle: BPE Pariyatti Editions, 1999), 743.

36. Eliade, *Yoga*, 194.

37. Rory Mackenzie, *New Buddhist Movements in Thailand: Toward an Understanding of Wat Phra Dhammakaya and Santi Asoke* (London: Routledge, 2012), 109–113; Kate Crosby, "Tantric Theravāda: A Bibliographic Essay on the Writings of François Bizot and Others on the Yogāvacara Tradition," *Contemporary Buddhism* 1, no. 2 (2000): 141–143; Kate Crosby, "History versus Modern Myth: The Abhayagirivihāra, the Vimuttimagga and Yogāvacara Meditation," *Journal of Indian Philosophy* 27, no. 6 (1999): 503–509.

38. Karl H. Potter, *Abhidharma Buddhism to 150 A.D.* (Princeton, NJ: Princeton University Press, 1991), 112.

39. Jonathan C. Gold, "Vasubandhu," in *The Stanford Encyclopedia of Philosophy*, ed. Edward N. Zalta, Summer 2018 (Metaphysics Research Lab, Stanford University, 2018), https://plato.stanford.edu/archives/sum2018/entries/vasubandhu

40. Koichi Yamashita, *Pātañjala Yoga Philosophy with Reference to Buddhism* (Calcutta: Firma KLM Private Limited, 1994), 166–175; Larson and Bhattacharya, *Encyclopedia of Indian Philosophies*, 42–45; Phillip A. Maas, "Sarvāstivāda Abhidharma and the Yoga of Patañjali" (Congress of the International Association of Buddhist Studies, Vienna, 2014); Karen O'Brien-Kop, "Classical Discourses of Liberation: Shared Botanical Metaphors in Sarvāstivāda Buddhism and the Yoga of Patañjali," *Religions of South Asia* 11, no. 2–3 (2017): 123–157; Stuart Ray

Sarbacker, "Meditation as Desired: Smṛti in the Yogasūtra and Cognate Buddhist Sources" (Association for Asian Studies Annual Conference, Honolulu, 2011).

41. Some of the intersections and differentiations between Buddhist Abhidharma and Sāṃkhya are explored in Johannes Bronkhorst, "Sāṃkhya in the Abhidharmakośa Bhāṣya," *Journal of Indian Philosophy* 25, no. 4 (August 1997): 393–400.

42. Luis O. Gomez, "Buddhism in India," in *The Religious Traditions of Asia*, ed. Joseph Mitsuo Kitagawa (New York & London: Macmillan Pub. Co. & Collier Macmillan, 2002), 63–64.

43. K.S. Bouthillette, "Like Ploughing: An Early Mādhyamikan Refutation of 'Vedic' Yoga" (17th World Sanskrit Conference, Vancouver, BC, 2018). This is in contrast to the more common refutation of Sāṃkhya metaphysics, which can be, presumably, extended to Pātañjala Yoga.

44. Alex Wayman, *Untying the Knots in Buddhism: Selected Essays* (Delhi: Motilal Banarsidass Publishers, 1997), 64–72.

45. Stephen C. Berkwitz, *South Asian Buddhism: A Survey* (London & New York: Routledge, 2010), 87–91.

46. Frederick J. Streng, "Śūnyam and Śūnyatā," in *Encyclopedia of Religion*, ed. Lindsay Jones, 2nd ed., vol. 13 (Detroit, MI: Macmillan Reference USA, 2005), 8855–8860.

47. Silk, "The Yogācāra Bhikṣu."

48. Discussed in Karen O'Brien-Kop, "The 'Other' Yogaśāstra: Reconfiguring the Category of Classical Yoga" (American Academy of Religion Annual Meeting, Denver, 2018).

49. Ulrich Timme Kragh, "The Yogācārabhūmi and Its Adaptation," in *The Foundation for Yoga Practitioners: The Buddhist Yogācārabhūmi Treatise and Its Adaptation in India, East Asia, and Tibet*, ed. Ulrich Timme Kragh (Cambridge, MA: Harvard University Press, 2013), 30–31. Again, this parallels the manner in which it is defined in Pātañjala Yoga in significant ways.

50. The *Lotus Sūtra* presentation of the *ekayāna* and variant Buddhist views are discussed at length in Donald S. Lopez, *The Lotus Sutra: A Biography* (Princeton, NJ: Princeton University Press, 2016).

51. Leslie S. Kawamura, "Atīśa," in *Encyclopedia of Religion* (Detroit, MI: Macmillan Reference USA, 2005).

52. Śāntideva, Kate Crosby, and Andrew Skilton, *The Bodhicaryāvatāra* (Oxford & New York: Oxford University Press, 2008), xiv–xvii.

53. Crosby, *Theravada Buddhism*, 27–28. See also *Mahāvastu* 1.231–239.

54. Śāntideva, Crosby, and Skilton, *The Bodhicaryāvatāra*, xvi.

55. Theravāda traditions have a separate list of ten perfections, mentioned in the *Jātaka* stories as part of the Bodhisattva's path to Buddhahood. Crosby,

Theravada Buddhism, 28. See also Naomi Appleton, *Jātaka Stories in Theravāda Buddhism: Narrating the Bodhisatta Path* (Farnham, Surrey, England & Burlington, VT: Ashgate Pub., 2010), 98–103.

56. Paul Williams, *Mahāyāna Buddhism: The Doctrinal Foundations* (London & New York: Routledge, 1998), 204–215.

57. Williams, *Mahāyāna Buddhism*, 206.

58. *Yogasūtra* 4.29. The attainment of *dharmamegha* is associated in the *Yogasūtra* with the destruction of *kleśa-* and *jñeyāvaraṇa*. *Yogasūtra* 4.31. This is clearly genealogically related to the Yogācāra view in the *Bodhisattvabhūmi*. On the latter, see the brief discussion in Robert E. Buswell and Donald S. Lopez, eds., *The Princeton Dictionary of Buddhism* (Princeton, NJ: Princeton University Press, 2014), 897.

59. The term *mahāsattva* is being drawn from the tradition but extended in its heuristic application here as referring to the elevated status of such Bodhisattvas. A discussion of the technical meaning of the term can be found in Linnart Mäll, *Studies in the Aṣṭasāhasrikā Prajñāpāramitā and Other Essays* (Delhi: Motilal Banarsidass, 2005), 56–62.

60. David L. Snellgrove, *Indo-Tibetan Buddhism: Indian Buddhists and Their Tibetan Successors* (Boston: Shambhala, 2002), 58–61; Williams, *Mahāyāna Buddhism: The Doctrinal Foundations*, 228–243.

61. Snellgrove, *Indo-Tibetan Buddhism*, 74–75.

62. Kenneth G. Zysk, *Asceticism and Healing in Ancient India Medicine in the Buddhist Monastery* (Delhi: Motilal Banarsidass, 2010), 67–69.

63. Snellgrove, *Indo-Tibetan Buddhism*, 141.

64. Koichi Shinohara, *Spells, Images, and Maṇḍalas: Tracing the Evolution of Esoteric Buddhist Rituals* (New York: Columbia University Press, 2014), xiv–xvii.

65. Samuel, *The Origins of Yoga and Tantra*, 211–28.

66. Samuel, *Origins*, 211–228.

67. Samuel, *Origins*, 211–228.

68. Mikel Burley, *Classical Samkhya and Yoga: An Indian Metaphysics of Experience* (London: Routledge, 2012), 82–90.

Chapter 7

1. Gavin D. Flood, "The Śaiva Traditions," in *The Blackwell Companion to Hinduism*, ed. Gavin D. Flood (Malden, MA: Blackwell, 2005), 204–205; Gérard Colas, "History of Vaiṣṇava Traditions: An Esquisse," in *The Blackwell Companion to Hinduism*, ed. Gavin D. Flood (Malden, MA: Blackwell, 2005), 230–233.

2. Flood, "The Śaiva Traditions," 207–208.

3. David N. Lorenzen, "Śaivism: An Overview," in *Encyclopedia of Religion*, ed. Lindsay Jones, 2nd ed., vol. 12 (Detroit, MI: Macmillan Reference USA, 2005), 8042.

4. Flood, "Śaiva Traditions," 207–208.

5. Flood, "Śaiva Traditions," 212.

6. Richard S. Weiss, *Recipes for Immortality. Healing, Religion, and Community in South India* (New York: Oxford University Press, 2009), 61; Mariasusai Dhavamony, "Śaivism: Śaiva Siddhānta," in *Encyclopedia of Religion*, ed. Lindsay Jones (Detroit, MI: Macmillan Reference USA, 2005), Gale Virtual Reference Library.

7. Francis X. Clooney and Tony K. Stewart, "Vaiṣṇava," in *The Hindu World*, ed. Sushil Mittal and Gene R Thursby (New York: Routledge, 2007), 162–165.

8. Colas, "History of Vaiṣṇava Traditions: An Esquisse," 261–262.

9. David N. Lorenzen, "Bhakti," in *The Hindu World*, ed. Sushil Mittal and Gene R Thursby (New York: Routledge, 2007), 185.

10. Robert C. Lester, *Rāmānuja on the Yoga* (Madras: The Adyar Library, 1976), 100–132.

11. Paul H. Sherbow, "Viśvanātha Cakravartī's View on Yoga," *Journal of Vaishnava Studies* 14, no. 1 (Fall 2005): 209–232; Jason D. Fuller, "Aṣṭāṅga-Yoga and Bhaktivinoda Thakura," *Journal of Vaishnava Studies* 14, no. 1 (Fall 2005): 233–242. See also the discussion of the Gauḍīya view on Pātañjala Yoga in Barbara A. Holdrege, *Bhakti and Embodiment: Fashioning Divine Bodies and Devotional Bodies in Krsna Bhakti* (New York: Routledge, 2015), 40–45.

12. Sushil Mittal, Gene R. Thursby, and Kathleen M. Erndl, eds., "Śākta," in *The Hindu World* (New York: Routledge, 2007), 154.

13. Mittal, Thursby, and Erndl, "Śākta," 147–152.

14. Mittal, Thursby, and Erndl, "Śākta," 149–150.

15. Mittal, Thursby, and Erndl, "Śākta," 154–155.

16. Mittal, Thursby, and Erndl, "Śākta," 156.

17. June McDaniel, *Offering Flowers, Feeding Skulls: Popular Goddess Worship in West Bengal* (New York: Oxford University Press, 2004), 89–97. One of the most important sacred sites or "seats" (*pīṭha*) of Śākta traditions is the Kāmākhyā temple in Assam, which demonstrates the integration of Kaula, Śaiva, Brāhmaṇical, and indigenous traditions in India, and the role of Śākta traditions in the establishment of political power in the medieval era.

18. Matthew Clark, "Sādhus and Sādhvīs," in *Encyclopedia of Religion*, ed. Lindsay Jones (Detroit, MI: Macmillan Reference USA, 2005), 8020.

19. Clark, "Sādhus and Sādhvīs," 1819.

20. Clark, "Sādhus and Sādhvīs," 8019–8020.

21. See, for example, the discussion of the formation of the Daśanāmi sect in Matthew James Clark, *The Daśanāmī-Saṃnyāsīs: The Integration of Ascetic Lineages into an Order* (Leiden: Brill, 2006).

22. Haripada Chakraborti, *Asceticism in Ancient India: In Brahmanical, Buddhist, Jaina and Ajivika Societies: From the Earliest Times to the Period of Śaṅkarāchārya* (Calcutta: Punthi Pustak, 1993), 179.

23. Chakraborti, 179. Translated as "hill," "city," "learning," "wood," "forest," "mountain," "ocean," "temple," "hermitage," and "true knowledge" by Chakraborti.

24. White, *Sinister Yogis*, 227–228. Shashank Chaturvedi, "Khichdi Mela in Gorakhnath Math: Symbols, Ideas and Motivations," *Society and Culture in South Asia* 3, no. 2 (July 1, 2017): 135–156.

25. Sondra L. Hausner, *Wandering with Sadhus: Ascetics in the Hindu Himalayas* (Bloomington: Indiana University Press), 85–88.

26. William R. Pinch, *Warrior Ascetics and Indian Empires* (Cambridge, NY: Cambridge University Press, 2012), 28–58; White, *Sinister*, 198–254.

27. Olivelle, "King and Ascetic: State Control of Asceticism in the Ārthaśāstra," 39–59; McKean, *Divine Enterprise*; Stuart Ray Sarbacker, "Swami Ramdev: Modern Yoga Revolutionary," in *Gurus of Modern Yoga*, ed. Mark Singleton and Ellen Goldberg (New York & London: Oxford University Press, 2014), 363–364.

28. Lorenzen, "Bhakti," 185.

29. Heidi Pauwels, "Who Are the Enemies of the Bhaktas? Testimony about 'Śāktas' and 'Others; from Kabīr, the Rāmānandīs, Tulsīdās, and Harirām Vyās," *Journal of the American Oriental Society* 130, no. 4 (2010): 509–539; Patton Burchett, "Bitten by the Snake: Early Modern Devotional Critiques of Tantra-Mantra," *The Journal of Hindu Studies* 6, no. 1 (2013): 1–20.

30. Lorenzen, "Bhakti," 204.

31. Lorenzen, "Bhakti," 185.

32. Karine Schomer, *The Sants: Studies in a Devotional Tradition of India* (Delhi: Motilal Banarsidass, 1987), 64–73.

33. Kamala E. Nayar, Jaswinder Singh Sandhu, and Nānak, *The Socially Involved Renunciate: Guru Nanak's Discourse to the Nāth Yogis* (Albany, NY: SUNY Press, 2007), 14–16, 50–58.

34. Nayar, Sandhu, and Nānak, *Socially*, 48–49. On the connections and disconnections between tantra and *bhakti*, see also Patton Burchett, *A Genealogy of Devotion: Bhakti, Tantra, Yoga, and Sufism in North India* (New York: Columbia University Press, 2019).

35. Nayar, Sandhu, and Nānak, *Socially*, 48–49.

36. Nayar, Sandhu, and Nānak, *Socially*, 57–58.

37. Pinch, *Warrior Ascetics and Indian Empires*, 38–41.

38. Davidson, *Indian Esoteric Buddhism*, 25–74; André Padoux, *The Hindu Tantric World: An Overview*, 26–27; Dowman, *Masters of Mahāmudrā*, 1–3. On the rise of Śaivism as a dominant political force in medieval India, see Alexis Sanderson, "The Śaiva Age: The Rise and Dominance of Śaivism during the Early

Medieval Period," in *Genesis and Development of Tantrism*, ed. Shingo Einoo (Japan: Sankibō Busshorin, 2009), 41–350.

39. David Gordon White, "Tantra in Practice: Mapping a Tradition," in *Tantra in Practice*, ed. David Gordon White (Princeton, NJ: Princeton University Press, 2000), 24–31; White, *Kiss of the Yogini*, 123–159.

40. Sarbacker, *Samādhi*, 111–126.

41. The case of Gautama as *tāntrika* is discussed in John Powers, *A Concise Introduction to Tibetan Buddhism* (Ithaca, NY: Snow Lion, 2008), 68.

42. White, *Kiss*, 67–93; Alexis Sanderson, "Śaivism and the Tantric Traditions," in *The World's Religions*, ed. Stewart Sutherland et al. (London: Routledge, 1988), 671–672.

43. Hatley, "What Is a Yoginī? Towards a Polythetic Definition," 23–24. Women's possession ritualism traditions are of significant import in Hinduism, in some cases representing a framework for spiritual authority parallel to that of priestly orthodoxy. See for example, Kathleen M. Erndl, *Victory to the Mother: The Hindu Goddess of Northwest India in Myth, Ritual, and Symbol* (New York: Oxford Univ. Press, 1993), 105–134; Smith, *The Self Possessed*, 68–75.

44. Sanderson, "Śaivism and the Tantric," 664.

45. Sanderson, "Śaivism and the Tantric," 668–669.

46. Flood, "The Śaiva Traditions," 208–209.

47. One practice that exemplifies Pāśupata antinomiansim is the emulation of animal behavior, such as a cow or deer. Andrew J. Nicholson, "Dialogue and Genre in Indian Philosophy," in *Dialogue in Early South Asian Religions: Hindu, Buddhist, and Jain Traditions*, ed. Brian Black and Laurie L. Patton (London & New York: Routledge, 2016), 165. Within Theravāda Buddhist narrative, such practices are critiqued by Gautama Buddha as leading to rebirth as an animal, but they also appear with a more positive appraisal in the *Mahābhārata*. Alexandra van der Geer, "Introduction," in *Animals in Stone: Indian Mammals Sculptured through Time*, ed. Alexandra van der Geer (Boston: Brill, 2008), 35.

48. Andrew J. Nicholson, "Is Yoga Hindu? On the Fuzziness of Religious Boundaries," *Common Knowledge* 19, no. 3 (2013): 494.

49. Sanderson, "Śaivism and the Tantric," 668, 690–696. Alexis Sanderson, "Śaivism: Trika Śaivism," in *Encyclopedia of Religion*, ed. Lindsay Jones (Detroit, MI: Macmillan Reference USA, 2005).

50. Douglas Renfrew Brooks, "The Ocean of the Heart: Selections from the Kulārṇava Tantra," in *Tantra in Practice*, ed. David Gordon White (Princeton, NJ: Princeton University Press, 2000), 347–360; Stuart Ray Sarbacker, "Indo-Tibetan Tantrism as Spirit Marriage," in *Perceiving the Divine through the Human Body: Mystical Sensuality*, ed. Thomas Cattoi and June McDaniel (New York: Palgrave Macmillan, 2011), 29–43; Paul E. Muller-Ortega, *The Triadic Heart of Śiva: Kaula*

Tantricism of Abhinavagupta in the Non-Dual Shaivism of Kashmir (Albany, NY: SUNY Press, 1989), 57–58. Dates follow those proposed in Gudrun Bühnemann, *Maṇḍalas and Yantras in the Hindu Traditions* (Leiden: Brill, 2003), 52; Gudrun Bühnemann, "On Puraścaraṇa: Kulārṇavatantra, Chapter 15," in *Ritual and Speculation in Early Tantrism: Studies in Honour of André Padoux*, ed. André Padoux and Teun Goudriaan (Albany, NY: SUNY Press, 1992), 61. The *Kubjikāmatatantra* is often viewed as formative in the development of tantric conceptions of *cakra* and *nāḍī*. Mallinson and Singleton, *Roots of Yoga*, xix–xx.

51. Gavin D. Flood, "The Purification of the Body," in *Tantra in Practice*, ed. David Gordon White (Princeton, NJ: Princeton University Press, 2000), 509.

52. D. Dennis Hudson, "Tantric Rites in Āṇṭāl's Poetry," in *Tantra in Practice*, ed. David Gordon White (Princeton, NJ: Princeton University Press, 2000), 211.

53. Sanjukta Gupta, "The Pāñcarātra Attitude to Mantra," in *Understanding Mantras*, ed. Harvey P Alper (Albany, NY: SUNY Press, 1989), 224–248; Sanjukta Gupta, "Yoga and Antaryāga in Pāñcarātra," in *Ritual and Speculation in Early Tantrism: Studies in Honour of André Padoux*, ed. André Padoux and Teun Goudriaan (Albany, NY: SUNY Press, 1992), 175–208.

54. Flood, "The Purification of the Body."

55. Marion Rastelli, "Yoga in the Daily Routine of the Pāñcarātrins," in *Yoga in Transformation*, ed. Phillip A. Maas and Karin Preisendanz (Göttingen: Vienna University Press, 2018), 225–252.

56. Mittal, Thursby, and Erndl, "Śākta," 154–155.

57. Sanderson, "Śaivism and the Tantric," 688–689.

58. Sanderson, "Śaivism and the Tantric," 688–689.

59. Sanderson, "Śaivism and the Tantric," 678.

60. Robert E. Buswell and Donald S. Lopez, eds., *The Princeton Dictionary of Buddhism* (Princeton, NJ: Princeton University Press, 2014), 55.

61. Lance S. Cousins, "Aspects of Esoteric Southern Buddhism," in *Indian Insights: Buddhism, Brahmanism and Bhakti*, ed. Peter Connolly and Sue Hamilton (London: Luzac Oriental, 1997), 185–207.

62. John Newman, "Vajrayoga in the Kālacakra Tantra," in *Tantra in Practice*, ed. David Gordon White (Princeton, NJ: Princeton University Press, 2000), 587.

63. David B. Gray, *The Cakrasamvara Tantra (the Discourse of Śrī Heruka), (Śrīherukābhidhāna): A Study and Annotated Translation* (New York: American Institute of Buddhist Studies, 2007), 35–54. On Śaiva imagery in Buddhist tantras, see also Snellgrove, *Indo-Tibetan Buddhism*, 152–160.

64. Paul Dundas, "The Jain Monk Jinapati Sūri Gets the Better of a Nāth Yogī," in *Tantra in Practice*, ed. David Gordon White (Princeton, NJ: Princeton University Press, 2000), 231–232. See also Paul Dundas, "Losing One's Mind and Becoming Enlightened: Some Remarks on the Concept of Yoga in Śvetāmbara

Jainism and Its Relations to the Nāth Siddha Tradition," in *Yoga: The Indian Tradition*, ed. David Carpenter and Ian Whicher (London: RoutledgeCurzon, 2003), 130–42; Paul Dundas, "Becoming Gautama: Mantra and History in Śvetāmbara Jainism," in *Open Boundaries: Jain Communities and Cultures in Indian History*, ed. John E. Cort (Albany, NY: SUNY Press, 2000), 231–338.

65. Olle Qvarnström, "Jain Tantra: Divinatory and Meditative Practices of the Twelfth-Century Yogaśāstra of Hemacandra," in *Tantra in Practice*, ed. David Gordon White (Princeton, NJ: Princeton University Press, 2000), 595–601. Somadeva Vasudeva, "The Śaiva Yogas and Their Relation to Other Systems of Yoga," *RINDAS Series of Working Papers: Traditional Indian Thoughts*, no. 26 (2017): 1–17.

66. Damien Keown et al., *Buddhism: A Dictionary Of* (Oxford: Oxford University Press, 2004), 293.

67. The term *sūkṣmaśarīra* is used here in a conventional sense to indicate conceptions of a "subtle body." Given alternate meanings of that expression in Indian literature, some authors use other terms, such as the "yogic body" (perhaps intimating the Sanskrit *yogaśarīra* or *yogadeha*). Mallinson and Singleton, *Roots of Yoga*, 171ff; Douglas Djurdjevic and Shukdev Singh, *Sayings of Goraknāth: Annotated Translation of the Gorakh Bānī* (New York: Oxford University Press, 2019), 9.

68. Anton Zigmund-Cerbu, "The Ṣaḍaṅgayoga," *History of Religions* 3, no. 1 (1963): 131–132. The example given in Zigmund-Cerbu shows the common *dhyāna*-factors to *sūtra* and *tantra* practice.

69. White suggests this list may have developed from an earlier three-word list, and that the term *maithuna* refers to sexual fluids, not the sexual act itself. White, *Kiss*, 83–85. The term *mudrā* may alternately refer to fermented grain (alcohol), a seal or gesture, possession, or a consort. Bruce M. Sullivan, *Historical Dictionary of Hinduism* (Lanham, MD & London: The Scarecrow Press, 1997), 78; Loriliai Biernacki and Oxford University Press, *Renowned Goddess of Desire Women, Sex, and Speech in Tantra* (New York: Oxford University Press, 2008), 97–98, 254 n.17.

70. White, *Kiss*, 219–257.

71. On the complexities of the dynamic between the literal and symbolic application of tantric ideology, see Christian K. Wedemeyer, *Making Sense of Tantric Buddhism: History, Semiology, and Transgression in the Indian Traditions* (New York: Columbia University Press, 2013).

72. Snellgrove, *Indo-Tibetan Buddhism*, 251.

73. Snellgrove, *Indo-Tibetan Buddhism*, 293–294.

74. Snellgrove, *Indo-Tibetan Buddhism*, 248.

75. Heinrich von Stietencron, "Cosmographic Buildings of India: The Circles of the Yoginīs," in *"Yogini" in South Asia: Interdisciplinary Approaches*, ed. István Keul (London & New York: Routledge, Taylor & Francis Group, 2013), 70; Sarbacker, *Samādhi*, 120.

76. Von Stietencron, "Cosmographic Buildings of India: The Circles of the Yoginīs," 72–73; Alexis Sanderson, "Vajrayāna: Origin and Function," in *Buddhism into the Year 2000: International Conference Proceedings* (Bangkok: Dhammakaya Foundation, 1994), 87–102.

77. Hatley, "What Is a Yoginī? Towards a Polythetic Definition," 23–24; Sarbacker, *Samādhi*, 119–26.

78. Hatley, "What Is a Yoginī?," 21–31.

79. Hausner, "The Category of the Yoginī as a Gendered Practitioner."

80. Serinity Young, *Courtesans and Tantric Consorts: Sexualities in Buddhist Narrative, Iconography and Ritual* (New York & London: Routledge, 2004), 140–142.

81. An argument articulated at length in Shaw, *Passionate Enlightenment*. On the notion of the *yoginī* as a "threshold" deity, see Sarbacker, *Samādhi*, 120.

82. Gudrun Bühnemann, "The Śāradātilakatantra on Yoga: A New Edition and Translation of Chapter 25," *Bulletin of the School of Oriental and African Studies, University of London* 74, no. 2 (2011): 205–235.

83. Navjivan Rastogi, "The Yogic Disciplines of the Monistic Śaiva Tantric Traditions of Kashmir: Threefold, Fourfold, and Six-Limbed," in *Ritual and Speculation in Early Tantrism: Studies in Honour of André Padoux*, ed. André Padoux and Teun Goudriaan (Albany, NY: SUNY Press, 1992), 257–258.

84. Friedrich Otto Schrader, *Introduction to the Pāñcarātra and the Ahirbudhnya Saṃhitā* (Madras: Adyar Library and Research Centre, 1973), 124.

85. Wallace, *The Inner Kālacakratantra*, 25–26.

86. Wallace, *Inner*, 25–28; Günter Grönbold, *The Yoga of Six Limbs: An Introduction to the History of Ṣaḍaṅgayoga*, trans. Robert L. Hütwohl (Santa Fe, NM: Spirit of the Sun Publications, 1996), 3–17. Two different texts appear under the title *Gorakṣaśataka*, one of which had been transmitted earlier as the *Vivekamārtaṇḍa*, which is the version indicated here. James Mallinson, "The Original Gorakṣaśataka," in *Tantra in Practice*, ed. David Gordon White (Princeton, NJ: Princeton University Press, 2000), 262–266.

87. Wallace, *Inner*, 26.

88. Grönbold, *Yoga of Six Limbs*, 11.

89. Wallace, *Inner*, 29.

90. Wallace, *Inner*, 27.

91. Rastogi, "Yogic Disciplines, 247; Paul E. Muller-Ortega, *Triadic Heart*, 38–39.

92. Paul E. Muller-Ortega, "Becoming Bhairava: Meditative Vision in Abhinavagupta's Parātrīśikā-Laghuvṛtti," in *The Roots of Tantra*, ed. Katherine Anne Harper and Robert L Brown (Albany, NY: SUNY Press, 2002), 213–230; Rastogi, "Yogic Disciplines," 265–270.

93. Paul E. Muller-Ortega, "'Tarko Yogāṅgam Uttamam': On Subtle Knowledge and the Refinement of Thought in Abhinavagupta's Liberative Tantric Method," in *Theory and Practice of Yoga: Essays in Honor of Gerald James Larson*, ed. Knut A. Jacobsen (Leiden & Boston: Brill, 2005), 181–212.

94. Muller-Ortega, "'Tarko,'" 186–192. On the first two grounds, the import of *jñāna* and the painfulness of yoga *sādhana*, Abhinavagupta appears to parallel Śaṅkara's critique of *aṣṭāṅgayoga*.

95. Muller-Ortega, "'Tarko,'" 186–192.

96. Rastogi, "Yogic Disciplines," 255–256.

97. James Mallinson, "The Yogī's Latest Trick," *Journal of the Royal Asiatic Society* 24, no. 1 (January 2014): 169–170.

98. Grönbold, *Yoga of Six Limbs*, 19–20.

99. McDaniel, *Offering Flowers, Feeding Skulls*, 9–10; Mani Rao, *Living Mantra: Mantra, Deity, and Visionary Experience Today* (Cham: Palgrave Macmillan, 2018), 5–8.

100. Gudrun Bühnemann, "The Six Rites of Magic," in *Tantra in Practice*, ed. David Gordon White (Princeton, NJ: Princeton University Press, 2000), 447–462.

101. Bühnemann, "Six Rites," 448.

102. Sanderson, "Śaivism and the Tantric," 694–699; Newman, "Vajrayoga in the Kālacakra Tantra," 593.

103. Per Kvaerne, "On the Concept of Sahaja in Indian Buddhist Tantric Literature," *Temenos* 11 (1975): 88–135. Buddhist and Vaiṣṇava traditions focused on the *sahaja* state are sometimes referred to as *sahajiyā* traditions, and both appear to have had sexual components. Colas, "History of Vaiṣṇava Traditions: An Esquisse," 263–264. The term *sahaja* was also used extensively by both Gorakṣanātha and Kabīr. David N. Lorenzen, Adrián Muñoz, and David N. Lorenzen, eds., "Religious Identity in Gorakhnath and Kabir," in *Yogi Heroes and Poets: Histories and Legends of the Nāths* (Albany, NY: SUNY Press, 2011), 19–49.

104. Though there are householder Nāths as well, which are discussed in David N. Lorenzen and Adrián Muñoz, eds., *Yogi Heroes and Poets: Histories and Legends of the Nāths* (Albany, NY: SUNY Press, 2011).

105. On the significance of the number 84, which also appears as an enumeration of forms of yoga *āsana*, see Gudrun Bühnemann, *Eighty-Four Āsanas in Yoga: A Survey of Traditions, with Illustrations* (New Delhi: D.K. Printworld, 2007), 26; Ron Davidson, *Indian Esoteric Buddhism: A Social History of the Tantric Movement* (New York & Chichester: Columbia University Press, 2005), 308–309.

106. Various classifications of *siddha* types and orders is discussed in David Gordon White, *The Alchemical Body: Siddha Traditions in Medieval India* (Chicago

& London: University of Chicago Press, 2007), 2–10. White is particularly interested in the Rasa Siddhas, who practiced alchemy and utilized a set of common disciplines and terminology shared with other Siddha lineages.

107. George Weston Briggs, *Gorakhnāth and the Kānphaṭa Yogīs* (Delhi: Motilal Banarsidass, 1998), 1–2. On the initiation of Nāth ascetics, see Véronique Bouillier, *Monastic Wanderers: Nāth Yogī Ascetics in Modern South Asia* (London: Routledge, 2018), 40–68.

108. Briggs, *Gorakhnāth and the Kānphaṭa Yogīs*, 21–22; Gorakṣanātha and M.L. Gharote, *Siddhasiddhāntapaddhatiḥ: A Treatise on the Nātha Philosophy* (Lonavla: The Lonavla Yoga Institute, 2005), vii.

109. Briggs, *Gorakhnāth and the Kānphaṭa Yogīs*, 15–16. *Cannabis* use among the Nāths is discussed in White, *The Alchemical Body*, 2007, 118–119, 412 n220.

110. James Mallinson, "Nāth Sampradāya," in *Brill's Encyclopedia of Hinduism*, ed. Knut Jacobsen et al. (Leiden & Boston: Brill, 2011), 410. See also Bouillier, *Monastic Wanderers*, 301–319.

111. *Haṭhapradīpikā* 1.5–9. Though these names vary in spelling considerably among manuscripts.

112. Kalyani Mallik, *Siddha-Siddhānta-Paddhati and Other Works of the Nātha Yogīs* (Poona: Poona Oriental Book House, 1954), 23; Sanderson, "Śaivism and the Tantric," 681.

113. Mallinson, "Nāth Sampradāya," 423. This "internalization" of the tantric ritual process is the larger focus of White, *Kiss of the Yogini*. Abhinavagupta refers to a figure named Matsyendra in his *Tantrāloka*. See Mallik, *Siddha-Siddhānta-Paddhati and Other Works of the Nātha Yogīs*, 9. For a discussion of the *Masyendrasaṃhitā* and its genealogical role in the development of the Nātha teachings, including a discussion of its usage of *yogāṅga*, see Csaba Kiss, "The Masyendrasaṃhitā: A Yoginī-Centered Thirteenth-Century Text from the South Indian Śāmbhava Cult," in *Yogi Heroes and Poets: Histories and Legends of the Naths*, ed. David N. Lorenzen and Adrián Muñoz (Albany, NY: SUNY Press, 2011), 143–162.

114. An overview of the formative figures and practices of the Nāths can be found in Bouillier, *Monastic Wanderers*, 11–39.

115. Mallik, *Siddha-Siddhānta-Paddhati and Other Works of the Nātha Yogīs*, 1–2.

116. Mallinson, "Nāth Sampradāya," 421.

117. Mallik, *Siddha-Siddhānta-Paddhati and Other Works of the Nātha Yogīs*, 4–5. Discussed at length in David N. Lorenzen and Muñoz, *Yogi Heroes and Poets*, 109–141.

118. Mallik, *Siddha-Siddhānta-Paddhati and Other Works of the Nātha Yogīs*, 3–4.

119. Mallinson, "The Yogī's Latest Trick," January 2014, 173. Mallinson argues that in its broadest sense the term *layayoga*, the "yoga of dissolution," may refer to a range of different practices of meditation, visualization, and *kuṇḍalinī*-raising. See James Mallinson, "Śāktism and Haṭhayoga," in *Goddess Traditions in Tantric Hinduism: History, Practice, and Doctrine*, ed. Bjarne Wernicke Oleson (London: Routledge, 2016), 115–119.

120. Mallinson, "The Yogī's Latest Trick," January 2014, 177. The *Amaraughaprabodha* is, in turn, likely largely derived from the Buddhist *Amṛtasiddhi*, as discussed below.

121. The Nāths are inheritors of the practice of the Dakṣināmnāya tradition of Kaula Śaivism, which is focused on worship of the goddesses Bālasundarī or Tripurāsundarī, having moved on from the earlier Paścimāmnāya tradition, which is no longer extant. Mallinson, "Nāth Sampradāya," 142.

122. Mallinson, "The Yogī's Latest Trick," January 2014, 174 n38.

123. One such appearance is in the *Yogabīja*. Jason Birch, "The Meaning of Hatha in Early Hathayoga," *Journal of the American Oriental Society* 131, no. 4 (2011): 527–534.

124. Birch, "Meaning of Hatha," 535.

125. Mallinson, "Yoga: Haṭha Yoga," 2011; Birch, "Meaning of Hatha," 545–546. As noted above, Mallinson argues that the Buddhist *Amṛtasiddhi* appears to be a primary source for much of the later *haṭhayoga* materials. James Mallinson, "The Amṛtasiddhi: Haṭhayoga's Tantric Buddhist Source Text," in *Śaivism and the Tantric Traditions: A Festschrift for Alexis Sanderson*, ed. Dominic Goodall, Shaman Hatley, and Harunaga Isaacson (Leiden: Brill, Forthcoming); James Mallinson, "Kālavañcana in the Konkan: How a Vajrayāna Haṭhayoga Tradition Cheated Buddhism's Death in India," *Religions* 10, no. 4 (April 2019): 273. Schaeffer has noted the fluidity of religious boundaries suggested by the notion that a Buddhist practitioner should seek to become "Śiva, lord of yogins," a central theme of the *Amṛtasiddhi*. Kurtis R. Schaeffer, "The Attainment of Immortality: From Nāthas in India to Buddhists in Tibet," *Journal of Indian Philosophy* 30, no. 6 (2002): 515–533.

126. Mallinson, "Yoga: Haṭha Yoga," 2011; Birch, "Meaning of Hatha," 545–546.

127. Mallinson, "Yoga: Haṭha Yoga," 2011; Birch, "Meaning of Hatha," 545–546.

128. Mallinson, "Nāth Sampradāya," 423–424; David N. Lorenzen, Muñoz, and Lorenzen, "Religious Identity in Gorakhnath and Kabir," 31–32.

129. James Mallinson, "Yoga: Haṭha Yoga," in *Brill's Encyclopedia of Hinduism*, ed. Knut Jacobsen et al. (Leiden & Boston: Brill, 2011), 773; Mallinson, "Śāktism and Haṭhayoga," 2016, 115–119. Mallinson notes the referencing of *laya* as a form of "dissolution" in *prakṛti* in *Yogasūtra* verse 1.19. Mallinson, 115 n55.

130. Birch, "Meaning of Hatha," 542–543; Birch, "Rājayoga," 404–407. However, the application of these terms is often inconsistent, one important example being the identification of Pātañjala Yoga alternately with *haṭhayoga* or *rājayoga*. Though it is common for Pātañjala Yoga to be referred to as *rājayoga* in the modern context, this identification appears to be relatively recent in origin. See Birch, "Rājayoga." Pātañjala Yoga can be argued to be genealogically related to both subtypes (*haṭha-* and *rājayoga*), given the instrumentality of the external *aṅga* (*yama*, *niyama*, *āsana*, *prāṇāyāma*, and *pratyāhāra*) in attaining a productive mental state, and emphasis in the system on the achievement of yogic mastery (*saṃyama*) through the cultivation of *samādhi* as a basis for yogic power (*vibhūti*) and liberation (*kaivalya*), the latter being associated with the cessation of mental activity (*cittavṛttinirodha*). In some cases, the terminology of Rājayoga refers instead to sexual practices. Birch, "Rājayoga," 409–412.

131. Birch refers to Svātmārāma's *Haṭhaprādipikā* as "dismantling" the fourfold system of yoga in order to create a "complete" system of *haṭhayoga*. Birch, "Meaning of Hatha," 527.

132. Mallinson, "Yoga: Haṭha Yoga," 2011, 771–772.

133. Larson and Bhattacharya, *Encyclopedia of Indian Philosophies*, 476. According to Birch, the *aṣṭāṅgayoga* model of the *Yogayājñavalkya* was, along with a similar system found in the *Vasiṣṭhasaṃhitā* (12th century CE), influential on the development of later *haṭhayoga* texts and practice. Birch, "Meaning of Hatha," 528, 548.

134. *Siddhasiddhāntapaddhati* 2.32–39. The introduction of the *aṣṭāṅgayoga* system is identical to *Yogasūtra* 2.29, though the *aṣṭāṅgayoga* factors themselves are defined in novel ways. Gorakṣanātha and Gharote, *Siddhasiddhāntapaddhatiḥ*, 43–47; Mallik, *Siddha-Siddhānta-Paddhati and Other Works of the Nātha Yogīs*, 60–61.

135. T.R. Srinivasa Ayyangar, *The Yoga Upanisads* (Fremont, CA: Jain Publ., 2006), 301–325.

136. Jean Varenne, *Yoga and the Hindu Tradition* (Chicago: University of Chicago Press, 1976), 195–222; Ayyangar, *The Yoga Upanisads*, 97, 448–449.

137. Birch, "Rājayoga," 540–541.

138. *Haṭhaprādipikā* 1.34–35. In some modern versions of the *Haṭhapradīpikā*, the practices of *yama* and *niyama* are presented as the foundation of yoga, numbered as 10 of each factor, expanding on those developed in *aṣṭāṅgayoga*, including terms such as faith (*āstikya*) and charity (*dāna*), following the expanded model found in medieval and Purāṇic texts. As was the case with the Purāṇic framing of yoga as six- (*ṣaḍ*) or eight-limbed (*aṣṭāṅga*), the utilization of limbed frameworks in broader *haṭhayoga* texts is interwoven with innovations in the practice of the limbs, expanding the *yama* and *niyama* factors, *āsana* repertoire, variations of

prāṇāyāma, and techniques associated with *bindu*-restriction and the awakening *śakti* or *kuṇḍalinī*, such as *mudrā* and *bandha*. For a larger discussion of post-Pātañjala Yoga systems of *yama* and *niyama*, see Jacqueline Hargreaves and Jason Birch, "The Yamas and Niyamas: Part 2—Medieval and Modern Views," *Yoga Scotland Magazine*, no. 50 (2016): 36–39.

139. Ayyangar, *The Yoga Upanisads*, 10.

140. *Haṭhapradīpikā*, 1.34, 38.

141. Seth Powell, "Etched in Stone: Sixteenth-Century Visual and Material Evidence of Śaiva Ascetics and Yogis in Complex Non-Seated Āsanas at Vijayanagara," *Journal of Yoga Studies* 1, no. 1 (2018): 45–106.

142. *Haṭhapradīpikā*, 1.33. Jason Birch, "The Proliferation of Āsana-s in Late-Medieval Yoga Texts," in *Yoga in Transformation*, ed. Phillip A. Maas and Karin Preisendanz (Göttingen: Vienna University Press, 2018), 101–170.

143. Birch, "Proliferation," 134–142.

144. *Haṭhapradīpikā* 2.73–77.

145. Guy Beck, "Sacred Music and Hindu Religious Experience: From Ancient Roots to the Modern Classical Tradition," *Religions* 10, no. 85 (February 2019): 1–15.

146. This is also referred to as *sarasvatīcālana*, and aims to rouse *kuṇḍalinī*. Mallinson notes the association of the goddess Sarasvatī with speech, and thus the tongue. Mallinson, "The Original Gorakṣaśataka," 257–258.

147. *Haṭhapradīpikā* 3.95, 98.

148. White, *The Alchemical Body*, 2007, 2–10. On the *Haṭhapradīpikā* and the retention of sexual fluids, see pp. 273–281.

149. It might be further noted that many Indian Sādhus and Sādhvīs, especially within Śaiva traditions, have and continue to use *cannabis* extensively as a sacramental substance in order to enhance relaxation, contemplation, and devotion, and as a catalyst for social bonding. The use of *cannabis* among Śaiva *sādhu* traditions in Nepal is documented in S.L. Acharya et al., "Cannabis, Lord Shiva and Holy Men: Cannabis Use Among Sadhus in Nepal," *Journal of Psychiatrists' Association of Nepal* 3, no. 2 (2014): 9–14. Hausner notes the particular import of the *cilam* pipe in social and ritual life surrounding the *sādhu*-domain fire pit (*dhūni*). Sondra L. Hausner, *Wandering with Sadhus: Ascetics in the Hindu Himalayas* (Bloomington: Indiana University Press, 2008), 120–123. See also Michael R. Aldrich, "Tantric Cannabis Use in India," *Journal of Psychedelic Drugs* 9, no. 3 (July 1977): 227–233; Theodore M. Godlaski, "Shiva, Lord of Bhang," *Substance Use & Misuse* 47, no. 10 (July 2012): 1067–1072. The use of *cannabis* and opium among contemporary Bāuls is discussed in Fabrizio M. Ferrari, "Mystic Rites For Permanent Class Conflict: The Bauls Of Bengal, Revolutionary Ideology and Post-Capitalism," *South Asia Research* 32, no. 1 (2012): 21–38.

150. *Haṭhapradīpikā*, 4.3–4.

151. Snellgrove, *Indo-Tibetan Buddhism*, 183.

152. Reginald Ray, "Mahāsiddhas," in *Encyclopedia of Religion* (Detroit, MI: Macmillan Reference USA, 2005).

153. Dowman, *Masters of Mahāmudrā*, 2, 313ff., 372ff.

154. Davidson, *Indian Esoteric Buddhism*, 170–171.

155. Sarbacker, "Swami Ramdev: Modern Yoga Revolutionary," 121–124.

156. Shashi Bhushan Dasgupta, *Obscure Religious Cults* (Calcutta: Firma KLM, 1995), 99–103.

157. Snellgrove, *Indo-Tibetan Buddhism*, 429–430. Tibetan literature associates Padmasambhava's arrival in Tibet with an appeal for assistance from the Indian monk Śāntarakṣita, whose attempt to establish the first Tibetan monastery, Samye, was facing natural disasters as a result of the opposition of local deities. Padmasambhava is said to have overcome the opposition of the local deities, which may be, in part, an allegory for the success of tantric and yogic methodologies over those of *sūtra* methodologies in propagating Buddhism in its early phase in Tibet.

158. Roger R. Jackson, "Saraha's Queen Dohās," in *Yoga in Practice*, ed. David Gordon White (Princeton, NJ: Princeton University Press, 2012), 163.

159. Jackson, "Saraha's Queen," 163.

160. Jackson, "Saraha's Queen," 164.

161. Jackson, "Saraha's Queen," 163.

162. Dasgupta, *Obscure*, 51–77.

163. Dasgupta, *Obscure*, 114–122. On the Bāul tradition, see Jeanne Openshaw, *Seeking Bāuls of Bengal* (Cambridge: Cambridge University Press, 2004), 26–28. On the connections between various sectarian Sahajiyā sects and their modes of ritual life, see also Richard Widdess, "Caryā and Cacā: Change and Continuity in Newar Buddhist Ritual Song," *Asian Music*, 2004, 7–41.

164. Rin-chen-rnam-rgyal, Herbert V. Guenther, and Nāḍapāda, *The Life and Teaching of Nāropa*, UNESCO Collection of Representative Works (Oxford: Clarendon Press, 1963), 131–248.

165. Rin-chen-rnam-rgyal, Guenther, and Nāḍapāda, 132–249.

166. Ringu Tulku, "Six Yogas of Naropa," *Bulletin of Tibetology*, no. 1–4 (1982): 40–44.

167. Ian A. Baker, "Tibetan Yoga: Somatic Practice in Vajrayāna Buddhism and Dzogchen," in *Yoga in Transformation*, ed. Phillip A. Maas and Karin Preisendanz (Göttingen: Vienna University Press, 2018), 345. A variant on the Sanskrit is *nāḍī-vāyu-adhisāra*. See Gnas-mdo Karma-chags-med, Rinpoche Gyatrul, and B. Alan Wallace, *A Spacious Path to Freedom: Pratical Instructions on the Union of Mahāmudrā and Atiyoga* (Ithaca, NY: Snow Lion, 1998), 222.

168. Bryan J. Cuevas, *The Hidden History of The Tibetan Book of the Dead* (New York: Oxford University Press, 2003), 53.

169. Alf Hiltebeitel, "Hinduism," in *Encyclopedia of Religion*, ed. Lindsay Jones (Detroit, MI: Macmillan Reference USA, 2005), 4007.

170. Hiltebeitel, "Hinduism." However, influence and integration did occur in numerous ways, directly and indirectly. Phillip B. Wagoner, " 'Sultan among Hindu Kings': Dress, Titles, and the Islamicization of Hindu Culture at Vijayanagara," *The Journal of Asian Studies* 55, no. 4 (1996): 851–880.

171. John Newman, "Islam in the Kālacakra Tantra," *Journal of the International Association of Buddhist Studies* 21, no. 2 (1998): 311–371.

172. Carl W. Ernst, "Muslim Interpreters of Yoga," in *Yoga: The Art of Transformation*, ed. Debra Diamond (Washington, DC: Arthur M. Sackler Gallery, Smithsonian Institution, 2013), 59–67.

173. Ernst, "Muslim Interpreters."

174. Clark, "Sādhus and Sādhvīs," 8021.

Chapter 8

1. Kulke and Rothermund, *A History of India*, 170–171.

2. For a discussion of the complex relationship between British colonialism and caste, see Nicholas B. Dirks, *Castes of Mind* (Princeton, NJ: Princeton University Press, 2011).

3. Kulke and Rothermund, *History of India*, 194–248.

4. Pinch, *Warrior Ascetics and Indian Empires*, 104–147; David Gordon White, *Sinister Yogis* (Chicago & London: University of Chicago Press, 2009), 198–254.

5. An overview of the impact of colonialism in India, including the impact of Christian monotheism on Hindu traditions, can be found in Sharada Sugirtharajah, "Colonialism," in *Studying Hinduism: Key Concepts and Methods*, ed. Sushil Mittal and Gene Thursby (New York: Routledge, 2009), 85–97. The critique of the colonial Orientalist model developed by Said and others is discussed in Carl Olson, "Orientalism," in *Studying Hinduism: Key Concepts and Methods*, ed. Sushil Mittal and Gene Thursby (New York: Routledge, 2009), 290–300.

6. Sarbacker, "Reclaiming the Spirit through the Body: The Nascent Spirituality of Modern Postural Yoga," 101–102.

7. Sarbacker, "Reclaiming," 108–111.

8. Alter, *Yoga in Modern India*, 73–108. Kuvalayananda pioneered laboratory research into the effects of practices such as posture (*āsana*) and breath control (*prāṇāyāma*) on physiological factors such as blood oxygen concentration. More recently, scientists have utilized technology such as electroencephalography (EEG)

and magnetic resonance imaging (MRI) to measure the neurobiological effects of yoga. See, for example, Dusana Dorjee, *Neuroscience and Psychology of Meditation in Everyday Life* (London: Taylor and Francis, 2017); Daniel Goleman and Richard J. Davidson, *Altered Traits: Science Reveals How Meditation Changes Your Mind, Brain, and Body* (New York: Avery, 2017); B. Alan Wallace, *Contemplative Science: Where Buddhism and Neuroscience Converge* (New York & Chichester: Columbia University Press, 2009).

9. See, for example, the discussion of "superstructures" in Frits Staal, *Exploring Mysticism: A Methodological Essay* (Berkeley: University of California Press, 1988), 168–189. Staal expresses considerable skepticism regarding the value of physiological models in the study of religious experience. See Staal, 102–120.

10. Jason Birch, "Premodern Yoga Traditions and Ayurveda: Preliminary Remarks on Shared Terminology, Theory, and Praxis," *History of Science in South Asia* 6 (2018): 1–83; Joseph S. Alter, "Yoga, Nature Cure, and 'Perfect' Health: The Purity of the Fluid Body in an Impure World," in *Yoga in Transformation*, ed. Phillip A. Maas and Karin Preisendanz (Göttingen: Vienna University Press, 2018), 439–461.

11. Mark Singleton, "Yoga, Eugenics, and Spiritual Darwinism in the Early Twentieth Century," *International Journal of Hindu Studies* 11, no. 2 (2007): 125–146. This might be further connected to interest in yoga in European fascism, including within the context of Nazi Germany. See, for example, Douglas T. McGetchin, *Indology, Indomania, and Orientalism: Ancient India's Rebirth in Modern Germany* (Madison, NJ: Fairleigh Dickinson University Press, 2009), 179; C.G. Jung, *The Psychology of Kundalini Yoga: Notes of the Seminar given in 1932*, ed. Sonu Shamdasani (London: Routledge, 2015), xl–xlii. A relationship parallels connections between gymnastics and fascist movements in midcentury Europe, especially in Italy and Germany. Singleton, "Yoga, Eugenics," 135, 137. Alessio Ponzio, *Shaping the New Man: Youth Training Regimes in Fascist Italy and Nazi Germany* (Madison: University of Wisconsin Press, 2015), 72, 100, 112; Hans Bonde, *Gymnastics and Politics: Niels Bukh and Male Aesthetics* (Copenhagen: Museum Tusculanum Press, University of Copenhagen, 2006), 127–164. With respect to related ideas of the "biomoral" in modern yoga, see Patrick McCartney, "Spiritual Bypass and Entanglement in Yogaland (योगस्तान): How Neoliberalism, Soft Hindutva, and Banal Nationalism Facilitate Yoga Fundamentalism," *Politics and Religion Journal* 13, no. 1 (March 2019): 137–175.

12. Sarah Strauss and Laura Mandelbaum, "Consuming Yoga, Conserving the Environment: Transcultural Discourses on Sustainable Living," in *Yoga Traveling: Bodily Practice in Transcultural Perspective* (Heidelberg: Springer, 2013).

13. Strauss and Mandelbaum, "Consuming Yoga," 184–187. Also discussed in Sarah Schrank, "American Yoga: The Shaping of Modern Body Culture in the United States," *American Studies* 53, no. 1 (May 2014): 169–181.

14. This was particularly inspired by William Broad, *The Science of Yoga: The Risks and the Rewards* (New York: Simon & Schuster, 2012). See also Joanna Walters, "'Yoga Can Damage Your Body' Article Throws Exponents off-Balance," *The Observer*, January 14, 2012, sec. Life and Style, https://www.theguardian.com/lifeandstyle/2012/jan/14/yoga-can-damage-body-row; Matthew Remski, "Yoga Can Injure You. Here's How to Find a Class That Won't," *The Guardian*, October 27, 2016, sec. Opinion, https://www.theguardian.com/commentisfree/2016/oct/27/yoga-injury-class-regulation-bad-practitioners. A more personal exploration of the ways in which modern postural yoga practitioners test the limits of their bodies can be found in Benjamin Lorr, *Hell-Bent: Obsession, Pain, and the Search for Something like Transcendence in Competitive Yoga* (New York: St. Martin's Press, 2014).

15. On yoga as a "science" in Vivekananda, see Vivekananda, Nikhilananda, and Ramakrishna Vedanta Centre, *Vivekananda: The Yogas and Other Works* (New York & Bourne End: Ramakrishna Vedanta Centre, 1984), 579–585. On India's material needs, see page 194.

16. According to Gandhi, political freedom and personal freedom are inseparable, with the control of a nation being dependent on people's ability exert self-control over themselves. Dennis Dalton, *Mahatma Gandhi: Nonviolent Power in Action* (New York: Columbia University Press, 2012), 12–29.

17. Singleton, "Yoga, Eugenics," 136–138.

18. Joseph S. Alter, *Gandhi's Body: Sex, Diet, and the Politics of Nationalism*, Critical Histories (Philadelphia: University of Pennsylvania Press, 2000), 83–112.

19. The popular yoga guru Swami Ramdev's teachings and writings bear the common thread of an uplifting of all of Indian society through the widespread and universal practice of yoga. Sarbacker, "Swami Ramdev: Modern Yoga Revolutionary," 367–369. With respect to transnational anglophone yoga, see, for example, Jois, *Yoga Mala*, 3–6.

20. Modi's affiliation with the Bharatiya Janata Party (BJP) situates him within a strong nationalist pro-Hindu ideological and political framework. The BJP's ideological partner, the Rashtriya Swayam Sevak Sangh (RSS), has actively included the practice of yoga within its system of physical discipline. Joseph S. Alter, "Yoga Shivir," in *Yoga in the Modern World: Contemporary Perspectives*, ed. Mark Singleton and Jean Byrne (New York: Routledge, Taylor & Francis, 2008), 36–48. Modi drew significant publicity for his public performance of yoga *āsana* among large crowds in New Delhi during the inaugural International Day of Yoga celebration. "Yoga Day: Origin, Theme, Importance, Celebrations, All FAQs Answered," NDTV.com, https://www.ndtv.com/india-news/fourth-international-yoga-day-theme-importance-celebrations-all-you-need-to-know-1870368. The underlying political implications, especially with respect modern Hindu Nationalist politics is discussed in Patrick McCartney, "The Unintended Consequences

of International Day of Yoga," *Daily O* (blog), June 21, 2018, https://www.dailyo.in/variety/international-yoga-day-soft-power-hindutva-narendra-modi-deen-dayal-upadhyaya-hedgewar/story/1/25021.html.

21. Vandana Shiva, "Nature as the Feminine Principle," in *This Sacred Earth Religion, Nature, Environment*, ed. Roger S. Gottlieb (New York: Routledge, 2004), 382–385. Shiva is particularly well known as an advocate for the preservation of India's delicate ecosystems.

22. Sarbacker, "Swami Ramdev: Modern Yoga Revolutionary," 364–367.

23. Discussed in Sallie B. King, *Socially Engaged Buddhism* (Honolulu, Hawai'i: University of Hawai'i Press, 2009); Christopher S. Queen, *Engaged Buddhism: Buddhist Liberation Movements in Asia* (Albany, NY: SUNY Press, 2011).

24. Strauss and Mandelbaum, "Consuming Yoga, Conserving the Environment: Transcultural Discourses on Sustainable Living," 194–197.

25. Andrea R. Jain, *Selling Yoga: From Counterculture to Pop Culture* (New York: Oxford University Press, 2015), 106–108.

26. Rageshri Ganguly, "Surya Namaskar in MP School Curriculum," *The Times of India*, January 21, 2016, https://timesofindia.indiatimes.com/city/bhopal/Surya-Namaskar-in-MP-school-curriculum/articleshow/50551191.cms; Agencies, "Despite Controversy, 50 Lakh MP Students Participate in 'Surya Namaskar,'" *Indian Express*, January 12, 2012, http://indianexpress.com/article/news-archive/regional/despite-controversy-50-lakh-mp-students-participate-in-surya-namaskar. The performance of the Sun Salutation and the chanting of the mantra *oṃ* were dropped from the agenda of the International Day of Yoga in India due to a similar controversy. Agencies; FP Staff, "No Surya Namaskar on International Yoga Day: Modi Govt Axes Asana to Soothe Irate Muslim Groups," *Firstpost*, June 9, 2015, http://www.firstpost.com/india/no-surya-namaskar-on-international-yoga-day-modi-govt-axes-asana-to-soothe-irate-muslim-groups-2286068.html; PTI, "Yoga Day 2016 Diluted: No 'Suryanamaskar,' Chanting of 'OM' Not Compulsory," *First post*, June 8, 2016, http://www.firstpost.com/india/yoga-day-2016-diluted-no-suryanamaskar-chanting-of-om-not-compulsory-2823704.html. Government officials in India have argued that over forty-seven Arab countries had endorsed the International Day of Yoga and that it was not, as some had claimed, an attempt to spread the Hindutva agenda. IANS, "'Why Are Indian Muslims Opposing Yoga When Muslim Countries Are Supporting It?,'" *The New Indian Express*, June 13, 2015, http://www.newindianexpress.com/nation/2015/jun/13/Why-Are-Indian-Muslims-Opposing-Yoga-When-Muslim-Countries-Are-Supporting-It-768643.html.

27. Anna Leach, "One of San Francisco's Toughest Schools Transformed by the Power of Meditation," *The Guardian*, November 24, 2015, https://www.theguardian.com/teacher-network/2015/nov/24/san-franciscos-toughest-schools-transformed-meditation; Sarah Augenstein, "The Introduction of Yoga in German

Schools: A Case Study," in *Yoga Traveling: Bodily Practice in Transcultural Perspective* (Heidelberg: Springer, 2013), 155–172; Amit Anand Choudhary, "Yoga in India: Supreme Court Says No to Compulsory Yoga Education in Schools," *Times of India*, August 8, 2017, http://timesofindia.indiatimes.com/india/supreme-court-says-no-to-compulsory-yoga-education-in-schools/articleshow/59967483.cms.

28. These legal actions against schools have found support, at times, from evangelical Christian organizations, such at the National Center for Law and Policy. Amanda Holpuch, "Evangelical Christian Group Helps Sue California School over Yoga Classes," *The Guardian*, January 10, 2013, sec. US news, http://www.theguardian.com/world/2013/jan/10/christian-parents-sue-california-school-yoga. One highly publicized case was decided in favor of proponents of a public school yoga program in Encinitas, California, sponsored by the Jois Foundation. In that case, the judge argued that while yoga does have religious roots, it can be sufficiently adapted to suit public education. Tony Perry, "Legal Fight against Yoga in Encinitas Schools Is Finished," *Los Angeles Times*, June 12, 2015, http://www.latimes.com/local/lanow/la-me-ln-yoga-legal-fight-20150612-story.html; Holpuch, "Evangelical Christian Group." See also Jain, *Selling Yoga*, 163–164.

29. Choudhary, "Yoga in India."

30. A question interrogated at length in David Gordon White, *The Yoga Sutra of Patanjali: A Biography* (Princeton, NJ & Oxford: Princeton University Press, 2014).

31. An important figure in the modern valorization of the *Yogasūtra* and its practice within a Sāṃkhya-Yoga lineage of monasticism is Hariharānanda Āraṇya (1869–1947), whose translation and interpretation of Sāṃkhya-Yoga literature was lauded by scholars as well as practitioners of yoga. Knut A. Jacobsen, "In Kapila's Cave," in *Theory and Practice of Yoga: Essays in Honour of Gerald James Larson*, ed. Knut A. Jacobsen (Leiden & Boston: Brill, 2005), 334. For a fuller discussion of Āraṇya's work, see Jacobsen, *Yoga in Modern Hinduism*.

32. Though it is difficult to differentiate which techniques early modern yoga figures learned from a *guru* and which they reconstituted from textual traditions or adapted from Indian and European physical culture, they brought a reconstructive coherence to modern yoga that helped make yoga accessible for modern and global audiences. See, for example, Sivananda's eclectic presentation of religion, philosophy, and postural practice in his work *Yoga Asanas*. Sivananda, *Yoga Asanas* (Sivanandanagar: Divine Life Society, 1979).

33. Mallinson, "Yoga: Haṭha Yoga," 2011, 9–11.

34. Sarbacker, "Swami Ramdev," 368–369.

35. A framing that was inspired, in part, by Vivekananda and the Vedanta Society. Leigh Eric Schmidt, *Restless Souls: The Making of American Spirituality* (Berkeley: University of California Press, 2012), 162–165. For further discussion of

yoga and the Spiritual-But-Not-Religious (SBNR) phenomenon, see William Barclay Parsons, ed., *Being Spiritual but Not Religious: Past, Present, Future(s)* (New York: Routledge, 2018); Robert C. Fuller, *Spiritual, but Not Religious: Understanding Unchurched America* (Oxford: Oxford University Press, 2010).

36. White, *Yoga Sutra of Patanjali*, 116.

37. Stephen N. Hay, *Sources of Indian Tradition: Volume Two, Modern India and Pakistan* (New Delhi: Penguin, 1992), 72–82. A similar line of thinking is found in Gandhi's writing and discourses, which emphasizes a universal and transcendent truth (*satya*) to be held to (*āgraha*) with intense discipline in order to obtain both spiritual and political freedom. According to Gandhi, this truth (*satya*) is also God, a transcendent and universal reality that is perceived in fragments by human beings who are limited in their capacity to know totality.

38. Such universalism is rooted, in part, in the conception that human psychology, the domain of meditation, is distinct from religion and culture. See, for example, Robert Wright, *Why Buddhism Is True: The Science and Philosophy of Meditation and Enlightenment* (New York: Simon & Schuster, 2017). On the larger of issues of the fluidity of the sacred/secular boundary, see Ann Gleig, *American Dharma: Buddhism Beyond Modernity* (New Haven, CT: Yale University Press, 2019). The universalism of Modern Buddhism also includes an emphasis on the universality of the teachings of the Buddha (*buddhadharma*), such as the pervasiveness of suffering (*duḥkha*) and the enduring value of cultivating kindness (*maitrī*), compassion (*karuṇā*), and wisdom (*prajñā*).

39. Richard Hughes Seager, *Buddhism in America* (New York: Columbia University Press, 2012), 257–263.

40. Singleton, *Yoga Body*, 81.

41. Elizabeth De Michelis, *A History of Modern Yoga: Patañjali and Western Esotericism* (London & New York: Continuum, 2005), 80–83; Arthur Versluis, *American Transcendentalism and Asian Religions* (New York: Oxford University Press, 1994), 55–82; Stefanie Syman, *The Subtle Body: The Story of Yoga in America* (New York: Farrar, Straus and Giroux, 2010), 26–36.

42. White, *Yoga Sutra*, 103–115.

43. "Harmonial Gymnastics" is a term coined by Singleton. See Singleton, *Yoga Body*, 143–162.

44. On the larger context and reception of Radhakrishnan's views, see Ann Taves, "Religious Experience," in *Encyclopedia of Religion*, ed. Lindsay Jones, 2nd ed., vol. 11 (Detroit, MI: Macmillan Reference USA, 2005), 7736–7750.

45. For a larger discussion of Huxley's countercultural role, see Morgan Shipley, *Psychedelic Mysticism: Transforming Conciousness, Religious Experiences, and Voluntary Peasants in Postwar America* (Lanham, MD: Lexington Books, 2015). On Huxley's experiments and their impact on Buddhist spirituality, see Douglas

Osto, *Altered States: Buddhism and Psychedelic Spirituality in America* (New York: Columbia University Press, 2018).

46. Paul Vitello, "Hindu Group Stirs Debate in Fight for Soul of Yoga," *The New York Times*, November 27, 2010, https://www.nytimes.com/2010/11/28/nyregion/28yoga.html. On the issue of yoga, spirituality, and cultural appropriation, see Mary Grace Antony, "'It's Not Religious, But It's Spiritual:' Appropriation and the Universal Spirituality of Yoga," *Journal of Communication & Religion* 37, no. 4 (Winter 2014): 63–81.

47. Michael Day, "Exorcists Warn Vatican over 'Beautiful Young Vampires' and Satanic Yoga," *Independent UK*, May 13, 2015, http://www.independent.co.uk/news/world/europe/exorcists-warn-vatican-over-beautiful-young-vampires-and-satanic-yoga-10174001.html; Cathy Lynn Grossman, "Yoga Poses Dangers to Genuine Christian Faith: Theologian," *USA Today*, September 20, 2010, http://content.usatoday.com/communities/Religion/post/2010/09/yoga-christian-mohler-palin/1#.WYt75oplCEI; Jalil Hamid, "Malaysia Backs down from Yoga Ban amid Backlash," *Reuters*, November 26, 2010, https://www.reuters.com/article/us-malaysia-islam-yoga-idUSTRE4AP2CA20081126; Fiona Connor, "Anglican Church Bans Yoga for 'Worshipping False Gods,'" *Daily Mail Online*, June 12, 2017, https://www.dailymail.co.uk/news/article-4597742/Anglican-Church-bans-yoga-worshipping-false-gods.html; Rebecca Allison, "Vicar in a Twist over Yoga Classes in Church Hall," *The Guardian*, August 28, 2002, sec. UK news, https://www.theguardian.com/uk/2002/aug/28/religion.world.

48. William Kremer, "Does Doing Yoga Make You a Hindu?," *BBC News*, November 21, 2013, http://www.bbc.com/news/magazine-25006926. The fact that Hindu identity is often "naturalistic" in nature (i.e., one is "born" a Hindu) further complicates this issue. On the larger issue of yoga and Hindu identity, see Nicholson, "Is Yoga Hindu?"

49. Sarbacker, "The Icon of Yoga: Patañjali as Serpent-King in Modern Yoga," 31–35; Sarbacker, "The Numinous and Cessative in Modern Yoga," 173–177. McCartney argues that such trappings are also potentially an entry point for anglophone yoga practitioners, knowingly or unknowingly, into Hindu nationalism. Patrick McCartney, "Politics beyond the Yoga Mat: Yoga Fundamentalism and the 'Vedic Way of Life,'" *Global Ethnographic*, no. 4 (May 2017): 1–18.

50. Philip Deslippe, "The Swami Circuit: Mapping the Terrain of Early American Yoga," *Journal of Yoga Studies* 1 (May 2018): 5–44. The formative Krishnamacharya tradition's success in Mysore and greater India was, in part, said to have been a function of the success of public performances by Krishnamacharya and by his disciples, such as B.K.S. Iyengar. T.K.V Desikachar and Richard H. Cravens, *Health, Healing and beyond: Yoga and the Living Tradition of Krishnamacharya*

(New York: Aperture, 1998), 87–96. Iyengar is particularly noteworthy, given that his publications, such as *Light on Yoga*, and numerous television appearances in Europe and the United States led to his considerable celebrity and the exposure of a wide international audience to postural yoga practice. Frederick M. Smith and Joan White, "Becoming an Icon: B.K.S. Iyengar as a Yoga Teacher and a Yoga Guru," in *Gurus of Modern Yoga*, ed. Mark Singleton and Ellen Goldberg (New York & London: Oxford University Press, 2014), 131; Suzanne Newcombe, "The Institutionalization of the Yoga Tradition: 'Gurus' B.K.S. Iyengar and Yogini Sunita in Britain," in *Gurus of Modern Yoga*, ed. Mark Singleton and Ellen Goldberg (New York & London: Oxford University Press, 2014), 155–156.

51. On the explosion of books on yoga in the post-Vivekananda era, see Alter, *Yoga in Modern India*, xvii–xx. On the importance of visual media in the twentieth and twenty-first centuries, see Singleton, *Yoga Body*, 163–174; Sarbacker, "Swami Ramdev," 355–358.

52. Sarbacker, "Numinous," 176–177; Sarbacker, "Power and Meaning in the Yogasūtra of Patañjali," 206–218.

53. On Pierre Bernard, Blanche DeVries, and Theos Bernard, see Hugh B. Urban, "The Omnipotent Oom: Tantra and Its Impact on Modern Western Esotericism," *Esoterica: Journal of Esoteric Studies* 3 (2001): 218–259; Joseph Laycock, "Yoga for the New Woman and the New Man: The Role of Pierre Bernard and Blanche DeVries in the Creation of Modern Postural Yoga," *Religion and American Culture: A Journal of Interpretation* 23, no. 1 (2013): 101–136; Paul G Hackett, *Theos Bernard, the White Lama: Tibet, Yoga, and American Religious Life* (New York: Columbia University Press, 2012); Stefanie Syman, *Subtle Body: The Story of Yoga in America* (New York: Farrar, Straus & Giroux, 2011), 80–141; Robert Love, *The Great Oom: The Improbable Birth of Yoga in America* (New York: Viking, 2010).

54. Elliott Goldberg, *The Path of Modern Yoga: The History of an Embodied Spiritual Practice* (Rochester, VT: Inner Traditions, 2016), 16–27. According to Goldberg, the rise of the Indian middle class is connected to the various factors (such as a focus on health and beauty) that characterize modern yoga.

55. Jain, *Selling Yoga*, 81. Multiple facets of the yoga industry are explored in Søren Askegaard and Giana M. Eckhardt, "Glocal Yoga: Re-Appropriation in the Indian Consumptionscape," *Marketing Theory* 12, no. 1 (March 2012): 45–60.

56. Suzanne Newcombe, "Spaces of Yoga: Towards a Non-Essentialist Understanding of Yoga," in *Yoga in Transformation*, ed. Phillip A. Maas and Karin Preisendanz (Göttingen: Vienna University Press, 2018), 549–573; Stuart Ray Sarbacker, "The Yoga Studio as Locus Numinous" (Yogascapes Japan, Kyoto, Japan, 2018).

57. Sarbacker, "Icon of Yoga," 32–34; Sarbacker, "Numinous," 176–177.

58. Mary Billard, "Yoga's New Wave," *The New York Times*, April 23, 2010, sec. Fashion & Style, https://www.nytimes.com/2010/04/25/fashion/25yoga.html.

59. "Yoga Alliance Designations," accessed August 9, 2017, https://www.yogaalliance.org/Credentialing; "Accreditation—International Association of Yoga Therapists (IAYT)," accessed February 8, 2019, https://www.iayt.org/page/AccreditationLanding. The Yoga Alliance also credentials programs, which serve as a primary basis for students to obtain authorization. There has been considerable debate in the anglophone yoga community with regards to the value of Yoga Alliance certification. See, for example, James Brown, "Yoga Alliance Is Ruining Yoga," *American Yoga School* (blog), January 7, 2014, https://americanyoga.school/yoga-alliance-ruining-yoga/; "A Response to James Brown," Yoga Alliance, January 9, 2014, https://www.yogaalliance.org/Home/A_Response_to_James_Brown.

60. "Scheme for Voluntary Certification of Yoga Professionals," accessed February 8, 2019, http://www.yogacertification.qci.org.in The Yoga Certification Board is advised by a number of prominent Indian yoga gurus, including Swami Ramdev, Sadhguru Jaggi Vasudev, and Swami Chidananda Saraswati. On the emergence of academic and vocational programs in the study of religion in India in the twenty-first century, see Christopher Chapple, "The Academic Study of Yoga in India," *Journal of Dharma Studies* 3 (2020): 107–120.

61. See, for example, "How to Become Certified Iyengar Yoga Teacher?," accessed August 9, 2017, http://bksiyengar.com/modules/Teacher/certeach.htm; "Certification Process: IYNAUS, Iyengar Yoga: National Association of the United States," accessed August 9, 2017, https://iynaus.org/teach/certification; Genny Wilkinson-Priest, "Does Authorization Matter?," *Elephant Journal*, November 13, 2013, https://www.elephantjournal.com/2013/11/does-authorization-matter-genny-wilkinson-priest.

62. Krishna Ravi Srinivas, "Intellectual Property Rights and Traditional Knowledge: The Case of Yoga," *Economic and Political Weekly* 42, no. 27/28 (2007): 2866–2871.

63. Samantha Masunaga, "YogaWorks Chain Stretches Its Reach in California with Deal," *Los Angeles Times*, June 4, 2015, http://www.latimes.com/business/la-fi-yogaworks-acquisition-20150604-story.html.

64. Mara Santilli, "Is Your Beat-Bumping Hip-Hop Yoga Class Still Considered 'Real' Yoga?," *Shape Magazine*, October 10, 2017, https://www.shape.com/fitness/trends/fast-paced-yoga-with-music-trend; Jake Panasevich, "Why Yoga Is More Than a Workout," *US News & World Report* (blog), March 11, 2015, https://health.usnews.com/health-news/blogs/eat-run/2015/03/11/why-yoga-is-more-than-a-workout. Even established modern yoga teachers take different positions as to what makes yoga distinct from gymnastics or calisthenics, whether it be, for

example, the observance of the *yama* and *niyama* factors or the use of *haṭha*-type practices such as *prāṇāyāma* and *bandha*. Sarbacker, "Reclaiming the Spirit through the Body: The Nascent Spirituality of Modern Postural Yoga," 103–104.

65. Jain, *Selling Yoga*, 95–98, 164.

66. Mark Singleton, "Transnational Exchange and the Genesis of Modern Postural Yoga," in *Yoga Traveling*, ed. Beatrix Hauser, Transcultural Research—Heidelberg Studies on Asia and Europe in a Global Context (Springer International Publishing, 2013), 39.

67. Eilidh Macrae, *Exercise in the Female Life-Cycle in Britain, 1930–1970* (London: Palgrave Macmillan, 2016), 22; David L Chapman, *Sandow the Magnificent: Eugen Sandow and the Beginnings of Bodybuilding* (Urbana; Chicago: University of Illinois Press, 2006), 190–91.

68. Singleton, "Transnational Exchange," 42–44.

69. Alter, *Gandhi's Body*, 83–112.

70. Goldberg, *Path of Modern Yoga*, 249–274; Mark Singleton, "Transnational Exchange," 47–48; Suzanne Newcombe, "The Revival of Yoga in Contemporary India," in *Oxford Research Encyclopedia of Religion* (Oxford University Press, May 24, 2017).

71. See, for example, Yoga Journal, Yoga Alliance, and Ipsos Public Affairs, "2016 Yoga in America Study," National Study, accessed September 10, 2017, https://www.yogaalliance.org/Portals/0/2016%20Yoga%20in%20America%20Study%20RESULTS.pdf. The study claims that as of 2015, 52% of yoga teachers in the United States were women and 48% are men. Among practitioners, 72% were women and 28% men.

72. See, for example, the discussion of Spiritualism and Theosophy in Ann Braude, *Radical Spirits: Spiritualism and Women's Rights in Nineteenth-Century America* (Bloomington, Ind: Indiana University Press, 2013).

73. An example of the latter being the "Yoga and Body Image Coalition." "Home," Yoga and Body Image Coalition, accessed August 10, 2017, http://ybicoalition.com The question of whether yoga is a "feminizing" enterprise, i.e. whether it is identified as a predominantly female gendered practice, is an interesting one, as it suggests the inversion of the principally male-gendered notions of yoga practice characteristic of Indian traditions. On the particular role of *Yoga Journal* in the construction of the "image" of yoga, see Pirkko Markula, "Reading Yoga: Changing Discourses of Postural Yoga on the Yoga Journal Covers," *Communication & Sport* 2, no. 2 (June 1, 2014): 143–71.

74. See, for example, the representation of Krishnamacharya's views in *Śrī Krishnamacharya the Pūrnācārya* (Chennai: Krishnamacharya Yoga Mandiram, 1997), 75.

75. Jois, *Yoga Mala*, 7–12; B.K.S. Iyengar, *Light on Pranayama: The Yogic Art of Breathing* (New York: Crossroad, 1981), 97.

76. Ruth Vanita, "'Free to Be Gay': Same-Sex Relations in India, Globalised Homophobia and Globalised Gay Rights," in *Human Rights in Postcolonial India*, ed. O.P. Dwivedi and V.G. Julie Rajan (Basingstoke: Taylor & Francis, 2016), 326.

77. Vanita, "'Free to Be Gay,'" 326. In this context, Shankar argues that Ayyappa, a popular deity in southern India, is considered a child of the male gods Śiva and Viṣṇu (in his female form as Mohinī), that all individuals have male and female components, and therefore that discrimination based upon sexual orientation does not make sense. Critics, however, have viewed Shankar's ideas that sexual orientation is malleable and that heterosexuality is "normal" as problematic. Shreya Thakur, "India Rejects Section 377: Sri Sri Ravi Shankar Comes Out In Support," *Republic World*, September 6, 2018, https://www.republicworld.com/india-news/general-news/india-rejects-section-377-sri-sri-ravi-shankar-comes-out-in-support.

78. A wide-ranging exploration of issues regarding sexual orientation, gender, and ethnic identity can be found in Beth Berila, Melanie Klein, and Chelsea Jackson Roberts, eds., *Yoga, the Body, and Embodied Social Change: An Intersectional Feminist Analysis* (Lanham, MD: Lexington Books, 2016).

79. Bhagwan Shree Rajneesh, *Tantra, Spirituality & Sex* (San Francisco; New York: The Rainbow Bridge, 1976).

80. The complexity of the relationship between yoga and sex in the United States is documented in Andrea R. Jain, "Subversive Spiritualities: Yoga's Complex Role in the Narrative of Sex and Religion in the Twentieth-Century United States," in *Devotions and Desires: Histories of Sexuality and Religion in the Twentieth-Century United States*, ed. Gillian Frank, Bethany Moreton, and Heather Rachelle White, 2018, 34–53.

81. Markula, "Reading Yoga."

82. Sarah Schrank, "Naked Yoga and Sexualization of Asana," in *Yoga, the Body, and Embodied Social Change: An Intersectional Feminist Analysis*, ed. Beth Berila, Melanie Klein, and Chelsea Jackson Roberts (Lanham, MD: Lexington Books, 2016), 155–74.

83. Vindu Goel, "India Offers Atypical Video Challenges," *The New York Times*, December 27, 2015, sec. Technology, https://www.nytimes.com/2015/12/28/technology/bollywood-and-us-media-giants-try-to-induce-indians-to-pay-for-video.html; "10 Bollywood Actresses Who Do YOGA to Stay Fit!," indiatimes.com, June 17, 2015, http://www.indiatimes.com/news/world/10-bollywood-actresses-who-do-yoga-to-stay-fit-294040.html.

84. Anya P Foxen, *Biography of a Yogi: Paramahansa Yogananda and the Origins of Modern Yoga*, 2017, 49–55; Robert Love, "Fear of Yoga," *Columbia Journalism Review* 45, no. 4 (2006): 80–90. In addition to Ramacharaka (Walter

Atkinson), famous occultists such as Alistair Crowley fashioned "yogi" personas. Laycock, "Yoga for the New Woman and the New Man," 115–16.

85. Emily S. Rueb, "Yoga Adjustments Tread a Fine Line of Personal Space," *The New York Times*, February 11, 2011, sec. N.Y. / Region, https://www.nytimes.com/2011/02/13/nyregion/13stretch.html; Antonia Blyth, "How #MeToo Shook the Yoga World," ELLE, March 29, 2018, https://www.elle.com/beauty/health-fitness/a19609192/how-metoo-shook-the-yoga-world/; Patrick McCartney, "Downward Facing Dogs, Core Indian Values and Institutionalised Rape of Children," *Sociology International Journal* 2, no. 6 (2018): 748–52; Matthew D. Remski, *Practice and All Is Coming: Abuse, Cult Dynamics and Healing in Yoga and Beyond* (New Zealand: Embodied Wisdom Publishing, 2019).

86. Amanda Lucia, "Guru Sex: Charisma, Proxemic Desire, and the Haptic Logics of the Guru-Disciple Relationship," *Journal of the American Academy of Religion* 86, no. 4 (November 29, 2018): 953–988.

87. Sarbacker, "Power and Meaning," 213. The potential for abuse by a *guru* is analogous in a number of ways to problem of transference in psychological therapy, in which the imbalance in power and authority between therapist and patient leads to a vulnerability and susceptibility of the patient to both psychological control and sexual abuse.

88. A topic discussed in Georg Feuerstein, *Holy Madness: Spirituality, Crazy-Wise Teachers, and Enlightenment* (Prescott, AZ: Hohm Press, 2006).

89. Bühnemann, *Eighty-Four Āsanas in Yoga*, 143–144; Birch, "The Proliferation of Āsana-s in Late-Medieval Yoga Texts."

90. Jayatarāma and Swāmī Maheśānanda, *Jogapradīpyakā of Jayatarāma* (Lonavla: Kaivalyadhama S.M.Y.M Samiti, 2006), 14.

91. In the modern Ashtanga Vinyasa Yoga system of K. Pattabhi Jois, for example, the standard duration of time a posture is held is five breaths, though it may be extended for pedagogical or therapeutic purposes. Jois, *Yoga Mala*, 48 n.40. Jois presented his system as an expression of traditional *aṣṭāṅgayoga*, though Singleton has noted the possibility that *aṣṭāṅga* may also refer to an eight-limbed prostration incorporated into Indian physical culture. Singleton, *Yoga Body*, 205–206. In contrast, in Iyengar yoga, it is common to hold an *āsana* for several minutes to deepen the experience of the posture and to find precise proprioception-based alignment within the posture. The focus on proprioception and relaxation in modern yoga may both point to a deeper "spiritual" dimension to the physicalism of postural yoga and further demonstrate postural yoga's connection to European physical culture. See Mark Singleton, "Salvation through Relaxation: Proprioceptive Therapy and Its Relationship to Yoga," *Journal of Contemporary Religion* 20, no. 3 (October 2005): 289–304.

92. Carrico Mara, "Contraindications of Yoga," in *Injury Prevention for Fitness Instructors* (San Diego: IDEA Health & Fitness Association, 2001), 38–44; "Yoga's

Growing Threat of Legal Liability," www.counterpunch.org, accessed February 8, 2019, https://www.counterpunch.org/2014/07/04/yogas-growing-threat-of-legal-liability.

93. The Śaiva-Śākta seven-*cakra* model appears extensively in modern traditions, in part due to its representation in Orientalist and New Age literature in the nineteenth and twentieth century, such as Sir John Woodroffe's *The Serpent Power* and the Theosophist C.W. Leadbetter's work, *The Chakras*. John George Woodroffe, *The Serpent Power: Being the Ṣaṭ-Cakra-Nirūpana and Pādukā-Pañcaka: Two Works on Laya-Yoga* (New York: Dover Publications, 2000); C.W. Leadbeater, *The Chakras* (Wheaton, IL: Quest Books/Theosophical Publishing House, 2013).

94. Lola Williamson, *Transcendent in America: Hindu-Inspired Meditation Movements as New Religion* (New York & London: New York University Press, 2010), 111; Ellen Goldberg, "Swami Kṛpālvānanda: The Man Behind Kripalu Yoga," in *Gurus of Modern Yoga*, ed. Mark Singleton and Ellen Goldberg (Oxford & New York: Oxford University Press, 2014), 177.

95. The larger notion that *āsana* and *prāṇāyāma* have positive, especially purificatory, effects on the subtle body and on latent emotional states is a pervasive conception in modern yoga traditions. In some cases, the use of a particular yoga *āsana* may be viewed as effecting a particular *cakra*, and thereby having both spiritual and physical effects, such as the plow posture (*halāsana*) having an effect on the "throat *cakra*" (*viśuddhicakra*), which is viewed as governing the power of speech, and on the thyroid gland in the neck, associated with physical metabolism. Lucy Lidell, Narayani, and Fausto Dorelli, *The Sivananda Companion to Yoga* (New York: Simon & Schuster, 1983), 34–64. See also, for example, the exploration of the body's role in trauma mechanisms discussed in David Emerson and Elizabeth K. Hopper, *Overcoming Trauma through Yoga: Reclaiming Your Body* (Berkeley, CA: North Atlantic Books, 2011).

96. An ethnographically oriented discussion of modern *satsaṅg* that focuses on its emotive dimension can be found in Patrick McCartney, "Suggesting Śāntarasa in Shanti Mandir's Satsaṅga: Ritual, Performativity and Ethnography in Yogaland," *Ethnologia Actualis* 17, no. 2 (December 2017): 81–122.

97. For a discussion of the dynamics of *sevā* in a contemporary, transnational organization, see Amanda J. Lucia, " 'Give Me Sevā Overtime': Selfless Service and Humanitarianism in Mata Amritanandamayi's Transnational Guru Movement," *History of Religions* 54, no. 2 (November 2014): 188–207.

98. On the role of *kīrtan* in anglophone, transnational yoga, see Stephen Jacobs, "Yoga Jam: Remixing Kīrtan in the Art of Living," *The Journal of Religion and Popular Culture*, March 17, 2017. For an examination of the social and political aspects of *kīrtan* in the Indian context, see Anna C. Schultz, *Singing a Hindu Nation: Marathi Devotional Performance and Nationalism* (New York: Oxford University Press, 2013).

99. See, for example, Peggy Cappy, *Yoga for All of Us: A Modified Series of Traditional Poses for Any Age and Ability* (New York: St. Martin's Press, 2007), 46; Glennon Doyle Melton, *Carry On, Warrior: Thoughts on Life Unarmed* (New York: Simon and Schuster, 2013), 190. One of the few textual references to a similar phrasing can be found in Adam Smith, *Powers of Mind* (New York: Summit Books: 1982), 379. Smith's work represents the phrase being spoken by a follower of Sri Aurobindo. The larger context of *namaste*, including with reference to the performance of worship (*pūjā*), which the reference to the divine may emulate, is discussed in A.K. Krishna Nambiar, *Namaste: Its Philosophy and Significance in Indian Culture* (Delhi: Spiritual India Pub. House, 1979).

100. This is not to say that postural systems of yoga are not contemplative in nature or do not contain an aspect of mental discipline. In fact, postural systems often have either an implicit or explicit meditative component. Traditional systems of yoga recognized the interdependence of physical and psychic life, acknowledging how physical practices affect mental states and how meditative practices affect the physical body. However, there is an important distinction in techniques that cultivate discipline of physical and of mental activities. This is illustrated, for example, by the distinction between the utilization of a plurality of *āsana* forms and *vinyāsa* and *prāṇāyāma* techniques as opposed to an emphasis upon seated, static meditation.

101. See, for example, the discussion of the meditation-science interface in B. Alan Wallace, *Contemplative Science: Where Buddhism and Neuroscience Converge* (New York & Chichester: Columbia University Press, 2009).

102. On Terapanth Jain traditions, see Jain, *Selling Yoga*, 58–62.

103. Jason Birch and Jaqueline Hargreaves, "Yoganidrā: An Understanding of the History and Context.," n.d., http://theluminescent.blogspot.co.uk/2015_01_01_archive.html.

104. De Michelis, *History of Modern Yoga*, 2005, 110–112.

105. Aravamudan uses the term "Guru English" to signify a distinct English language variant or "register" developed by Vivekananda and others in the propagation of Hindu-based spirituality and yoga in Europe and the United States in the late nineteenth and early twentieth century. Srinivas Aravamudan, *Guru English: South Asian Religion in a Cosmopolitan Language* (Princeton, NJ: Princeton University Press, 2011), 16–21.

106. De Michelis, *History of Modern Yoga*, 149–180.

107. White, *Yoga Sutra*, 116–142.

108. Gwilym Beckerlegge, "Eknath Ranade, Gurus, and Jīvanvrats: The Vivekananda Kendra's Promotion of the 'Yoga Way of Life,'" in *Gurus of Modern Yoga*, ed. Mark Singleton and Ellen Goldberg (New York & London: Oxford University Press, 2014), 327–350.

109. Alter, *Yoga in Modern India*, 26–28.

110. Ann Gleig and Charles I. Flores, "Remembering Sri Aurobindo and the Mother: The Forgotten Lineage of Integral Yoga," in *Gurus of Modern Yoga*, ed. Mark Singleton and Ellen Goldberg (New York & London: Oxford University Press, 2014), 40–44.

111. Kusumita P. Pedersen, "Sri Chinmoy's Work at the United Nations: Spirituality and the Power of Silence," *CrossCurrents* 60, no. 3 (September 2010): 339–351.

112. Mohandas Karamchand Gandhi, *Non-Violent Resistance (Satyagraha)* (Mineola, NY: Dover Publications, 2001), 37–46.

113. Vinay Lal, "Nakedness, Nonviolence, and Brahmacharya: Gandhi's Experiments in Celibate Sexuality," *Journal of the History of Sexuality* 9, no. 1–2 (April 2000): 105–136.

114. Richard H. Davis, *The Bhagavad Gita: A Biography* (Princeton, NJ: Princeton University Press, 2016), 82–105.

115. Davis, *Bhagavad Gita*, 82–105. These may be, in turn, contrasted with the critique offered by neo-Buddhist and Dalit activist B.K. Ambedkar. Meera Nanda, "Ambedkar's Gita," *Economic and Political Weekly* 51, no. 49 (2016): 38–45.

116. Anthony Parel, *Gandhi's Philosophy and the Quest for Harmony* (Cambridge: Cambridge University Press, 2008), 118; Gandhi, *Non-Violent Resistance*, 93–94.

117. Singleton, "Transnational Exchange," 46; "Madhavdas Ji," KaivalyaDham Yoga Institute, https://kdham.com/madhavdas-ji.

118. Alter, *Yoga in Modern India*, 73–108.

119. Svātmārāma and Swami Digambara, *Haṭhapradīpikā* (Lonavla, Maharashtra, India: Kaivalyadhama S.M.Y.M Samiti, 1980); Swami Maheshanandaji et al., eds., *Yoga Concordance*, 4 vols. (Lonavla, Maharashtra, India: Kaivalyadhama S.M.Y.M Samiti, 2001); "Specialised Yoga Certificate Course," KaivalyaDham Yoga Institute, https://kdham.com/specialised-yoga-certificate-course.

120. Alter, *Yoga in Modern India*, 87–88.

121. "Sri OP Tiwari Ji–IYA Governing Council," Indian Yoga Association, http://www.yogaiya.in/profile/sri-op-tiwari-ji.

122. Goldberg, *Path*, 16–27; Joseph S. Alter, "Shri Yogendra: Magic, Modernity, and the Burden of the Middle-Class Yogi," in *Gurus of Modern Yoga*, ed. Mark Singleton and Ellen Goldberg (New York & London: Oxford University Press, 2014), 62–63.

123. Alter, "Shri Yogendra: Magic, Modernity, and the Burden of the Middle-Class Yogi," 62–63; Mark Singleton, "Yoga and Physical Culture: Transnational History and Blurred Discursive Contexts," in *Routledge Handbook of Contemporary India*, ed. Knut A. Jacobsen (Abingdon, UK: Routledge, 2016), 177–178.

124. Alter, "Shri Yogendra: Magic, Modernity, and the Burden of the Middle-Class Yogi," 64.

125. Alter, "Shri Yogendra," 65.

126. Alter, "Shri Yogendra," 74–75; Santan Rodrigues, *The Householder Yogi: Life of Shri Yogendra* (Bombay: Yogendra Publications Fund, The Yoga Inst., 2008), 218–223.

127. Williamson, *Transcendent in America*, 72. Williamson notes that in addition to its success in North America, particularly in California, the SRF currently has centers in fifty-four countries.

128. Lola Williamson, *Transcendent in America: Hindu-Inspired Meditation Movements as New Religion* (New York & London: New York University Press, 2010), 66–78; Catherine Wessinger, "Hinduism Arrives in America: The Vedanta Movement and the Self-Realization Fellowship," in *America's Alternative Religions*, ed. Timothy Miller (Albany, NY: SUNY Press, 1995), 173–190.

129. Mark Singleton, "Yoga and Physical Culture: Transnational History and Blurred Discursive Contexts," in *Routledge Handbook of Contemporary India*, ed. Knut A. Jacobsen (Abingdon, UK: Routledge, 2016), 178. Walter Isaacson writes about the pervasive influence that *Autobiography of a Yogi* had on Steve Jobs, the co-founder of Apple Computer, in his biography. Walter Isaacson, *Steve Jobs* (New York: Simon & Schuster, 2015), 35, 46–47, 527.

130. Singleton, *Yoga Body*, 132–133.

131. Singleton, *Yoga Body*, 132–133.

132. And, following that, taught in the Ghosh lineage for decades. Jerome Armstrong, *Calcutta Yoga: Buddha Bose & the Yoga Family of Bishnu Ghosh and Yogananda* (US: Webstrong LLC Publishing, 2018), 244–323, 573.

133. Choudhury also claimed to have recovered from a severe knee injury under Ghosh's supervision through the practice of yoga. The Japanese origin narrative attributes the emergence of the warmed room method to a response to the Japanese winter. Armstrong, *Calcutta Yoga:* 529–538; Bikram Choudhury, *Bikram Yoga: The Guru Behind Hot Yoga Shows the Way to Radiant Health and Personal Fulfillment* (New York: HarperCollins, 2007), 24–25.

134. Jain, *Selling Yoga*, 144–146.

135. Sarah Larson, "'Bikram' and the Fraught, Telling Tale of a Yoga Phenomenon," June 27, 2018, https://www.newyorker.com/culture/podcast-dept/bikram-and-the-fraught-telling-tale-of-a-yoga-phenomenon.

136. "International Yoga Sports Federation—Rajashree Choudhury," http://www.iysf.org/about-iysf/board/rajashree-choudhur.

137. Beatrix Hauser, "Touching the Limits, Assessing Pain: On Language Peformativity, Health, and Well-Being in Yoga Classes," in *Yoga Traveling: Bodily Practice in Transcultural Perspective* (Heidelberg: Springer, 2013), 114 n.14.

138. Alter, *Gandhi's Body*, 95. Pant considered the Sun Salutation a perfect form of exercise, being universally accessible as it requires no special environment or equipment and avoids the excesses of other physical culture systems.

139. Goldberg, *Path*, 185–188.

140. Dattatraya Chintaman Mujumdar, ed., *Encyclopedia of Indian Physical Culture; a Comprehensive Survey of the Physical Education in India, Profusely Illustrating Various Activities of Physical Culture, Games, Exercises, Etc., as Handed over to Us from Our Fore-Fathers and Practised in India* (Baroda: Good Companions, 1950), 18–19, 453–458.

141. In 4.6, Rāmdās encourages the reader to perform *namaskār*, particularly to *sūrya* and the *guru*, but also to the various forms of the gods and to holy persons. It is viewed as a way of reducing enmity and guilt, and as facilitating spiritual knowledge and liberation.

142. Bhawanrao Srinivasrao Pant and Louise Morgan, *The Ten-Point Way to Health: Surya Namaskars* (London: Dent, 1956), 23–25.

143. Pant and Morgan, *The Ten-Point Way*, 33.

144. Pant and Morgan, 55–60. Though such admonitions may have been additions by Louise Morgan (see below). He recommends that women suspend practice during menstruation, adapt the practice after the fifth month of pregnancy, and suspend practice after the eighth month of pregnancy, resuming it one or more months after childbirth.

145. The section on the use of the Sun Salutation in schools correlates with the larger social and nationalist vision of Pant's work, expressed in the mass performance of the Sun Salutation by his followers in Aundh. See Alter, *Gandhi's Body*, 94–101. Pant's enthusiasm for the group performance of the Sun Salutation anticipated the contemporary mass performance of yoga in India and around the world in celebration of the International Day of Yoga.

146. Alter, *Gandhi's Body*, 94–101. Goldberg notes that Swami Sivananda viewed the Sun Salutation as a form of "sun therapy" and a warm-up exercise for yoga, as opposed to yoga proper. Goldberg, *Path*, 327–332. Birch notes that the nineteenth-century *Jyotsnā* commentary of Brahmānanda on the *Haṭhapradīpikā* warns against the practice of *sūrya-namaskāra*, due to the risk of harm to the body. Birch, "Proliferation," 139, 139 n.98.

147. Goldberg, *Path*, 275–284.

148. Goldberg, *Path*, 275–284.

149. Goldberg, *Path*, 285–294.

150. Goldberg, *Path*, 289. Pant and Morgan, *Ten-Point Way*, 36. The more recent history of the yoga mat is often associated with Angela Farmer, a student of B.K.S. Iyengar, who adapted carpet padding for use as a non-slip surface. Fernando Pagés Ruiz, "The Sticky Business + History of Yoga Mats," *Yoga Journal*, August 28, 2007, https://www.yogajournal.com/yoga-101/sticky-business. The use of the yoga mat might be compared, on some level, to the use of Tiger, Antelope, and other animal skins as a "mat" by premodern yoga practitioners. See, for example,

the qualities of various "mats" given in the fifteenth-century text of the *Puraścaraṇacandrikā* discussed in Jason Birch and Jaqueline Hargreaves, "The Religiosity of the Yoga Mat," April 18, 2016, https://www.theluminescent.org/2016/04/the-religiosity-of-yoga-mat.html.

151. Sarbacker, "Swami Ramdev," 352–355.

152. Sarbacker, "Swami Ramdev," 357. The Patañjali Yogpeeth consists of a yoga auditorium, a yoga research center, an *āyurveda* hospital and dispensary, vision and dental clinics, visitor residences and cafeterias, and an extensive library.

153. Sarbacker, "Swami Ramdev," 368.

154. Sarbacker, "Swami Ramdev," 364–367.

155. Sarbacker, "Swami Ramdev," 363–364.

156. Joanne Punzo Waghorne, "Engineering an Artful Practice: On Jaggi Vasudev's Isha Yoga and Sri Sri Ravi Shankar's Art of Living," in *Gurus of Modern Yoga*, ed. Mark Singleton and Ellen Goldberg (New York & London: Oxford University Press, 2014), 285. Vasudev's Isha Yoga system draws heavily on the language of his previous career as an engineer. See, for example, Jaggi Vasudev, *Inner Engineering: A Yogi's Guide to Joy* (New York: Spiegel & Grau, 2016).

157. "On the Ground—Sadhguru's Mission," http://isha.sadhguru.org/mission.

158. "About Us," Art of Living (India), https://www.artofliving.org/in-en/about-us.

159. Aditya Iyer, "Maha Shivratri: Protesters Urge Modi Not to Attend Isha Foundation Event," *Hindustan Times*, February 24, 2017, https://www.hindustantimes.com/india-news/maha-shivratri-protesters-urge-modi-not-to-attend-isha-foundation-event/story-LR9F1JjnIwE9uQ5je7gkJP.html.

160. White, *Yoga Sutra*, 197–224. The variations in narratives among biographies of Krishnamacharya, at minimum, convey the sense of the "multiple perspectives" possible on the life of this influential teacher.

161. Desikachar and Cravens, *Health, Healing and Beyond*, 37–39.

162. Desikachar and Cravens, *Health*, 43.

163. Singleton, *Yoga Body*, 184–190.

164. The hybridity of Krishnamacharya's system was first explored in N.E. Sjoman, *The Yoga Tradition of the Mysore Palace* (New Delhi: Abhinav Publications, 1999), 35–68.

165. Mark Singleton, M. Narasimhan, and M.A. Jayashree, "Yoga Makaranda of T. Krishnamacharya," in *Yoga in Practice*, ed. David Gordon White (Princeton, NJ: Princeton University Press, 2012), 337–342. Though drawing upon the physicalism of *haṭhayoga*, Krishnamacharya largely abandons the more visceral practices of *ṣaṭkarman*.

166. Sarbacker, "Icon of Yoga," 17–22.

167. White, *Yoga Sutra*, 211–219.

168. Newcombe, "Institutionalization," 155–157.

169. B.K.S. Iyengar, *Light on Yoga: Yoga Dipika* (New York: Schocken Books, 1979), 19–53.

170. Iyengar discourages performing *prāṇāyāma* with *āsana*, and suggests that Sūrya Namaskār can be utilized to "develop the chest" in those so desiring. Iyengar, *Light on Yoga*, 468.

171. Newcombe, "Institutionalization," 153.

172. Iyengar, like his teacher Krishnamacharya, was known to be strict and demanding of his students, sometimes striking them in the process of making adjustments, which earned him the moniker "Beat, Kick, and Slap" (i.e., B.K.S.) Iyengar. Malini Nair, "The Guru with a Stick," *The Times of India*, August 24, 2014, https://timesofindia.indiatimes.com/home/sunday-times/deep-focus/The-guru-with-a-stick/articleshow/40839884.cms.

173. Smith and White, "Becoming an Icon: B.K.S. Iyengar as a Yoga Teacher and a Yoga Guru," 129–131.

174. Smith and White, "Becoming," 131.

175. Sarbacker, "Icon of Yoga," 20–21.

176. "Patricia Walden: Lighting the Way | IYNAUS | Iyengar Yoga: National Association of the United States," https://iynaus.org/yoga-samachar/fall-2011 winter-2012/patricia-walden-lighting-way; Holly Hammond, "Meet the Innovators: Judith Hanson Lasater," *Yoga Journal*, https://www.yogajournal.com/lifestyle/meet-the-innovators-judith-hanson-lasater.

177. Singleton, *Yoga Body*, 175–210.

178. Mark Singleton and Tara Fraser, "T. Krishnamacharya, Father of Modern Yoga," in *Gurus of Modern Yoga*, ed. Mark Singleton and Ellen Goldberg, 2014, 185. Singleton, *Yoga Body*, 175–210.

179. Singleton suggests the term may be Gurkhali in origin, if not a modification of the Sanskrit *grantha*. Singleton, *Yoga Body*, 184–185; Singleton and Fraser, "T. Krishnamacharya," 92. Burley follows the Sanskrit *kuruṇṭa*, referring to a yellow flower (perhaps as an *āyurvedic* herb?). Mikel Burley, *Haṭha-Yoga: Its Context, Theory, and Practice* (Delhi: Motilal Banarsidass Publishers, 2000), 16. Smith notes Sjoman's argument that the Sanskrit term *kuruṇṭa* refers to the idea of a "puppet," and thus the quick movement of postures utilizing ropes, a practice found in Iyengar Yoga. Benjamin Richard Smith, "With Heat Even Iron Will Bend: Discipline and Authority in Ashtanga Yoga," in *Yoga in the Modern World: Contemporary Perspectives*, ed. Mark Singleton and Jean Byrne (New York: Routledge, 2008), 157 n5.

180. Birch has argued that it is possible the name *kuruṇṭa* may be derived from the author of a late medieval–early modern text of the *Haṭhābhyāsapaddhati* who was named Kapālakuraṇṭaka. The *Haṭhābhyāsapaddhati* may have been a source

for a Mysore Palace text, the *Śrītattvanidhi*, which Krishnamacharya would have been familiar with. Jaqueline Hargreaves, "Asanas Old and New," *The Luminescent* (blog), October 8, 2013, http://theluminescent.blogspot.com/2013/10. See also Birch, "Proliferation."

181. Topics discussed at length in Remski, *Practice and All Is Coming.*

182. See, for example, Richard Freeman, *The Mirror of Yoga: Awakening the Intelligence of Body and Mind* (Boston: Shambhala, 2012); Gregor Maehle, *Yoga Meditation: Through Mantra, Chakras and Kundalini to Spiritual Freedom* (Crabbes Creek, NSW: Kaivalya Publications, 2013); Stuart Ray Sarbacker and Kevin Kimple, *The Eight Limbs of Yoga: A Handbook for Living Yoga Philosophy* (New York: North Point Press, 2015).

183. Jean-Claude Garnier, "Ashtanga Yoga Research Institute," Ashtanga Yoga Institute, http://yoga-ashtanga.net/en/tag/ashtanga-yoga-research-institute.

184. Smith, "With Heat," 141–142.

185. "AYRI," http://www.astanga.it/eng/?pagina=ayri.php.

186. Beryl Bender Birch, *Power Yoga: The Total Strength and Flexibility Workout* (New York: Touchstone, 2014), 15–34.

187. Gaiam, "About Gaiam," https://www.gaiam.com/pages/about-gaiam.

188. Christopher Chapple, *Yoga and the Luminous: Patanjali's Spiritual Path to Freedom* (Albany, NY: SUNY Press, 2008), 250; Singleton, "Yoga and Physical Culture: Transnational History and Blurred Discursive Contexts," 178–179; Susan Jacobs, "Magana Baptiste," *Yoga Journal,* December 1986. Walt Baptiste was also a former Mr. America.

189. Larson and Bhattacharya, *Encyclopedia of Indian Philosophies,* 154; "Core Philosophy," Jivamukti Yoga, August 10, 2015, https://jivamuktiyoga.com/core-philosophy; Sharon Gannon and David Life, *Jivamukti Yoga* (New York: Ballantine Books, 2002).

190. Shiva Rea, *Tending the Heart Fire: Living in Flow with the Pulse of Life* (Boulder, CO: Sounds True, 2014). Another popular California-based "Flow Yoga" tradition is that of White Lotus Yoga, founded by Ganga White and Tracy Rich. Gerald James Larson and Ram Shankar Bhattacharya, *Encyclopedia of Indian Philosophies: India's Philosophy of Meditation. Yoga. Volume XII* (Motilal Banarsidass Publishe, 2008), 159.

191. Andreĭ Lappa, *Yoga, Tradition of Unification* (Kyiv: A. Lappa, 2000).

192. Sarbacker, "Yoga Studio."

193. Sarbacker, "Yoga Studio."

194. Sarbacker, "Icon of Yoga," 27–31. The icon of Patañjali is similar to a well-known one found at the Śiva temple at Chidambaram in Tamil Nadu.

195. Kausthub's role in the KYM and KHFY was impacted by allegations of improper relationships with students in 2012. Singleton and Fraser, "T. Krishnamacharya, Father of Modern Yoga," 103 n3.

196. "Teachers and Staff," Krishnamacharya Healing and Yoga Foundation, http://www.khyf.net/team.

197. See, for example T.K.V. Desikachar and Desikachar, Mekhala, *Patanjali's Yogasutra: An Exploration* (Chennai, India: Krishnamacharya Yoga Mandiram and Swathi Soft Solutions, 2000).

198. "American Viniyoga Institute—About Founder Gary Kraftsow," http://viniyoga.businesscatalyst.com/about/who-we-are/about-gary-kraftsow. See also Gary Kraftsow, "Defining Yoga Therapy: A Call to Action," *International Journal of Yoga Therapy* 20, no. 1 (October 2010): 27–29.

199. "DVDs and Videos Archives," *American Viniyoga Institute* (blog), https://www.viniyoga.com/product-category/video.

200. Michelle Goldberg, *The Goddess Pose: The Audacious Life of Indra Devi, the Woman Who Helped Bring Yoga to the West* (New York: Vintage, 2016), 14.

201. Goldberg, *The Path of Modern Yoga*, 338–340.

202. Goldberg, *Path* 342–343.

203. Goldberg, *Path* 346, 351. Goldberg, *The Goddess Pose*, 168–171.

204. Goldberg, *Path*, 348.

205. Kenneth Liberman, "The Reflexivity of the Authenticity of Haṭha Yoga," in *Yoga in the Modern World: Contemporary Perspectives*, ed. Mark Singleton and Jean Byrne (New York: Routledge, 2008), 107.

206. On the legacy of Sai Baba and his community, see Smriti Srinivas, "Sathya Sai Baba and the Repertoire of Yoga," in *Gurus of Modern Yoga*, ed. Mark Singleton and Ellen Goldberg (New York: Oxford University Press, 2014), 261–282; Hugh B. Urban, "Avatar for Our Age: Sathya Sai Baba and the Cultural Contradictions of Late Capitalism," *Religion* 33, no. 1 (January 2003): 73–93; Tulasi Srinivas, "Doubtful Illusions: Magic, Wonder and the Politics of Virtue in the Sathya Sai Movement," *Journal of Asian and African Studies* 52, no. 4 (June 2017): 381–411.

207. Strauss, *Positioning Yoga*, 36.

208. Strauss, *Positioning*, 37.

209. Strauss, *Positioning*, 37.

210. Strauss, *Positioning*, 39. "His Holiness Sri Swami Sivananda Saraswati Maharaj," http://www.dlshq.org/saints/siva.htm.

211. A summary of Sivananda's overarching views on yoga can be found in Swami Sivananda, *Essence of Yoga* (Theri-Garhwal, UP: Divine Life Society, 1988). On yoga *āsana*, see Swami Sivananda, *Yoga Asanas*, 2nd ed., Himalayan Yoga Series, no. 14 (Madras: P.K. Vinayagam, 1935).

212. Sivananda, *Yoga Asanas*.

213. Swami Sivananda, "Yoga," http://www.dlshq.org/teachings/yoga.htm.

214. Strauss, *Positioning*, 42–43.

215. McKean, *Divine Enterprise*, 164.

216. "His Holiness Sri Swami Chidananda Saraswati Maharaj," http://www.dlshq.org/saints/chida.htm; McKean, *Divine Enterprise*, 164.

217. "Welcome to Bihar Yoga Bharati—Bihar Yoga," http://www.biharyoga.net/uncategorized/welcome.

218. "Welcome to Satyananda Yoga ~ Bihar Yoga—Bihar Yoga," http://www.biharyoga.net. McCartney, "Downward Facing Dogs." These parallel recent accusations of sexual abuse directed at Swami Vishnu Devananda in Canada. See Matthew Remski, "How a #MeToo Facebook Post Toppled a Yoga Icon," https://gen.medium.com/how-a-metoo-facebook-post-toppled-a-yoga-icon-c25577185e40.

219. Integral Yoga is also the name of Satchidananda's yoga system.

220. Dean Ornish, *Dr. Dean Ornish's Program for Reversing Heart Disease* (New York: Ballantine Books).

221. Building on the success of Richard Hittleman's earlier TV series, *Yoga for Health* (1970). Jain, *Selling Yoga*, 70.

222. Strauss, *Positioning*, 41–42.

223. Strauss, *Positioning*, 41–42.

224. "Yogi Gupta | Dharma Yoga Center New York City," https://dharmayogacenter.com/resources/yogi-gupta/; "Master Yoga Chart | Dharma Yoga Center New York City," accessed February 15, 2019, https://dharmayogacenter.com/resources/yoga-poses/master-yoga-chart.

225. Finger cites his father, Kavi Yogiraj Mani Finger (1908–1998), as his principal teacher. Mani was a student of Yogananda before taking initiation from Swami Sivananda. Holly Hammond, "Meet the Innovators!," *Yoga Journal*, October 2000, 80–89; "About Ishta | ISHTA Yoga," http://ishtayoga.com/aboutishta; Stephanie Golden, "Like Father, Like Son," *Yoga Journal*, August 1994, 36–40.

226. Strauss, *Positioning*, 38–41; Eliade, *Yoga*, xvii–xix.

227. Initially published in French as *Yoga: Immortalité et Liberté* (1954). Eliade was a formative figure in the academic study of religion in the twentieth century. A summary and analysis of Eliade's work, including his controversial role in Romanian nationalist politics, can be found in Bryan S. Rennie, *Reconstructing Eliade: Making Sense of Religion* (Albany, NY: SUNY Press, 1996).

228. Eliade, *Yoga*, xvii.

229. Eliade, *Yoga*, xxxi.

230. Strauss, *Positioning*, 38–40.

231. Strauss, *Positioning*, 38–40.

232. Eliade appears to have viewed Ramakrishna as the more authentic of the two. Strauss, *Positioning*, 40.

233. Williamson, *Transcendent in America*, 83.

234. Williamson, *Transcendent*, 83.

235. Williamson, *Transcendent*, 90.

236. Williamson, *Transcendent*, 93.

237. Herbert Benson and Miriam Z. Klipper, *The Relaxation Response* (New York: Avon Books, 1975); Williamson, *Transcendent*, 100–103.

238. Williamson, *Transcendent*, 95; Craig Pearson, *The Complete Book of Yogic Flying: The Program of His Holiness Maharishi Mahesh Yogi to Enjoy Bubbling Bliss, Develop Total Brain Functioning and Higher States of Consciousness, and Create National Invincibility and World Peace* (Fairfield, IA: Maharishi University of Management Press, 2008).

239. "MERU Vlodrop," http://meru-mvu.org/vlodrop.

240. Samonway Dattagupta, "Uttarakhand Reopens The Beatles Ashram in Rishikesh as an Eco-Friendly Tourist Spot," *India Today*, December 9, 2015, http://indiatoday.intoday.in/story/uttarakhand-reopens-the-beatles-ashram-in-rishikesh-as-an-eco-friendly-tourist-spot/1/542082.html.

241. Williamson, *Transcendent*, 81.

242. Hans Baer, *Toward an Integrative Medicine: Merging Alternative Therapies with Biomedicine* (Walnut Creek, CA: AltaMira Press, 2004), 119–136.

243. See, for example, Deepak Chopra, David Simon, and Leanne Backer, *The Chopra Center Cookbook: Nourishing Body and Soul* (Hoboken, NJ: John Wiley & Sons, 2002).

244. "Welcome to Swami Dayananda Ashram–Arsha Vidya Pitham–Rishikesh," https://www.dayananda.org/; PTI, "Modi Mourns Death of Swami Dayananda Saraswati—Times of India," *The Times of India*, September 24, 2015, http://timesofindia.indiatimes.com/india/Modi-mourns-death-of-Swami-Dayananda-Saraswati/articleshow/49084779.cms. Another of Modi's gurus, Swami Atmasthanandaji Maharaj, a prominent member of the Ramakrishna Mission, passed away in 2017. PTI, "Swami Atmasthanandaji Maharaj Passes Away, PM Modi Says Personal Loss," *Hindustan Times*, June 19, 2017, http://www.hindustantimes.com/india-news/swami-atmasthanandaji-maharaj-passes-away-pm-modi-says-personal-loss/story-RvTH8E3UpMVMTjsrXbPQVL.html.

245. Br. Ramaswamy, "Swami Dayananda Saraswati," Newsletter, August 2009, http://www.arshavidya.in/Newsletter/Aug09/swamiji-his-life-and-work.pdf.

246. "H.H. Pujya Swami Chidanand Saraswatiji Ceaseless Service," http://www.pujyaswamiji.org/seva.

247. IANS, "PM Modi Hails Yoga, Says It Will Lead to New Era of Harmony and Togetherness," https://www.hindustantimes.com/, March 2, 2017, https://www.hindustantimes.com/india-news/pm-modi-hails-yoga-says-it-will-lead-to-new-era-of-harmony-and-togetherness/story-AMHGnbJXQYjJxaVItEMdiM.html. According to McCartney, these intersections bring non-Indian students into the sphere of Indian nationalist politics. McCartney, "Politics beyond the Yoga Mat."

248. Rajmani Tigunait, *At the Eleventh Hour: The Biography of Swami Rama* (Honesdale: Himalayan Institute Press, 2001).

249. Philip Goldberg, *American Veda: From Emerson and the Beatles to Yoga and Meditation—How Indian Spirituality Changed the West* (New York: Three Rivers Press, 2013), 211.

250. "Pandit Rajmani Tigunait, PhD," Himalayan Institute, August 25, 2017, https://www.himalayaninstitute.org/presenter/pandit-rajmani-tigunait. One of Tigunait's well-known North American students is Rod Stryker, formerly a student of the ISHTA yoga system of Mani and Alan Finger, and who founded the ParaYoga system. "Rod Stryker," Himalayan Institute, February 15, 2019, https://www.himalayaninstitute.org/presenter/rod-stryker.

251. Hugh B. Urban, *Tantra: Sex, Secrecy Politics, and Power in the Study of Religions* (Berkeley, CA: University of California, 2003), 134–147. On Pierre and Theos Bernard, see this chapter's note 53.

252. Hugh B. Urban, "Osho, From Sex Guru to Guru of the Rich: The Spiritual Logic of Late Capitalism," in *Gurus in America*, ed. Thomas A. Forsthoefel and Cynthia Ann Humes (Albany, NY: SUNY Press, 2005), 171.

253. Urban, "Osho," 171.

254. Urban, "Osho," 172–173.

255. Urban, "Osho," 182.

256. Margot Anand, *The Art of Sexual Ecstasy: The Path of Sacred Sexuality for Western Lovers* (Los Angeles: J.P. Tarcher, 1989), 27–46.

257. M.U. Hatengdi, *Nityananda: The Divine Presence* (Cambridge, MA: Rudra Press, 1984); Williamson, *Transcendent*, 108–109. See also Patrick McCartney, "Śāntamūrti: The Legitimate Disposition(s) of the 'Temple of Peace' Social Network," *Annual Papers of the Anthropological Institute* 8 (2018): 65–104.

258. See, for example, Douglas Renfrew Brooks, ed., *Meditation Revolution: A History and Theology of the Siddha Yoga Lineage* (New Delhi: Motilal Banarsidass Publishers, 2000).

259. Williamson, *Transcendent*, 109; Andrea R. Jain, "Muktananda: Entrepreneurial Godman, Tantric Hero," in *Gurus of Modern Yoga*, ed. Mark Singleton and Ellen Goldberg (New York & London: Oxford University Press, 2014), 190–191.

260. Williamson, *Transcendent*, 111. An early American disciple of Muktananda, Adi Da (Franklin Albert Jones, 1939–2008), also known as Da Free John, founded the separate tradition of Adidam after leaving Siddha Yoga, and was known for using unconventional, if not extreme, methods with disciples, leading to scrutiny and criticism of his work and organization. Scott Lowe, "Adidam," in *Introduction to New and Alternative Religions in America*, ed. Eugene V. Gallagher and W. Michael Ashcraft, vol. 4 (Westport, CT: Greenwood Press, 2006), 85–109. The popular yoga

scholar Georg Feuerstein was a disciple of Adi Da for a time, and discusses Adi Da's legacy in Feuerstein, *Holy Madness* (Prescott, AZ: Hohm Press, 2006).

261. Williamson, *Transcendent*, 114–116, 126–129.

262. Goldberg, "Swami Kṛpālvānanda: The Man Behind Kripalu Yoga," 171–176.

263. Goldberg, "Swami," 182.

264. Ellen Goldberg, "Amrit Desai and the Kripalu Center," in *Homegrown Gurus: From Hinduism in America to American Hinduism*, ed. Ann Gleig and Lola Williamson (Albany: SUNY Press, 2014), 65–69.

265. Goldberg, "Amrit Desai," 72–73.

266. Goldberg, "Amrit Desai," 80.

267. Referring to the refrain of "Hare Krishna" in Gauḍīya-style mantra-based *kīrtana*.

268. Harrison donated a seventeen-acre estate to ISKCON in 1973, which was subsequently renamed Bhaktivedanta Manor and has since served as a hub for ISKCON in Europe. Richard J. Cole, "Forty Years of Chanting: A Study of the Hare Krishna Movement From Its Foundation to the Present Day," in *The Hare Krishna Movement: Forty Years of Chant and Change*, ed. Graham Dwyer and Richard J. Cole (Londres: I.B. Tauris, 2007), 32.

269. Thomas S. Bremer, *Formed from This Soil: An Introduction to the Diverse History of Religion in America* (Hoboken: Wiley, 2014), 393–394.

270. See, for example, Rusty Wells, *Bhakti Flow Yoga: A Training Guide for Practice and Life* (Boston: Shambhala, 2015).

271. "Wai Lana Biography, Age, Birth Place, Personal Life & 'Oh My Sweet Lord'—Kowaliw.Net," http://kowaliw.net/wailana-bio; "Wai Lana Yoga TV Series," Text, Wai Lana, July 17, 2013, https://www.wailana.com/yoga/wai-lana-yoga-tv-series.

272. "Yoga—The Silk Road to Happiness—Interview with Wai Lana," *Asana–International Yoga Journal* (blog), August 17, 2016, https://www.asanajournal.com/yoga-the-silk-road-to-happiness-interview-with-wailana; "Jagad Guru Siddhaswarupananda Paramahamsa," http://www.scienceofidentityfoundation.net/about-us/jagad-guru-siddhaswarupananda-paramahamsa-chris-butler. Butler has been given additional media attention due to his connection with Hawaii Congressperson Tulsi Gabbard. James Cave, "Tulsi Gabbard Still Dogged By Krishna Cult Rumors," *Huffington Post*, March 16, 2015, sec. Politics, http://www.huffingtonpost.com/2015/03/16/tulsi-gabbard-krishna-cult-rumors_n_6879588.html.

273. Himani Kumar Sanagaram, "Padma Shri Winner Wai Lana Revolutionising Yoga in USA," *NewsGram*, February 4, 2016, https://www.newsgram.com/padma-shri-winner-wai-lana-revolutionising-yoga-in-usa/; Yatish Yadav, "Superstar in Top Padma League," *The New Indian Express*, January 26, 2016, http://www.new

indianexpress.com/nation/2016/jan/26/Superstar-in-Top-Padma-League-873638.html; Avarnita Mathur, "Full List of Padma Awardees 2016," January 25, 2016, http://indiatoday.intoday.in/story/full-list-of-padma-awardees-2016/1/579218.html. Sri Sri Ravi Shankar was awarded the higher Padma Vibhushan award the same year.

274. As per a press release authored by her organization. "Wai Lana's 'Namaste' Music Video Played at United Nations in Celebration of International Yoga Day," *PRWeb*, http://www.prweb.com/releases/2015/Namaste-Wailana/prweb12802457.htm.

275. Constance A. Jones and James D. Ryan, *Encyclopedia of Hinduism* (New York: Checkmark Books, 2008), 310, 357.

276. Jones and Ryan, *Encyclopedia*, 285–287.

277. Karen Pechelis, "Introduction: Hindu Female Gurus in Historical and Philosophical Context," in *The Graceful Guru: Hindu Female Gurus in India and the United States*, ed. Karen Pechilis (New York: Oxford University Press, 2004), 31–36. Amma, in particular, developed a close relationship with Indian Prime Minister Narendra Modi. Ariel Sophia Bardi, "The Soft Nationalism of Amma, India's Hugging Saint," *Los Angeles Review of Books*, August 6, 2019, https://lareviewofbooks.org/article/the-soft-nationalism-of-amma-indias-hugging-saint. See also Amanda Lucia, "Innovative Gurus: Tradition and Change in Contemporary Hinduism," *International Journal of Hindu Studies* 18, no. 2 (August 2014): 221–263.

278. Carol S. Anderson, "The Life of Gauri Ma," in *The Graceful Guru: Hindu Female Gurus in India and the United States*, ed. Karen Pechilis (New York: Oxford University Press, 2004), 70–71; Catherine Cornille, "Mother Meera, Avatar," in *The Graceful Guru*, 131–135.

279. Gombrich, *Theravada Buddhism*, 186–192.

280. Gombrich, *Theravada Buddhism*, 186–192.

281. Daniel M. Stuart, "Insight Transformed: Coming to Terms with Mindfulness in South Asian and Global Frames," *Religions of South Asia* 11, no. 2–3 (August 2018): 158–181.

282. Ingrid Jordt, *Burma's Mass Lay Meditation Movement Buddhism and the Cultural Construction of Power* (Athens: Ohio University Press, 2007), 22–23; Joanna Cook, *Meditation in Modern Buddhism: Renunciation and Change in Thai Monastic Life* (Cambridge: Cambridge University Press, 2014), 26–27; Erik Braun, *The Birth of Insight: Meditation, Modern Buddhism, and the Burmese Monk Ledi Sayadaw*, Buddhism and Modernity (Chicago & London: University of Chicago Press, 2013), 4–5.

283. Cook, *Meditation*, 27.

284. Braun, *Birth of Insight*, 57–59, 123.

285. Cook, *Meditation*, 42.

286. Braun, *Birth of Insight*, 162.

287. Braun, 166–167.

288. Sarah Powers, *Insight Yoga* (Boston, MA: Shambhala, 2009); Paul Grilley, *Yin Yoga: Outline of a Quiet Practice* (Ashland, OR: White Cloud Press, 2002); Active Interest Media Inc, "OM Page: Talking Shop with Paul Grilley," *Yoga Journal*, June 2003, 24.

289. "Vipassana," https://www.dhamma.org/en/schedules/schgiri; "Vipassana Meditation Center—Dhamma Dharā | Vipassana International," https://www.dhara.dhamma.org/about/international.

290. Shaila Catherine, *Focused and Fearless: A Meditator's Guide to States of Deep Joy, Calm, and Clarity* (Somerville, MA: Wisdom Publications, 2008); Stephen Snyder and Tina Rasmussen, *Practicing the Jhanas: Traditional Concentration Meditation as Presented by the Venerable Pa Auk Sayadaw* (Boston: Shambhala, 2009); Ajahn Brahm, *Mindfulness, Bliss, and beyond: A Meditator's Handbook* (Boston: Wisdom Publications, 2006).

291. "Mission," Mind & Life Institute, https://www.mindandlife.org/mission.

292. Charles S. Prebish, Kenneth K. Tanaka, and Amy Lavine, eds., "Tibetan Buddhism in America," in *The Faces of Buddhism in America* (Berkeley: University of California Press, 1999), 102–103.

293. Prebish, Tanaka, and Lavine, "Tibetan Buddhism," 102–103.

294. Dan Montgomery, "Samaya and the World of Shambhala," *Tricycle: The Buddhist Review*, August 6, 2018, https://tricycle.org/trikedaily/shambhala-samaya/; Matthew Abrahams, "Two Embattled Buddhist Leaders Pressured to Stop Teaching," *Tricycle: The Buddhist Review*, February 22, 2019, https://tricycle.org/trikedaily/sakyong-levine-teaching.

295. Ana Cristina Lopes, *Tibetan Buddhism in Diaspora: Cultural Re-Signification in Practice and Institutions* (London & New York: Routledge, 2015), 105.

296. Lopes, *Tibetan Buddhism in Diaspora*, 105.

297. Namkhai Norbu and Adriano Clemente, *Yantra Yoga: The Tibetan Yoga of Movement* (Ithaca, NY: Snow Lion, 2008), 1.

298. Namkhai Norbu and Clemente, *Yantra Yoga*, 3–5.

299. "About Ligmincha," http://www.ligmincha.org/index.php/en/about-us-ligmincha-institute/mission-statement.html.

300. Tenzin Wangyal and Marcy Vaughn, *Awakening the Sacred Body* (Carlsbad, CA: Hay House, Inc., 2011). One of Wangyal's students, Alejandro Chaoul-Reich, served as a yoga teacher and co-author in government-sponsored research on the use of Wangyal's Tibetan yoga system as a therapeutic intervention for cancer patients in the United States. Kavita D. Chandwani et al., "Randomized, Controlled Trial of Yoga in Women with Breast Cancer Undergoing Radiotherapy," *Journal of Clinical Oncology* 32, no. 10 (April 2014): 1058–1065.

301. Tarthang Tulku, *Tibetan Relaxation: The Illustrated Guide to Kum Nye Massage and Movement—A Yoga from the Tibetan Tradition* (London: Duncan Baird, 2007).

302. Thomas A. Tweed, "United States," in *Encyclopedia of Buddhism*, ed. Robert Buswell (New York: Macmillan Reference, 2003), 2: 864–870.

303. The revival of Buddhism in the People's Republic of China in the wake of the liberalization of government policies on religion has been marked by enthusiasm for both lay and monastic Ch'an meditation programs and the construction of retreat centers and temples designed to accommodate large national and international audiences. Mario Poceski, "Contemporary Chinese Buddhist Traditions," in *Oxford Handbook of Contemporary Buddhism*, ed. Michael Kessler Jerryson (New York: Oxford University Press, 2017), 79–99.

304. "Order of Interbeing History," *Order of Interbeing | Tiep Hien* (blog), July 12, 2011, https://orderofinterbeing.org/about/our-history/; "Plum Village," Plum Village, January 3, 2013, https://plumvillage.org/about/plum-village.

305. Jain, *Selling Yoga*, 56–65.

306. Jain, *Selling Yoga*, 56–65.

307. Jain, *Selling Yoga*, 56–65. Mahapragya appears to have been very familiar with Goenka's *vipassanā* method, in particular. Stuart, "Insight Transformed," 168–171.

308. Smita Kothari, "Prekṣā Dhyāna in Jaina Yoga," in *Yoga in Jainism*, ed. Christopher Chapple (New York: Routledge, 2015), 210–228.

309. James R. Lewis, "Autobiography of a Schism," *Marburg Journal of Religion* 15, no. 1 (2015): 1.

310. Philip Deslippe, "From Maharaj to Mahan Tantric: The Construction of Yogi Bhajan's Kundalini Yoga," *Sikh Formations* 8, no. 3 (December 2012): 369–376.

311. Deslippe, "Maharaj to Mahan Tantric," 373.

312. Deslippe, "Maharaj to Mahan Tantric," 373. "Sant Hazara Singh—Yogi Bhajan's First Teacher," Sikh Dharma International, September 13, 2017, https://www.sikhdharma.org/sant-hazara-singh-yogi-bhajans-first-teacher.

313. Lewis, "Autobiography," 3–4.

314. Lewis, "Autobiography," 3–4. Bhajan's Sikh convert disciples were critical of Punjabi Sikhs for what they observed as a lax observance of Sikh lifestyle regulations. See Lewis, "Autobiography," 5–6.

315. Sherri Buri McDonald, "Yogi's Legacy in Question," *The Register-Guard*, May 9, 2010, http://projects.registerguard.com/csp/cms/sites/web/news/cityregion/24671927-41/yogi-khalsa-bhajan-leaders-members.csp.

316. "Preparing for Sadhana," 3HO—Happy, Healthy, Holy, https://www.3ho.org/kundalini-yoga/sadhana/preparing-sadhana. Bhajan had a vision of a utopian

"Aquarian Age" to be ushered in through dedicated spiritual practice. The *Gurū Granth Sāhib* is also known as the *Ādi Granth*, or "First Book."

317. "About IKYTA | IKYTA—International Kundalini Yoga Teachers Association," https://www.ikyta.org/about-ikyta.

318. Dharam S. Khalsa and Darryl O'Keeffe, *The Kundalini Yoga Experience: Bringing Body, Mind, and Spirit Together* (New York: Simon & Schuster, 2002).

319. Constance Waeber Elsberg, *Graceful Women: Gender and Identity in an American Sikh Community* (Knoxville: University of Tennessee Press, 2003), 50–52.

320. Margot Dougherty, "Twist & Shout: Touching Your Toes Means Different Things to Different People. An Essential Guide to L.A.'s Yoga Schools," *Los Angeles Magazine*, January 2001, 93.

321. Elsberg, *Graceful Women*, 166.

322. K. Kavanaugh and M.B. Pennington, "Spirituality, Christian (History Of)," in *New Catholic Encyclopedia* (Detroit, MI: Gale, 2003), 13: 443–451.

323. Michal Chelbin, "Yoga Poses in Israel," *The New York Times*, March 7, 2014, sec. Magazine, https://www.nytimes.com/2014/03/09/magazine/yoga-poses-in-israel.html; Taffy Brodesser-Akner, "A Modern Orthodox Jew Asks: Is Yoga Kosher?," *Tablet Magazine*, January 5, 2010, http://www.tabletmag.com/jewish-life-and-religion/23099/is-yoga-kosher; Sarah Maslin Nir, "In Queens, Seeking to Clear a Path Between Yoga and Islam," *The New York Times*, April 8, 2012, sec. N.Y. / Region, https://www.nytimes.com/2012/04/09/nyregion/in-queens-seeking-to-clear-a-path-between-yoga-and-islam.html.

324. Laurette Willis, *Praisemoves: The Christian Alternative to Yoga* (Eugene, OR: Harvest House, 2006); Diane Bloomfield, *Torah Yoga = תורה יוגה: Experiencing Jewish Wisdom through Classic Postures* (San Francisco: Jossey-Bass, 2004).

325. Jain, *Selling Yoga*, 125–126.

326. Jain, *Selling Yoga*, 125–126.

327. Jain, *Selling Yoga*, 125–126. PTI, "Surya Namaskar Similar to Namaz: Yogi Adityanath," *The Indian Express*, March 29, 2017, http://indianexpress.com/article/india/surya-namaskar-similar-to-namaz-yogi-adityanath-4591630.

328. James Gaddy, "When Yoga Meets CrossFit, It's More Burn, Less Om," *Bloomberg.Com*, January 9, 2017, https://www.bloomberg.com/news/articles/2017-01-09/-mashup-yoga-classes-mix-crossfit-boxing-and-cardio-with-oms.

329. Sarah Toland, "The Rise of Yoga in the NBA and Other Pro Sports," *SI.Com*, https://www.si.com/edge/2014/06/27/rise-yoga-nba-and-other-pro-sports; Lynn Zinser, "Title for the Seahawks Is a Triumph for the Profile of Yoga," *The New York Times*, February 4, 2014, sec. Pro Football, https://www.nytimes.com/2014/02/05/sports/football/title-for-the-seahawks-is-a-triumph-for-the-profile-of-yoga.html.

330. Melissa D'costal, "Yoga as a Sport in Olympics?—Times of India," *The Times of India*, October 3, 2012, http://timesofindia.indiatimes.com/life-style/health-

fitness/fitness/Yoga-as-a-sport-in-Olympics/articleshow/16639916.cms; CBS/AP, "Yoga Poses as Olympic Sport: Is That a Stretch?," February 28, 2012, https://www.cbsnews.com/news/yoga-poses-as-olympic-sport-is-that-a-stretch; Singleton, *Yoga Body*, 209–210.

331. "Yoga Federation of India: Rules for National Yoga Sports Championship," http://www.yogafederationofindia.com/rules_nyc.html; Joseph S. Alter, *Moral Materialism: Sex and Masculinity in Modern India* (New Delhi: Penguin Books, 2011), 149–177.

332. Chandrima Chakraborty, "The Hindu Ascetic as Fitness Instructor: Reviving Faith in Yoga," *International Journal of the History of Sport* 24, no. 9 (n.d.): 1172–1186; Charles S. Prebish, *Religion and Sport: The Meeting of Sacred and Profane* (Westport CT: Greenwood Press, 1993).

333. James Mallinson, "The Yogī's Latest Trick," *Journal of the Royal Asiatic Society* 24, no. 1 (January 2014): 174 n38.

334. See, for example, Brooke Schedneck, *Thailand's International Meditation Centers: Tourism and the Global Commodification of Religious Practices* (London & New York: Routledge, Taylor & Francis, 2017).

Works Cited

"10 Bollywood Actresses Who Do YOGA to Stay Fit!" indiatimes.com, June 17, 2015. http://www.indiatimes.com/news/world/10-bollywood-actresses-who-do-yoga-to-stay-fit-294040.html

"A Response to James Brown." *Yoga Alliance*, January 9, 2014. https://www.yogaalliance.org/Home/A_Response_to_James_Brown

Abhayadatta, and Keith Dowman. *Masters of Mahamudra: Songs and Histories of the Eight-Four Buddhist Siddhas*. Albany, NY: SUNY Press, 1985.

"About IKYTA | IKYTA—International Kundalini Yoga Teachers Association." https://www.ikyta.org/about-ikyta

"About Ishta | ISHTA Yoga." http://ishtayoga.com/aboutishta

"About Ligmincha." http://www.ligmincha.org/index.php/en/about-us-ligmincha-institute/mission-statement.html

"About Us." Art of Living (India). https://www.artofliving.org/in-en/about-us

Abrahams, Matthew. "Two Embattled Buddhist Leaders Pressured to Stop Teaching." *Tricycle: The Buddhist Review*, February 22, 2019. https://tricycle.org/trikedaily/sakyong-levine-teaching

"Accreditation—International Association of Yoga Therapists (IAYT)." https://www.iayt.org/page/AccreditationLanding

Acharya, S.L., J. Howard, S.B. Panta, S.S. Mahatma, and J. Copeland. "Cannabis, Lord Shiva and Holy Men: Cannabis Use among Sadhus in Nepal." *Journal of Psychiatrists Association of Nepal* 3, no. 2 (2014): 9–14.

Acri, Andrea. "Dharma Pātañjala: A Śaiva Scripture from Ancient Java; Studied in the Light of Related Old Javanese and Sanskrit Texts." Gonda Indological Studies, vol. 16. Gronigen: Egbert Forsten, 2012.

Active Interest Media, Inc. "OM Page: Talking Shop with Paul Grilley." *Yoga Journal*, June 2003, 24.

Agencies. "Despite Controversy, 50 Lakh MP Students Participate in 'Surya Namaskar.'" *Indian Express*. January 12, 2012. http://indianexpress.com/article/

news-archive/regional/despite-controversy-50-lakh-mp-students-participate-in-surya-namaskar

Ajahn Brahm. *Mindfulness, Bliss, and beyond: A Meditator's Handbook*. Boston: Wisdom Publications, 2006.

Aldrich, Michael R. "Tantric Cannabis Use in India." *Journal of Psychedelic Drugs* 9, no. 3 (July 1977): 227–233.

Allison, Rebecca. "Vicar in a Twist over Yoga Classes in Church Hall." *The Guardian*, August 28, 2002, sec. UK news. https://www.theguardian.com/uk/2002/aug/28/religion.world

Alter, Joseph S. *Gandhi's Body: Sex, Diet, and the Politics of Nationalism*. Critical Histories. Philadelphia: University of Pennsylvania Press, 2000.

———. *Moral Materialism: Sex and Masculinity in Modern India*. New Delhi: Penguin Books, 2011.

Alter, Joseph S. "Shri Yogendra: Magic, Modernity, and the Burden of the Middle-Class Yogi." In *Gurus of Modern Yoga*, edited by Mark Singleton and Ellen Goldberg, 60–79. New York & London: Oxford University Press, 2014.

Alter, Joseph S. *Yoga in Modern India: The Body between Science and Philosophy*. Princeton, NJ: Princeton University Press, 2004.

Alter, Joseph S. "Yoga, Nature Cure, and 'Perfect' Health: The Purity of the Fluid Body in an Impure World." In *Yoga in Transformation*, edited by Phillip A. Maas and Karin Preisendanz, 439–461. Göttingen: Vienna University Press, 2018.

———. "Yoga Shivir." In *Yoga in the Modern World: Contemporary Perspectives*, edited by Mark Singleton and Jean Byrne, 36–48. New York: Routledge, Taylor & Francis Group, 2008.

"American Viniyoga Institute—About Founder Gary Kraftsow." http://viniyoga.businesscatalyst.com/about/who-we-are/about-gary-kraftsow

Anand, Margot. *The Art of Sexual Ecstasy: The Path of Sacred Sexuality for Western Lovers*. Los Angeles: J.P. Tarcher, 1989.

Anderson, Carol S. "The Life of Gauri Ma." In *The Graceful Guru: Hindu Female Gurus in India and the United States*, edited by Karen Pechilis, 65–84. New York: Oxford University Press, 2004.

Antony, Mary Grace. " 'It's Not Religious, But It's Spiritual:' Appropriation and the Universal Spirituality of Yoga." *Journal of Communication & Religion* 37, no. 4 (Winter 2014): 63–81.

Appleton, Naomi. *Jātaka Stories in Theravāda Buddhism: Narrating the Bodhisatta Path*. Farnham, Surrey, England & Burlington, VT: Ashgate, 2010.

Aravamudan, Srinivas. *Guru English: South Asian Religion in a Cosmopolitan Language*. Princeton, NJ: Princeton University Press, 2011.

Arbel, Keren. *Early Buddhist Meditation: The Four Jhānas as the Actualization of Insight*. New York: Routledge, 2017.

Armstrong, Jerome. *Calcutta Yoga: Buddha Bose & the Yoga Family of Bishnu Ghosh and Yogananda*. United States: Webstrong LLC Publishing, 2018.

Askegaard, Søren, and Giana M. Eckhardt. "Glocal Yoga: Re-Appropriation in the Indian Consumptionscape." *Marketing Theory* 12, no. 1 (March 2012): 45–60.

Aśvaghoṣa, and Patrick Olivelle. *Life of the Buddha*. New York: New York University Press, 2009.

Augenstein, Sarah. "The Introduction of Yoga in German Schools: A Case Study." In *Yoga Traveling: Bodily Practice in Transcultural Perspective*, 155–172. Heidelberg: Springer, 2013.

"AYRI." http://www.astanga.it/eng/?pagina=ayri.php

Ayyangar, T. R. Srinivasa. *The Yoga Upanisads*. Fremont, CA: Jain, 2006.

Baer, Hans. *Toward an Integrative Medicine: Merging Alternative Therapies with Biomedicine*. Walnut Creek, CA: AltaMira Press, 2004.

Bailey, Greg, and Ian Mabbett. *The Sociology of Early Buddhism*. Cambridge: Cambridge University Press, 2006.

Baker, Ian A. "Tibetan Yoga: Somatic Practice in Vajrayāna Buddhism and Dzogchen." In *Yoga in Transformation*, edited by Phillip A. Maas and Karin Preisendanz, 335–384. Göttingen: Vienna University Press, 2018.

Bapat, P.V. *Vimuttimagga and Visuddhimagga: A Comparative Study*. Calcutta: Calcutta Oriental Press, Ltd., 1937.

Bardi, Ariel Sophia. "The Soft Nationalism of Amma, India's Hugging Saint." *Los Angeles Review of Books*, August 6, 2019. https://lareviewofbooks.org/article/the-soft-nationalism-of-amma-indias-hugging-saint

Beck, Guy. "Sacred Music and Hindu Religious Experience: From Ancient Roots to the Modern Classical Tradition." *Religions* 10, no. 85 (February 2019): 1–15.

Beckerlegge, Gwilym. "Eknath Ranade, Gurus, and Jīvanvrats: The Vivekananda Kendra's Promotion of the 'Yoga Way of Life.'" In *Gurus of Modern Yoga*, edited by Mark Singleton and Ellen Goldberg, 327–50. New York & London: Oxford University Press, 2014.

Bedekar, V.M. "Dhyānayoga in the Mahābhārata." *Bharatiya Vidya Bhavan* 20–21 (1960–1961): 116–125.

Benson, Herbert, and Miriam Z. Klipper. *The Relaxation Response*. New York: Avon Books, 1975.

Benton, Catherine. *God of Desire: Tales of Kāmadeva in Sanskrit Story Literature*. Albany, NY: SUNY Press, 2006.

Berila, Beth, Melanie Klein, and Chelsea Jackson Roberts, eds. *Yoga, the Body, and Embodied Social Change: An Intersectional Feminist Analysis*. Lanham, MD: Lexington Books, 2016.

Berkwitz, Stephen C. *South Asian Buddhism: A Survey*. London & New York: Routledge, 2010.

Bharati, Agehananda. "Indian Expatriates in North America and Neo-Hindu Movements." In *The Communication of Ideas*, edited by J.S. Yadava and Vinayshil Gautam, 245–255. New Delhi: Concept Publishing, 1980.

Bhattacharya, Ram Shankar, and Gerald James Larson. *Samkhya: A Dualist Tradition in Indian Philosophy*. Princeton, NJ: Princeton University Press, 1987.

Biernacki, Loriliai, and Oxford University Press. *Renowned Goddess of Desire Women, Sex, and Speech in Tantra.* New York: Oxford University Press, 2008.

Billard, Mary. "Yoga's New Wave." *The New York Times*, April 23, 2010, sec. Fashion & Style. https://www.nytimes.com/2010/04/25/fashion/25yoga.html

Birch, Beryl Bender. *Power Yoga: The Total Strength and Flexibility Workout*. New York: Touchstone, 2014.

Birch, Jason. "Premodern Yoga Traditions and Ayurveda: Preliminary Remarks on Shared Terminology, Theory, and Praxis." *History of Science in South Asia* 6 (2018): 1–83.

———. "Rājayoga: The Reincarnations of the King of All Yogas." *International Journal of Hindu Studies* 17, no. 3 (December 2013): 399–442.

———. "The Meaning of Hatha in Early Hathayoga." *Journal of the American Oriental Society* 131, no. 4 (2011): 527–554.

———. "The Proliferation of Āsana-s in Late-Medieval Yoga Texts." In *Yoga in Transformation*, edited by Phillip A. Maas and Karin Preisendanz, 101–170. Göttingen: Vienna University Press, 2018.

Birch, Jason, and Jaqueline Hargreaves. "The Religiosity of the Yoga Mat," April 18, 2016. https://www.theluminescent.org/2016/04/the-religiosity-of-yoga-mat.html

———. "Yoganidrā: An Understanding of the History and Context.," n.d. http://theluminescent.blogspot.co.uk/2015_01_01_archive.html

Bloomfield, Diane. *Torah Yoga = תורה יוגה: Experiencing Jewish Wisdom through Classic Postures*. San Francisco: Jossey-Bass, 2004.

Blyth, Antonia. "How #MeToo Shook the Yoga World." ELLE, March 29, 2018. https://www.elle.com/beauty/health-fitness/a19609192/how-metoo-shook-the-yoga-world

Bonde, Hans. *Gymnastics and Politics: Niels Bukh and Male Aesthetics*. Copenhagen: Museum Tusculanum Press, University of Copenhagen, 2006.

Bouillier, Véronique. *Monastic Wanderers: Nāth Yogī Ascetics in Modern South Asia*. London: Routledge, 2018.

Bouthillette, K.S. "Like Ploughing: An Early Mādhyamikan Refutation of 'Vedic' Yoga." Vancouver, BC, 2018.

Bouy, Christian. *Les Nātha-yogin et les Upaniṣads: étude d'histoire de la littérature hindoue*. Paris: Diffusion De Boccard, 1994.

Braude, Ann. *Radical Spirits: Spiritualism and Women's Rights in Nineteenth-Century America*. Bloomington: Indiana University Press, 2013.

Braun, Erik. *The Birth of Insight: Meditation, Modern Buddhism, and the Burmese Monk Ledi Sayadaw*. Buddhism and Modernity Series. Chicago & London: University of Chicago Press, 2013.

Bremer, Thomas S. *Formed from This Soil: An Introduction to the Diverse History of Religion in America*, Hoboken: Wiley, 2014.

Briggs, George Weston. *Gorakhnāth and the Kānphaṭa Yogīs*. Delhi: Motilal Banarsidass, 1998.

Broad, William. *The Science of Yoga the Risks and the Rewards*. New York: Simon & Schuster, 2012.

Brockington, John. "Sūrya Ivāparaḥ: Exemplary Deaths in the Mahābhārata." In *Release from Life–Release in Life*, edited by Andreas Bigger and Peter Schreiner, 21–35. New York: P. Lang, 2010.

———. "Yoga in the Mahābhārata." In *Yoga: The Indian Tradition*, edited by Ian Whicher and David Carpenter, 13–24. London & New York: Routledge-Curzon, 2003.

Brockington, John, and Mary Brockington, eds. "Re-Creation, Refashioning, Rejection, Response . . . How the Narrative Developed." In *The Other Ramayana Women: Regional Rejection and Response*, 1–16. New York: Taylor & Francis, 2016.

Brockington, John L. *The Sanskrit Epics*. Leiden: Brill, 1998.

Brodesser-Akner, Taffy. "A Modern Orthodox Jew Asks: Is Yoga Kosher?" *Tablet Magazine*, January 5, 2010. http://www.tabletmag.com/jewish-life-and-religion/23099/is-yoga-kosher

Bronkhorst, Johannes. *Greater Magadha: Studies in the Culture of Early India*. Leiden & Boston: Brill, 2007.

———. "Sāṃkhya in the Abhidharmakośa Bhāṣya." *Journal of Indian Philosophy* 25, no. 4 (August 1997): 393–400.

———. "The Reliability of Tradition." In *Boundaries, Dynamics and Construction of Traditions in South Asia*, edited by Federico Squarcini, 62–76. Firenze, Italy: Firenze University Press, 2005.

———. *The Two Sources of Indian Asceticism*. New Delhi: Motilal Banarsidass, 1998.

———. *The Two Traditions of Meditation in Ancient India*. Delhi: Motilal Banarsidass, 1993.

———. "Yoga and Seśvara Sāṃkhya." *Journal of Indian Philosophy* 9, no. 3 (1981): 309–320.

Brooks, Douglas Renfrew, ed. *Meditation Revolution: A History and Theology of the Siddha Yoga Lineage*. New Delhi: Motilal Banarsidass Publishers, 2000.

———. "The Ocean of the Heart: Selections from the Kulārṇava Tantra." In *Tantra in Practice*, edited by David Gordon White, 347–360. Princeton, NJ: Princeton University Press, 2000.

Brown, James. "Yoga Alliance Is Ruining Yoga." *American Yoga School* (blog), January 7, 2014. https://americanyoga.school/yoga-alliance-ruining-yoga

Bryant, Edwin F. *In Quest of the Origins of Vedic Culture: The Indo-Aryan Migration Debate*. New York: Oxford University Press, 2000.

———. "Patañjali's Theistic Preference, or, Was the Author of the Yoga Sūtras a Vaishnava?" *Journal of Vaishnava Studies* 14, no. 1 (Fall 2005): 7–28.

Bryant, Edwin F., and Laurie L. Patton. *The Indo-Aryan Controversy: Evidence and Inference in Indian History*. London & New York: Routledge, 2005.

Bucknell, Roderick S. "The Buddhist Path to Liberation: An Analysis of the Listing of Stages." *Journal of the International Association of Buddhist Studies* 7, no. 2 (1984): 7–40.

Buddhaghosa, and Ñāṇamoli. *The Path of Purification: Visuddhimagga*. Seattle: BPE Pariyatti Editions, 1999.

Bühnemann, Gudrun. *Eighty-Four Āsanas in Yoga: A Survey of Traditions, with Illustrations*. New Delhi: D.K. Printworld, 2007.

———. *Maṇḍalas and Yantras in the Hindu Traditions*. Leiden: Brill, 2003.

———. "Nāga, Siddha, and Sage: Visions of Patañjali as an Authority on Yoga." In *Yoga in Transformation*, edited by Phillip A. Maas and Karin Preisendanz, 575–622. Göttingen: Vienna University Press, 2018.

———. "On Puraścaraṇa: Kulārṇavatantra, Chapter 15." In *Ritual and Speculation in Early Tantrism: Studies in Honour of André Padoux*, edited by André Padoux and Teun Goudriaan, 61–106. Albany, NY: SUNY Press, 1992.

———. "The Śāradātilakatantra on Yoga: A New Edition and Translation of Chapter 25." *Bulletin of the School of Oriental and African Studies, University of London* 74, no. 2 (2011): 205–35.

———. "The Six Rites of Magic." In *Tantra in Practice*, edited by David Gordon White, 447–462. Princeton, NJ: Princeton University Press, 2000.

Buitenen, J.A.B. van. *The Maitrāyaṇīya Upanisad: A Critical Essay with Text, Translation and Commentary*. Boston: De Gruyter Mouton, 2017.

Burchett, Patton. *A Genealogy of Devotion: Bhakti, Tantra, Yoga, and Sufism in North India*. New York: Columbia University Press, 2019.

———. "Bitten by the Snake: Early Modern Devotional Critiques of Tantra-Mantra." *The Journal of Hindu Studies* 6, no. 1 (2013): 1–20.

Buri McDonald, Sherri. "Yogi's Legacy in Question." *The Register-Guard*. May 9, 2010. http://projects.registerguard.com/csp/cms/sites/web/news/cityregion/24671927-41/yogi-khalsa-bhajan-leaders-members.csp

Burley, Mikel. *Classical Sāṃkhya and Yoga: An Indian Metaphysics of Experience.* London: Routledge, 2012.

———. *Haṭha-Yoga: Its Context, Theory, and Practice.* Delhi: Motilal Banarsidass Publishers, 2000.

Buswell, Robert E., and Donald S. Lopez, eds. *The Princeton Dictionary of Buddhism.* Princeton, NJ: Princeton University Press, 2014.

———, eds. *The Princeton Dictionary of Buddhism.* Princeton, NJ: Princeton University Press, 2014.

Cahoudharyl, Amit Anand. "Yoga in India: Supreme Court Says No to Compulsory Yoga Education in Schools." *Times of India,* August 8, 2017. http://timesofindia.indiatimes.com/india/supreme-court-says-no-to-compulsory-yoga-education-in-schools/articleshow/59967483.cms

Cappy, Peggy. *Yoga for All of Us: A Modified Series of Traditional Poses for Any Age and Ability.* New York: St. Martin's Press, 2007.

Carman, John B. "Rāmānuja." In *Encyclopedia of Religion,* edited by Lindsay Jones, 2nd ed., 11:7614–7616. Detroit, MI: Macmillan Reference USA, 2005.

Catherine, Shaila. *Focused and Fearless a Meditator's Guide to States of Deep Joy, Calm, and Clarity.* Somerville, MA: Wisdom Publications, 2008.

Cave, James. "Tulsi Gabbard Still Dogged by Krishna Cult Rumors." *Huffington Post,* March 16, 2015, sec. Politics. http://www.huffingtonpost.com/2015/03/16/tulsi-gabbard-krishna-cult-rumors_n_6879588.html

CBS/AP. "Yoga Poses as Olympic Sport: Is That a Stretch?," February 28, 2012. https://www.cbsnews.com/news/yoga-poses-as-olympic-sport-is-that-a-stretch

"Certification Process: IYNAUS, Iyengar Yoga: National Association of the United States." https://iynaus.org/teach/certification

Chakraborti, Haripada. *Asceticism in Ancient India: In Brahmanical, Buddhist, Jaina and Ajivika Societies: From the Earliest Times to the Period of Śaṅkarāchārya.* Calcutta: Punthi Pustak, 1993.

Chakraborty, Chandrima. "The Hindu Ascetic as Fitness Instructor: Reviving Faith in Yoga." *International Journal of the History of Sport* 24, no. 9 (n.d.): 1172–1186.

Chandwani, Kavita D., George Perkins, Hongasandra Ramarao Nagendra, Nelamangala V. Raghuram, Amy Spelman, Raghuram Nagarathna, Kayla Johnson, et al. "Randomized, Controlled Trial of Yoga in Women With Breast Cancer Undergoing Radiotherapy." *Journal of Clinical Oncology* 32, no. 10 (April 2014): 1058–1065.

Chapman, David L. *Sandow the Magnificent: Eugen Sandow and the Beginnings of Bodybuilding.* Urbana & Chicago: University of Illinois Press, 2006.

Chapple, Christopher. *Nonviolence to Animals, Earth, and Self in Asian Traditions.* Albany, NY: SUNY Press, 1993.

———. *Yoga and the Luminous: Patanjali's Spiritual Path to Freedom.* Albany, NY: SUNY Press, 2008.

Chapple, Christopher Key. The Academic Study of Yoga in India. *Journal of Dharma Studies* 3 (2020), 107–120.

———. "Introduction." In *Yoga in Jainism*, edited by Christopher Key Chapple, 1–13. New York: Routledge, 2016.

———. "The Sevenfold Yoga of the Yogavāsiṣṭha." In *Yoga in Practice*, edited by David Gordon White, 117–139. Princeton, NJ: Princeton University Press, 2012.

Chapple, Christopher Key, Haribhadra Sūri, and John Thomas Casey. *Reconciling Yogas: Haribhadra's Collection of Views on Yoga*. Albany, NY: SUNY Press, 2003.

Chelbin, Michal. "Yoga Poses in Israel." *The New York Times*, March 7, 2014, sec. Magazine. https://www.nytimes.com/2014/03/09/magazine/yoga-poses-in-israel.html

Chopra, Deepak, David Simon, and Leanne Backer. *The Chopra Center Cookbook: Nourishing Body and Soul*. Hoboken, NJ: John Wiley & Sons, 2002.

Choudhury, Bikram. *Bikram Yoga: The Guru Behind Hot Yoga Shows the Way to Radiant Health and Personal Fulfillment*. New York: HarperCollins, 2007.

Clark, Matthew. "Sādhus and Sādhvīs." In *Encyclopedia of Religion*, edited by Lindsay Jones, 8019–8022. Detroit, MI: Macmillan Reference USA, 2005.

Clark, Matthew James. *The Daśanāmī-Saṃnyāsīs: The Integration of Ascetic Lineages into an Order*. Leiden: Brill, 2006.

———. *The Tawny One: Soma, Haoma, and Ayahuasca*. New York: Muswell Hill Press, 2017.

Clooney, Francis X., and Tony K. Stewart. "Vaiṣṇava." In *The Hindu World*, edited by Sushil Mittal and Gene R Thursby, 162–184. New York: Routledge, 2007.

Cohen, Signe. "The Upaniṣads and Early Buddhism." In *The Upaniṣads: A Complete Guide*, edited by Signe Cohen, 73–80. New York: Routledge, 2018.

———. "The Yoga Upaniṣads." In *The Upaniṣads: A Complete Guide*, edited by Signe Cohen, 405–411. New York: Routledge, 2018.

Colas, Gérard. "History of Vaiṣṇava Traditions: An Esquisse." In *The Blackwell Companion to Hinduism*, edited by Gavin D. Flood, 200–270. Malden, MA: Blackwell, 2005.

Cole, Richard J. "Forty Years of Chanting: A Study of the Hare Krishna Movement from Its Foundation to the Present Day." In *The Hare Krishna Movement: Forty Years of Chant and Change*, edited by Graham Dwyer and Richard J. Cole, 26–53. London: I.B. Tauris, 2007.

Connor, Fiona. "Anglican Church Bans Yoga for 'Worshipping False Gods.' " *Daily Mail Online*, June 12, 2017. https://www.dailymail.co.uk/news/article-4597742/Anglican-Church-bans-yoga-worshipping-false-gods.html

Cook, Joanna. *Meditation in Modern Buddhism: Renunciation and Change in Thai Monastic Life*. Cambridge: Cambridge University Press, 2014.

"Core Philosophy." Jivamukti Yoga, August 10, 2015. https://jivamuktiyoga.com/core-philosophy

Cornille, Catherine. "Mother Meera, Avatar." In *The Graceful Guru: Hindu Female Gurus in India and the United States*, edited by Karen Pechilis, 129–147. New York: Oxford University Press, 2004.

Cort, John E. *Jains in the World: Religious Values and Ideology in India*. Oxford & New York: Oxford University Press, 2001.

Cousins, Lance S. "Aspects of Esoteric Southern Buddhism." In *Indian Insights: Buddhism, Brahmanism and Bhakti*, edited by Peter Connolly and Sue Hamilton, 185–207. London: Luzac Oriental, 1997.

Cousins, L.S. "Scholar Monks and Meditator Monks Revisited." In *Destroying Mara Forever: Buddhist Ethics Essays in Honor of Damien Keown*, edited by Damien Keown, John Powers, and Charles S Prebish, 31–46. Ithaca, NY: Snow Lion, 2010.

Crangle, Edward Fitzpatrick. *The Origin and Development of Early Indian Contemplative Practices*. Wiesbaden: Harrassowitz Verlag, 1994.

Crosby, Kate. "History versus Modern Myth: The Abhayagirivihāra, the Vimuttimagga and Yogāvacara Meditation." *Journal of Indian Philosophy* 27, no. 6 (1999): 503–550.

———. "Tantric Theravāda: A Bibliographic Essay on the Writings of François Bizot and Others on the Yogāvacara Tradition." *Contemporary Buddhism* 1, no. 2 (2000): 141–198.

———. *Theravada Buddhism: Continuity, Diversity, and Identity*. Chichester, West Sussex & Malden, MA: Wiley Blackwell, 2014.

Cuevas, Bryan J. *The Hidden History of The Tibetan Book of the Dead*. New York: Oxford University Press, 2003.

Dalton, Dennis. *Mahatma Gandhi: Nonviolent Power in Action*. New York: Columbia University Press, 2012.

Dandekar, R.N. "Vedānta." In *Encyclopedia of Religion*, edited by Lindsay Jones, 2nd ed., 14:9543–9549. Detroit, MI: Macmillan Reference USA, 2005.

D'Aquili, Eugene G., and Andrew B. Newberg. *The Mystical Mind: Probing the Biology of Religious Experience*. Minneapolis, MN: Fortress Press, 1999.

Dasgupta, Shashi Bhushan. *Obscure Religious Cults*. Calcutta: Firma KLM, 1995.

Dasgupta, Surendranath. *A History of Indian Philosophy*. Cambridge: Cambridge University Press, 1961.

Dattagupta, Samonway. "Uttarakhand Reopens The Beatles Ashram in Rishikesh as an Eco-Friendly Tourist Spot." *India Today*, December 9, 2015. http://indiatoday.

intoday.in/story/uttarakhand-reopens-the-beatles-ashram-in-rishikesh-as-an-eco-friendly-tourist-spot/1/542082.html

David N. Lorenzen, and Adrián Muñoz, eds. *Yogi Heroes and Poets: Histories and Legends of the Naths*. Albany, NY: SUNY Press, 2011.

David N. Lorenzen, Adrián Muñoz, and David N. Lorenzen, eds. "Religious Identity in Gorakhnath and Kabir." In *Yogi Heroes and Poets: Histories and Legends of the Naths*, 19–49. Albany, NY: SUNY Press, 2011.

Davids, T.W. Rhys, and William Stede. *The Pali Text Society's Pali-English Dictionary*. Chipstead, Surrey: Pali Text Society: 1921.

Davidson, Ron. *Indian Esoteric Buddhism: A Social History of the Tantric Movement*. New York & Chichester: Columbia University Press, 2005.

Davis, Richard H. *The Bhagavad Gita: A Biography*. Princeton, NJ: Princeton University Press, 2016.

Day, Michael. "Exorcists Warn Vatican over 'Beautiful Young Vampires' and Satanic Yoga." *Independent UK*, May 13, 2015. http://www.independent.co.uk/news/world/europe/exorcists-warn-vatican-over-beautiful-young-vampires-and-satanic-yoga-10174001.html

D'costal, Melissa. "Yoga as a Sport in Olympics?—Times of India." *The Times of India*, October 3, 2012. http://timesofindia.indiatimes.com/life-style/health-fitness/fitness/Yoga-as-a-sport-in-Olympics/articleshow/16639916.cms

De Michelis, Elizabeth. *A History of Modern Yoga: Patañjali and Western Esotericism*. London & New York: Continuum, 2005.

Desikachar, T.K.V, and Richard H Cravens. *Health, Healing and beyond: Yoga and the Living Tradition of Krishnamacharya*. New York: Aperture, 1998.

Desikachar, T.K.V, and Desikachar, Mekhala. *Patanjali's Yogasutra: An Exploration*. Chennai, India: Krishnamacharya Yoga Mandiram and Swathi Soft Solutions, 2000.

Deslippe, Philip. "From Maharaj to Mahan Tantric: The Construction of Yogi Bhajan's Kundalini Yoga." *Sikh Formations* 8, no. 3 (December 2012): 369–387.

———. "The Swami Circuit: Mapping the Terrain of Early American Yoga." *Journal of Yoga Studies* 1 (May 2018): 5–44.

Dhand, Arti. *Woman as Fire, Woman as Sage: Sexual Ideology in the Mahābhārata*. Albany, NY: SUNY Press, 2008.

Dhavamony, Mariasusai. "Śaivism: Śaiva Siddhānta." In *Encyclopedia of Religion*, edited by Lindsay Jones, 12:8042–8043. Detroit, MI: Macmillan Reference USA, 2005. Gale Virtual Reference Library.

Dīkshitar, Ramachandra. "Yoga." In *The Purana Index*, 3:36. Madras: University of Madras, 55 1951–55.

Dirks, Nicholas B. *Castes of Mind*. Princeton, NJ: Princeton University Press, 2011.

Djurdjevic, Gordon, and Shukdev Singh. *Sayings of Goraknāth: Annotated Translation of the Gorakh Bānī.* New York: Oxford University Press, 2019.
Doniger, Wendy. *Śiva, the Erotic Ascetic.* New York: Oxford University Press, 1981.
Dorjee, Dusana. *Neuroscience and Psychology of Meditation in Everyday Life.* London: Taylor and Francis, 2017.
Dougherty, Margot. "Twist & Shout: Touching Your Toes Means Different Things to Different People. An Essential Guide to L.A.'s Yoga Schools." *Los Angeles Magazine*, January 2001.
Dowman, Keith. *Masters of Mahāmudrā: Songs and Histories of the Eighty-Four Buddhist Siddhas.* Albany, NY: SUNY Press, 2010.
Dundas, Paul. "A Digambara Jain Prescription of the Yogic Path to Deliverance." In *Yoga in Practice*, edited by David Gordon White, 143–161. Princeton, NJ: Princeton University Press, 2012.
———. "Becoming Gautama: Mantra and History in Śvetāmbara Jainism." In *Open Boundaries: Jain Communities and Cultures in Indian History*, edited by John E. Cort, 231–338. Albany, NY: SUNY Press, 2000.
———. "Losing One's Mind and Becoming Enlightened: Some Remarks on the Concept of Yoga in Śvetāmbara Jainism and Its Relations to the Nāth Siddha Tradition." In *Yoga: The Indian Tradition*, edited by David Carpenter and Ian Whicher, 130–142. London: RoutledgeCurzon, 2003.
———. "The Jain Monk Jinapati Sūri Gets the Better of a Nāth Yogī." In *Tantra in Practice*, edited by David Gordon White, 231–238. Princeton, NJ: Princeton University Press, 2000.
———. *The Jains.* London and New York: Routledge, 2002.
"DVDs and Videos Archives." *American Viniyoga Institute* (blog). https://www.viniyoga.com/product-category/video
Eliade, Mircea. *Yoga: Immortality and Freedom.* Translated by Willard Ropes Trask. Princeton, NJ: Princeton University Press, 2009.
Elsberg, Constance Waeber. *Graceful Women: Gender and Identity in an American Sikh Community.* Knoxville: University of Tennessee Press, 2003.
Emerson, David, and Elizabeth K Hopper. *Overcoming Trauma through Yoga: Reclaiming Your Body.* Berkeley, CA: North Atlantic Books, 2011.
Erndl, Kathleen M. *Victory to the Mother: The Hindu Goddess of Northwest India in Myth, Ritual, and Symbol.* New York: Oxford University Press, 1993.
Ernst, Carl W. "Accounts of Yogis in Arabic and Persian Historical and Travel Texts." *Jerusalem Studies in Arabic and Islam* 33 (2007): 409–426.
———. "Muslim Interpreters of Yoga." In *Yoga: The Art of Transformation*, edited by Debra Diamond, 59–67. Washington, DC: Arthur M. Sackler Gallery, Smithsonian Institution, 2013.

———. "Situating Sufism and Yoga." *Journal of the Royal Asiatic Society* 15, no. 1 (2005): 15–43.

Falk, Harry. "Soma I and II." *Bulletin of the School of Oriental and African Studies, University of London* 52, no. 1 (1989): 77–90.

Farmer, Steve, Richard Sproat, and Michael Witzel. "The Collapse of the Indus-Script Thesis: The Myth of a Literate Harappan Civilization." *Electronic Journal of Vedic Studies* 11, no. 2 (2016): 19–57.

Feeney, Kevin. "Revisiting Wasson's Soma: Exploring the Effects of Preparation on the Chemistry of Amanita Muscaria." *Journal of Psychoactive Drugs* 42, no. 4 (December 2010): 499–506.

Ferrari, Fabrizio M. "Mystic Rites for Permanent Class Conflict: The Bauls of Bengal, Revolutionary Ideology and Post-Capitalism." *South Asia Research* 32, no. 1 (2012): 21–38.

Feuerstein, Georg. *Holy Madness: Spirituality, Crazy-Wise Teachers, and Enlightenment.* Prescott, AZ: Hohm Press, 2006.

Fitzgerald, James L. "A Prescription for Yoga and Power in the Mahābhārata." In *Yoga in Practice*, edited by David Gordon White, 43–50. Princeton, NJ: Princeton University Press, 2012.

Fitzgerald, James L., Sushil Mittal, and Gene Thursby. "Mahābhārata." In *The Hindu World*, 52–74. New York: Routledge, 2004.

Flood, Gavin D. *The Ascetic Self: Subjectivity, Memory and Tradition*. Cambridge: Cambridge University Press, 2005.

———. *An Introduction to Hinduism*. Cambridge: Cambridge University Press, 1996.

———. "The Purification of the Body." In *Tantra in Practice*, edited by David Gordon White, 509–520. Princeton, NJ: Princeton University Press, 2000.

———. "The Śaiva Traditions." In *The Blackwell Companion to Hinduism*, edited by Gavin D. Flood, 200–228. Malden, MA: Blackwell, 2005.

Fort, Andrew O. *Jivanmukti in Transformation: Embodied Liberation in Advaita and Neo-Vedanta*. Albany, NY: SUNY Press, 1998.

———. "On Destroying the Mind: The Yogasūtras in Vidyāranya's Jīvanmuktiviveka." *Journal of Indian Philosophy* 27, no. 4 (1999): 377–395.

Fort, Andrew O., and Patricia Y Mumme. *Living Liberation in Hindu Thought.* Albany, NY: SUNY Press, 1996.

Foxen, Anya P. *Biography of a Yogi: Paramahansa Yogananda and the Origins of Modern Yoga*, New York: Oxford University Press, 2017.

FP Staff. "No Surya Namaskar on International Yoga Day: Modi Govt Axes Asana to Soothe Irate Muslim Groups." *Firstpost*. June 9, 2015. http://www.firstpost.com/india/no-surya-namaskar-on-international-yoga-day-modi-govt-axes-asana-to-soothe-irate-muslim-groups-2286068.html

Freeman, Richard. *The Mirror of Yoga: Awakening the Intelligence of Body and Mind*. Boston: Shambhala, 2012.

Fuller, Jason D. "Aṣṭāṅga-Yoga and Bhaktivinoda Thakura." *Journal of Vaishnava Studies* 14, no. 1 (Fall 2005): 233–242.

Fuller, Robert C. *Spiritual, but Not Religious: Understanding Unchurched America*. Oxford: Oxford University Press, 2010.

Funes Maderey, Ana Laura. "Kuṇḍalinī Rising and Liberation in the Yogavāsiṣṭha: The Story of Cūḍālā and Śikhidhvaja." *Religions* 8, no. 11 (November 2017): 248–263.

Gaddy, James. "When Yoga Meets CrossFit, It's More Burn, Less Om." *Bloomberg.Com*, January 9, 2017. https://www.bloomberg.com/news/articles/2017-01-09/-mashup-yoga-classes-mix-crossfit-boxing-and-cardio-with-oms

Gaiam. "About Gaiam." https://www.gaiam.com/pages/about-gaiam

Gandhi, Mohandas Karamchand. *Non-Violent Resistance (Satyagraha)*. Mineola: Dover, 2001.

Ganguly, Rageshri. "Surya Namaskar in MP School Curriculum—Times of India." *The Times of India*, January 21, 2016. https://timesofindia.indiatimes.com/city/bhopal/Surya-Namaskar-in-MP-school-curriculum/articleshow/50551191.cms

Gannon, Sharon, and David Life. *Jivamukti Yoga*. New York: Ballantine Books, 2002.

Garnier, Jean-Claude. "Ashtanga Yoga Research Institute." Ashtanga Yoga Institute. http://yoga-ashtanga.net/en/tag/ashtanga-yoga-research-institute

Geer, Alexandra van der. "Introduction." In *Animals in Stone: Indian Mammals Sculptured through Time*, edited by Alexandra van der Geer, 1–53. Boston: Brill, 2008.

Gerety, Finnian M.M. "This Whole World Is OM: Song, Soteriology, and the Emergence of the Sacred Syllable." PhD Thesis. Harvard University: Graduate School of Arts & Sciences, 2015.

Glasenapp, Helmuth von, and Shridhar B. Shrotri. *Jainism: An Indian Religion of Salvation*. Delhi: Motilal Banarsidass Publishers, 1999.

Gleig, Ann. *American Dharma: Buddhism Beyond Modernity*. New Haven, CT: Yale University Press, 2019.

Gleig, Ann, and Charles I. Flores. "Remembering Sri Aurobindo and the Mother: The Forgotten Lineage of Integral Yoga." In *Gurus of Modern Yoga*, edited by Mark Singleton and Ellen Goldberg, 38–59. New York & London: Oxford University Press, 2014.

Godlaski, Theodore M. "Shiva, Lord of Bhang." *Substance Use & Misuse* 47, no. 10 (July 5, 2012): 1067–1072.

Goel, Vindu. "India Offers Atypical Video Challenges." *The New York Times*, December 27, 2015, sec. Technology. https://www.nytimes.com/2015/12/28/technology/bollywood-and-us-media-giants-try-to-induce-indians-to-pay-for-video.html

Gold, Jonathan C. "Vasubandhu." In *The Stanford Encyclopedia of Philosophy*, edited by Edward N. Zalta, Summer 2018. Metaphysics Research Lab, Stanford University, 2018. https://plato.stanford.edu/archives/sum2018/entries/vasubandhu

Goldberg, Ellen. "Amrit Desai and the Kripalu Center." In *Homegrown Gurus: From Hinduism in America to American Hinduism*, edited by Ann Gleig and Lola Williamson, 63–86. Albany, NY: SUNY Press, 2014.

———. "Swami Kṛpālvānanda: The Man Behind Kripalu Yoga." In *Gurus of Modern Yoga*, edited by Mark Singleton and Ellen Goldberg, 171–189. Oxford & New York: Oxford University Press, 2014.

Goldberg, Elliott. *The Path of Modern Yoga: The History of an Embodied Spiritual Practice*. Rochester, VT: Inner Traditions, 2016.

Goldberg, Michelle. *The Goddess Pose: The Audacious Life of Indra Devi, the Woman Who Helped Bring Yoga to the West*. New York: Vintage, 2016.

Goldberg, Philip. *American Veda: From Emerson and the Beatles to Yoga and Meditation—How Indian Spirituality Changed the West*. New York: Three Rivers Press, 2013.

Golden, Stephanie. "Like Father, Like Son." *Yoga Journal*, August 1994, 36–40.

Goldman, R.P., and S.J. Sutherland Goldman. "Rāmāyaṇa." In *The Hindu World*, edited by Sushil Mittal and Gene Thursby, 75–96. New York: Routledge, 2004.

Goleman, Daniel, and Richard J Davidson. *Altered Traits: Science Reveals How Meditation Changes Your Mind, Brain, and Body*. New York: Avery, 2017.

Gombrich, Richard F. *Theravāda Buddhism: A Social History from Ancient Benares to Modern Colombo*. New York: Routledge, 2006.

Gombrich, Richard, and Gananath Obeyesekere. *Buddhism Transformed: Religious Change in Sri Lanka*. Delhi: Motilal Banarsidass, 1990.

Gomez, Luis O. "Buddhism in India." In *The Religious Traditions of Asia*, edited by Joseph Mitsuo Kitagawa, 41–95. New York & London: Macmillan & Collier Macmillan, 2002.

Gonda, J. *The Vision of Vedic Poets*. Berlin & New York: De Gruyter Mouton, 2011.

Gorakṣanātha, and M. L. Gharote. *Siddhasiddhāntapaddhatiḥ: A Treatise on the Nātha Philosophy*. Lonavla: The Lonavla Yoga Institute, 2005.

Gray, David B. *The Cakrasamvara Tantra (the Discourse of Śrī Heruka), (Śrīherukābhidhāna): A Study and Annotated Translation*. New York: American Institute of Buddhist Studies, 2007.

Grilley, Paul. *Yin Yoga: Outline of a Quiet Practice*. Ashland, OR: White Cloud Press, 2002.

Grönbold, Günter. *The Yoga of Six Limbs: An Introduction to the History of Ṣaḍaṅgayoga*. Translated by Robert L. Hütwohl. Santa Fe, NM: Spirit of the Sun Publications, 1996.

Grossman, Cathy Lynn. "Yoga Poses Dangers to Genuine Christian Faith: Theologian." *USA Today*, September 20, 2010. http://content.usatoday.com/communities/Religion/post/2010/09/yoga-christian-mohler-palin/1#.WYt75oplCEI

Gunaratana, Henepola. *The Path of Serenity and Insight: An Explanation of the Buddhist Jhānas*. Delhi: Motilal Banarsidass, 1985.

Gupta, Sanjukta. "The Pāñcarātra Attitude to Mantra." In *Understanding mantras*, edited by Harvey P Alper, 224–248. Albany, NY: SUNY Press, 1989.

———. "Yoga and Antaryāga in Pāñcarātra." In *Ritual and Speculation in Early Tantrism: Studies in Honour of André Padoux*, edited by André Padoux and Teun Goudriaan, 175–208. Albany, NY: SUNY Press, 1992.

Hackett, Paul G. *Theos Bernard, the White Lama: Tibet, Yoga, and American Religious Life*. New York: Columbia University Press, 2012.

Halbfass, Wilhelm. *Tradition and Reflection: Explorations in Indian Thought*. Albany, NY: SUNY Press, 1991.

Hamid, Jalil. "Malaysia Backs down from Yoga Ban amid Backlash." *Reuters*, November 26, 2010. https://www.reuters.com/article/us-malaysia-islam-yoga-idUSTRE4AP2CA20081126

Hammond, Holly. "Meet the Innovators!" *Joga Journal*, October 2000, 80–89.

———. "Meet the Innovators: Judith Hanson Lasater." Yoga Journal. https://www.yogajournal.com/lifestyle/meet-the-innovators-judith-hanson-lasater

Hargreaves, Jacqueline, and Jason Birch. "The Yamas and Niyamas: Part 2—Medieval and Modern Views." *Yoga Scotland Magazine*, no. 50 (2016): 36–39.

Hargreaves, Jaqueline. "Asanas Old and New." *The Luminescent* (blog), October 8, 2013. http://theluminescent.blogspot.com/2013/10

Harimoto, Kengo, and Śaṅkara. *God, Reason and Yoga: A Critical Edition and Translation of the Commentary Ascribed to Śaṅkara on Pātañjalayogaśāstra 1.23–28*. Hamburg: Department of Indian and Tibetan Studies, Universität Hamburg, 2014.

Harvey, Peter. "The Dynamics of Paritta Chanting in Southern Buddhism." In *Love Divine: Studies in Bhakti and Devotional Mysticism*, edited by Karel Werner, 53–84. London & New York: Routledge, Taylor & Francis Group, 1993.

Hatengdi, M.U. *Nityananda: The Divine Presence*. Cambridge, MA: Rudra Press, 1984.

Hatley, Shaman. "What Is a Yoginī? Towards a Polythetic Definition." In *"Yoginī" in South Asia: Interdisciplinary Approaches*, edited by István Keul, 21–31. London & New York: Routledge, Taylor & Francis Group, 2013.

Hauser, Beatrix. "Touching the Limits, Assessing Pain: On Language Peformativity, Health, and Well-Being in Yoga Classes." In *Yoga Traveling: Bodily Practice in Transcultural Perspective*, 109–134. Heidelberg: Springer, 2013.

Hausner, Sondra L. "The Category of the Yoginī as a Gendered Practitioner." In *"Yoginī" in South Asia: Interdisciplinary Approaches*, edited by István Keul, 32–43. London & New York: Routledge, Taylor & Francis Group, 2013.

Hausner, Sondra L. *Wandering with Sadhus: Ascetics in the Hindu Himalayas*. Bloomington & Chesham: Indiana University Press & Combined Academic, 2008.

Hawley, John Stratton, and Juergensmeyer, Mark. *Songs of the Saints of India*. New York: Oxford University Press, 2004.

Hay, Stephen N. *Sources of Indian Tradition: Volume Two, Modern India and Pakistan*. New Delhi: Penguin, 1992.

Healy, John Paul. *Yearning to Belong: Discovering a New Religious Movement*. Farnham: Ashgate, 2013.

Heesterman, Johannes C. *The Broken World of Sacrifice: An Essay in Ancient Indian Ritual*. Chicago: University of Chicago Press, 1993.

Heesterman, Johannes Cornelius. *The Inner Conflict of Tradition: Essays in Indian Ritual, Kingship, and Society*. Chicago: University of Chicago Press, 1985.

Hemacandra, and Olle Qvarnström. *The Yogaśāstra of Hemacandra: A Twelfth Century Handbook of Śvetāmbara Jainism*. Cambridge, MA: Harvard University Press, 2002.

"H.H. Pujya Swami Chidanand Saraswatiji Ceaseless Service." http://www.pujyaswamiji.org/seva

Hiltebeitel, Alf. "Hinduism." In *Encyclopedia of Religion*, edited by Lindsay Jones, 3988–4009. Detroit, MI: Macmillan Reference USA, 2005.

"His Holiness Sri Swami Chidananda Saraswati Maharaj." http://www.dlshq.org/saints/chida.htm

"His Holiness Sri Swami Sivananda Saraswati Maharaj." http://www.dlshq.org/saints/siva.htm

Holdrege, Barbara A. *Bhakti and Embodiment: Fashioning Divine Bodies and Devotional Bodies in Krsna Bhakti*. New York: Routledge, 2015.

———. *Veda and Torah: Transcending the Textuality of Scripture*. Albany, NY: SUNY Press, 1996.

Holpuch, Amanda. "Evangelical Christian Group Helps Sue California School over Yoga Classes." *The Guardian*, January 10, 2013, sec. US news. http://www.theguardian.com/world/2013/jan/10/christian-parents-sue-california-school-yoga

"Home." Yoga and Body Image Coalition. http://ybicoalition.com

Hopkins, Thomas J. "Saura Hinduism." In *Encyclopedia of Religion*, 8135–8136. Detroit, MI: Macmillan Reference USA, 2005.

Hoskote, Ranjit. *I, Lalla: The Poems of Lal Dēd*. New Delhi: Penguin Books, 2013.

"How to Become a Certified Iyengar Yoga Teacher?" http://bksiyengar.com/modules/Teacher/certeach.htm

Hudson, D. Dennis. "Tantric Rites in Āṇṭāl's Poetry." In *Tantra in Practice*, edited by David Gordon White, 206–227. Princeton, NJ: Princeton University Press, 2000.

Hume, Robert Ernest, and George C. O Haas. *The Thirteen Principal Upanishads*. London: Oxford University Press, 1968.

Huntington, Susan L. *The Art of Ancient India: Buddhist, Hindu, Jain*. New York: Weatherhill, 1985.

IANS. "PM Modi Hails Yoga, Says It Will Lead to New Era of Harmony and Togetherness." https://www.hindustantimes.com/, March 2, 2017. https://www.hindustantimes.com/india-news/pm-modi-hails-yoga-says-it-will-lead-to-new-era-of-harmony-and-togetherness/story-AMHGnbJXQYjJxaVItEMdiM.html

———. " 'Why Are Indian Muslims Opposing Yoga When Muslim Countries Are Supporting It?' " *The New Indian Express*, June 13, 2015. http://www.newindianexpress.com/nation/2015/jun/13/Why-Are-Indian-Muslims-Opposing-Yoga-When-Muslim-Countries-Are-Supporting-It-768643.html

"International Yoga Sports Federation—Rajashree Choudhury."http://www.iysf.org/about-iysf/board/rajashree-choudhury

Isaacson, Walter. *Steve Jobs*. New York: Simon & Schuster, 2015.

Iyengar, B.K.S. *Light on Pranayama: The Yogic Art of Breathing*. New York: Crossroad, 1981.

———. *Light on Yoga: Yoga Dipika*. New York: Schocken Books, 1979.

———. *Yoga for Sports: A Journey towards Health and Healing*, Chennai: Westland, 2015.

Iyer, Aditya. "Maha Shivratri: Protesters Urge Modi Not to Attend Isha Foundation Event." *Hindustan Times*. February 24, 2017. https://www.hindustantimes.com/india-news/maha-shivratri-protesters-urge-modi-not-to-attend-isha-foundation-event/story-LR9F1JjnIwE9uQ5je7gkJP.html

Jackson, Roger R. "Saraha's Queen Dohās." In *Yoga in Practice*, edited by David Gordon White, 161–184. Princeton, NJ: Princeton University Press, 2012.

Jacobi, Hermann. "Uber Das Ursprüngliche Yoga-System." *Sitzungsberichte Der Preusischen Akademie Der Wissenschaften*, 1929, 581–624.

Jacobs, Stephen. "Yoga Jam: Remixing Kīrtan in the Art of Living." *The Journal of Religion and Popular Culture* 29, no. 1 (Spring 2017), 1–18.

Jacobs, Susan. "Magana Baptiste." *Yoga Journal*, December 1986.

Jacobsen, Knut A. "In Kapila's Cave." In *Theory and Practice of Yoga: Essays in Honour of Gerald James Larson*, edited by Knut A. Jacobsen, 333–349. Leiden & Boston: Brill, 2005.

———. "Introduction: Yoga Traditions." In *Theory and Practice of Yoga: Essays in Honor of Gerald James Larson*, edited by Knut A. Jacobsen, 1–27. Leiden & Boston: Brill, 2005.

———. *Yoga in Modern Hinduism: Hariharānanda Āraṇya and Sāṃkhyayoga*. Abingdon: Routledge, 2018.

"Jagad Guru Siddhaswarupananda Paramahamsa." http://www.scienceofidentityfoundation.net/about-us/jagad-guru-siddhaswarupananda-paramahamsa-chris-butler

Jain, Andrea R. "Muktananda: Entrepreneurial Godman, Tantric Hero." In *Gurus of Modern Yoga*, edited by Mark Singleton and Ellen Goldberg, 190–209. New York & London: Oxford University Press, 2014.

———. *Selling Yoga: From Counterculture to Pop Culture*, New York: Oxford University Press, 2015.

———. "Subversive Spiritualities: Yoga's Complex Role in the Narrative of Sex and Religion in the Twentieth-Century United States." In *Devotions and Desires: Histories of Sexuality and Religion in the Twentieth-Century United States*, edited by Gillian Frank, Bethany Moreton, and Heather Rachelle White, 34–53, 2018.

Jaini, Padmanabh S. "On the Sarvajñatva (Omniscience) of Mahāvīra and the Buddha." In *Buddhist Studies in Honour of I.B. Horner*, edited by L. Cousins, Arnold Kunst, and K. R. Norman, 71–90. Dordrecht: Springer Netherlands, 1974.

Jaini, Padmanabh S. *The Jaina Path of Purification*. Delhi: M. Banarsidass, 2001.

Jamison, Stephanie W., and Joel P. Brereton. *The Rigveda: The Earliest Religious Poetry of India*. New York: Oxford University Press, 2014.

Jayatarāma and Swāmī Maheśānanda. *Jogapradīpyakā of Jayatarāma*. Lonavla: Kaivalyadhama S.M.Y.M Samiti, 2006.

Jha, D.N. *The Myth of the Holy Cow*. London: Verso, 2004.

Jois, K. Pattabhi. *Yoga Mala*. New York: North Point Press, 2002.

Jones, Constance A., and James D. Ryan. *Encyclopedia of Hinduism*. New York: Checkmark Books, 2008.

Jordt, Ingrid. *Burma's Mass Lay Meditation Movement Buddhism and the Cultural Construction of Power*. Athens: Ohio University Press, 2007.

Jung, C.G. *The Psychology of Kundalini Yoga: Notes of the Seminar given in 1932*. Edited by Sonu Shamdasani. London: Routledge, 2015.

Kaelber, Walter O. *Tapta Mārga: Ascetism and Initiation in Vedic India*. Albany, NY: SUNY Press, 1989.

Kakar, Sudhir. *Shamans, Mystics, and Doctors: A Psychological Inquiry into India and Its Healing Traditions*. New Delhi: Oxford, 2012.

Karen Pechilis, ed. *The Graceful Guru: Hindu Female Gurus in India and the United States*. New York: Oxford University Press, 2004.

Karma-chags-med, Gnas-mdo, Rinpoche Gyatrul, and B. Alan Wallace. *A Spacious Path to Freedom: Pratical Instructions on the Union of Mahāmudrā and Ati-yoga*. Ithaca, NY: Snow Lion, 1998.

Kauṭalya, and L.N. Rangarajan. *The Arthashastra*. New Delhi & London: Penguin Books, 1992.

Kavanaugh, K., and M.B. Pennington. "Spirituality, Christian (History Of)." In *New Catholic Encyclopedia*, 13:443–451. Detroit, MI: Gale, 2003.

Kawamura, Leslie S. "Atīśa." In *Encyclopedia of Religion*, 592–593. Detroit, MI: Macmillan Reference USA, 2005.

Kenoyer, Jonathan M. *Ancient Cities of the Indus Valley Civilization*. Karachi & Islamabad: Oxford University Press & American Institute of Pakistan Studies, 2011.

Keown, Damien, Charles Jones, Stephen Hodge, and Paolo Tinti. *Buddhism: A Dictionary Of.* Oxford: Oxford University Press, 2004.

Keul, István. *"Yoginī" in South Asia: Interdisciplinary Approaches*. London & New York: Routledge, Taylor & Francis Group, 2013.

Khalsa, Dharam S., and Darryl O'Keeffe. *The Kundalini Yoga Experience: Bringing Body, Mind, and Spirit Together*. New York: Simon & Schuster, 2002.

Killingley, Dermot. "The Upaniṣads and Yoga." In *The Upaniṣads: A Complete Guide*, edited by Signe Cohen, 174–185. New York: Routledge, 2018.

King, Sallie B. *Socially Engaged Buddhism*. Honolulu: University of Hawai'i Press, 2009.

Kinsley, David. "Avatāra." In *Encyclopedia of Religion*, edited by Lindsay Jones, 2nd ed., 2:707–708. Detroit, MI: Macmillan Reference USA, 2005.

———. *Hindu Goddesses: Visions of the Divine Feminine in the Hindu Religious Tradition; with a New Preface*. Berkeley: University of California Press, 1997.

Kiss, Csaba. "The Masyendrasaṃhitā: A Yoginī-Centered Thirteenth-Century Text from the South Indian Śāmbhava Cult." In *Yogi Heroes and Poets: Histories and Legends of the Nāths*, edited by David N. Lorenzen and Adrián Muñoz, 143–162. Albany, NY: SUNY Press, 2011.

Kloppenborg, Ria. *The Paccekabuddha: A Buddhist Ascetic: A Study of the Concept of the Paccekabuddha in Pali Canonical and Commentarial Literature*. Leiden: Brill, 1974.

Knipe, David M. "Becoming a Veda in the Godavari Delta." In *India and Beyond: Aspects of Literature, Meaning, Ritual, and Thought. Essays in Honor of Frits Staal*, edited by Dick van der Meij, 306–322. Leiden: International Institute for Asian Studies, 1997.

Knipe, David M. "One Fire, Three Fires, Five Fires: Vedic Symbols in Transition." *History of Religions* 12, no. 1 (August 1972): 28–41.

Knipe, David M. *Vedic Voices: Intimate Narratives of a Living Andhra Tradition*, New York: Oxford University Press, 2015.

Kohn, Livia. *Chinese Healing Exercises: The Tradition of Daoyin*. Honolulu: University of Hawai'i Press, 2008.

———. *Daoist Body Cultivation: Traditional Models and Contemporary Practices.* Magdalena, NM: Three Pines Press, 2006.

Kothari, Smita. "Prekṣā Dhyāna in Jaina Yoga." In *Yoga in Jainism*, edited by Christopher Chapple, 210–228. New York: Routledge, 2015.

Kraftsow, Gary. "Defining Yoga Therapy: A Call to Action." *International Journal of Yoga Therapy* 20, no. 1 (October 2010): 27–29.

Kragh, Ulrich Timme. "The Yogācārabhūmi and Its Adaptation." In *The Foundation for Yoga Practitioners: The Buddhist Yogācārabhūmi Treatise and Its Adaptation in India, East Asia, and Tibet*, edited by Ulrich Timme Kragh, 22–287. Cambridge, MA: Harvard University Press, 2013.

Kremer, William. "Does Doing Yoga Make You a Hindu?" *BBC News*, November 21, 2013. http://www.bbc.com/news/magazine-25006926

Krishna Nambiar, A.K. *Namaste: Its Philosophy and Significance in Indian Culture.* Delhi: Spiritual India Pub. House, 1979.

Krishnamurti, Bhadriraju. "Introduction." In *The Dravidian Languages*, edited by Bhadriraju Krishnamurti, 1–47. Cambridge: Cambridge University Press, 2003.

Kulke, Hermann, and Dietmar Rothermund. *A History of India.* London & New York: Routledge, 2016.

Kvaerne, Per. "On the Concept of Sahaja in Indian Buddhist Tantric Literature." *Temenos* 11 (1975): 88–135.

La Vallée Poussin, Louis de. "Le Bouddhisme et Le Yoga de Patañjali." *Mélanges Chinois et Bouddhiques* 5 (1937): 223–241.

Lal, Vinay. "Nakedness, Nonviolence, and Brahmacharya: Gandhi's Experiments in Celibate Sexuality." *Journal of the History of Sexuality* 9, no. 1–2 (April 2000): 105–136.

Lappa, Andreĭ. *Yoga, Tradition of Unification*. Kyiv: A. Lappa, 2000.

Larson, Gerald James, and Ram Shankar Bhattacharya. *Encyclopedia of Indian Philosophies: India's Philosophy of Meditation. Yoga. Volume XII.* Motilal Banarsidass Publishers, 2008.

Larson, Gerald James, and Knut A Jacobsen. *Theory and Practice of Yoga: Essays in Honour of Gerald James Larson*. Leiden & Boston: Brill, 2005.

Larson, Sarah. "'Bikram' and the Fraught, Telling Tale of a Yoga Phenomenon," June 27, 2018. https://www.newyorker.com/culture/podcast-dept/bikram-and-the-fraught-telling-tale-of-a-yoga-phenomenon

Latey, Penelope. "The Pilates Method: History and Philosophy." *Journal of Bodywork and Movement Therapies* 5, no. 4 (October 2001): 275–282.

Laycock, Joseph. "Yoga for the New Woman and the New Man: The Role of Pierre Bernard and Blanche DeVries in the Creation of Modern Postural Yoga." *Religion and American Culture: A Journal of Interpretation* 23, no. 1 (2013): 101–136.

Leach, Anna. "One of San Francisco's Toughest Schools Transformed by the Power of Meditation." *The Guardian*. November 24, 2015. https://www.theguardian.com/teacher-network/2015/nov/24/san-franciscos-toughest-schools-transformed-meditation

Leadbeater, C.W. *The Chakras*. Wheaton, IL: Quest Books/Theosophical Publishing House, 2013.

Lester, Robert C. *Rāmānuja on the Yoga*. Madras: The Adyar Library, 1976.

Levitt, Stephen Hillyer. "New Considerations Regarding the Identity of the Vedic Sóma as the Mushroom Fly-Agaric." In *Studia Orientalia, Volume 111*, edited by Lotta Aunio, 105–118. Helsinki: Finnish Oriental Society, 2011.

Lewis, I.M. *Arguments with Ethnography: Comparative Approaches to History, Politics & Religion*. London & New Brunswick: The Athlone Press, 1999.

Lewis, James R. "Autobiography of a Schism." *Marburg Journal of Religion* 15, no. 1 (2015): 1–19.

Liberman, Kenneth. "The Reflexivity of the Authenticity of Haṭha Yoga." In *Yoga in the Modern World: Contemporary Perspectives*, edited by Mark Singleton and Jean Byrne, 100–116. New York: Routledge, 2008.

Lidell, Lucy, Narayani, and Fausto Dorelli. *The Sivananda Companion to Yoga*. New York: Simon & Schuster, 1983.

Long, Jeffery D. *Jainism: An Introduction*. London & New York: I.B. Tauris, 2009.

Lopes, Ana Cristina. *Tibetan Buddhism in Diaspora: Cultural Re-Signification in Practice and Institutions*. London & New York: Routledge, 2015.

Lopez, Donald S. *The Lotus Sutra: A Biography*. Princeton, NJ: Princeton University Press, 2016.

Lorenzen, David N. "Bhakti." In *The Hindu World*, edited by Sushil Mittal and Gene R. Thursby, 185–209. New York: Routledge, 2007.

———. "Śaivism: An Overview." In *Encyclopedia of Religion*, edited by Lindsay Jones, 2nd ed., 12:8038–8042. Detroit, MI: Macmillan Reference USA, 2005.

Lorr, Benjamin. *Hell-Bent: Obsession, Pain, and the Search for Something like Transcendence in Competitive Yoga*, New York: St. Martin's Press, 2014.

Love, Robert. "Fear of Yoga." *Columbia Journalism Review* 45, no. 4 (2006): 80–90.

———. *The Great Oom: The Improbable Birth of Yoga in America*. New York: Viking, 2010.

Lowe, Scott. "Adidam." In *Introduction to New and Alternative Religions in America*, edited by Eugene V. Gallagher and W. Michael Ashcraft, 4:85–109. Westport, CT: Greenwood Press, 2006.

Lucia, Amanda. "Guru Sex: Charisma, Proxemic Desire, and the Haptic Logics of the Guru-Disciple Relationship." *Journal of the American Academy of Religion* 86, no. 4 (November 2018): 953–988.

———. " 'Give Me Sevā Overtime': Selfless Service and Humanitarianism in Mata Amritanandamayi's Transnational Guru Movement." *History of Religions* 54, no. 2 (November 2014): 188–207.

———. "Innovative Gurus: Tradition and Change in Contemporary Hinduism." *International Journal of Hindu Studies* 18, no. 2 (August 2014): 221–263.

Maas, Philipp A. *Samādhipāda: Das erste Kapitel des Pātañjalayogaśātra zum ersten Mal kritisch ediert*. Aachen: Shaker Verlag, 2006.

———. "Sarvāstivāda Abhidharma and the Yoga of Patañjali." Paper presented at the 17th Congress of the International Association of Buddhist Studies. Vienna, Austria, August 18–23, 2014.

———. "Sthirasukham Āsanam: Posture and Performance in Classical Yoga and Beyond." In *Yoga in Transformation*, edited by Phillip A. Maas and Karin Preisendanz, 49–100. Göttingen: Vienna University Press, 2018.

Macdonell, Arthur Anthony. *Vedic Mythology*. New Delhi: Munshiram Manoharlal, 2000.

Mackenzie, Rory. *New Buddhist Movements in Thailand: Toward an Understanding of Wat Phra Dhammakaya and Santi Asoke*. London: Routledge, 2012.

Macrae, Eilidh. *Exercise in the Female Life-Cycle in Britain, 1930–1970*. London: Palgrave Macmillan, 2016.

"Madhavdas Ji." KaivalyaDham Yoga Institute. https://kdham.com/madhavdas-ji

Maehle, Gregor. *Yoga Meditation: Through Mantra, Chakras and Kundalini to Spiritual Freedom*. Crabbes Creek, NSW: Kaivalya Publications, 2013.

Maheshanandaji, Swami, B.R. Sharma, G.S. Sahay, and R.K. Bodhe, eds. *Yoga Concordance*. 4 vols. Lonavla, Maharashtra, India: Kaivalyadhama S.M.Y.M Samiti, 2001.

Makransky, John J., ed. *Buddhahood Embodied: Sources of Controversy in India and Tibet*. Albany, NY: SUNY Press, 1997.

Malalasekera, G.P., Dhammavihari, W.G. Vīraratna, Buddhist Council of Ceylon, Ceylon, Ministry of Cultural Affairs, Sri Lanka, and Bauddha Kaṭayutu Depārtamēntuva. *Encyclopaedia of Buddhism*. Colombo: Govt. of Ceylon, 1961.

Malinar, Angelika. *The Bhagavadgītā: Doctrines and Contexts*. Cambridge: Cambridge University Press, 2009.

Mäll, Linnart. *Studies in the Aṣṭasāhasrikā Prajñāpāramitā and Other Essays*. Delhi: Motilal Banarsidass, 2005.

Mallik, Kalyani. *Siddha-Siddhānta-Paddhati and Other Works of the Nātha Yogīs*. Poona: Poona Oriental Book House, 1954.

Mallinson, James. "Kālavañcana in the Konkan: How a Vajrayāna Haṭhayoga Tradition Cheated Buddhism's Death in India." *Religions* 10, no. 4 (April 2019): 273.

———. "Nāth Sampradāya." In *Brill's Encyclopedia of Hinduism*, edited by Knut Jacobsen, Helene Basu, Angelika Malinar, and Vasudha Narayanan, 3:407–428. Leiden & Boston: Brill, 2011.

———. "Śāktism and Haṭhayoga." In *Goddess Traditions in Tantric Hinduism: History, Practice, and Doctrine*, edited by Bjarne Wernicke Oleson, 109–140. London: Routledge, 2016.

———. "The Amṛtasiddhi: Haṭhayoga's Tantric Buddhist Source Text." In *Śaivism and the Tantric Traditions: A Festschrift for Alexis Sanderson*, edited by Dominic Goodall, Shaman Hatley, and Harunaga Isaacson. Leiden: Brill, Forthcoming.

———. "The Original Gorakṣaśataka." In *Tantra in Practice*, edited by David Gordon White, 257–272. Princeton, NJ: Princeton University Press, 2000.

———. "The Yogī's Latest Trick." *Journal of the Royal Asiatic Society* 24, no. 1 (January 2014): 165–180.

———. "Yoga: Haṭha Yoga." In *Brill's Encyclopedia of Hinduism*, edited by Knut Jacobsen, Helene Basu, Angelika Malinar, and Vasudha Narayanan, 3:770–781. Leiden & Boston: Brill, 2011.

Mallinson, James, and Mark Singleton. *Roots of Yoga*. London: Penguin Books, 2017.

Mara, Carrico. "Contraindications of Yoga." In *Injury Prevention for Fitness Instructors*, 38–44. San Diego: IDEA Health & Fitness Association, 2001.

Markula, Pirkko. "Reading Yoga: Changing Discourses of Postural Yoga on the Yoga Journal Covers." *Communication & Sport* 2, no. 2 (June 2014): 143–171.

"Master Yoga Chart | Dharma Yoga Center New York City." https://dharmayoga-center.com/resources/yoga-poses/master-yoga-chart

Masunaga, Samantha. "YogaWorks Chain Stretches Its Reach in California with Deal." *Los Angeles Times*, June 4, 2015. http://www.latimes.com/business/la-fi-yogaworks-acquisition-20150604-story.html

Matchett, Freda. "The Purāṇas." In *The Blackwell Companion to Hinduism*, edited by Gavin D. Flood, 129–143. Malden, MA: Blackwell, 2007.

Mathur, Avarnita. "Full List of Padma Awardees 2016," January 25, 2016. http://indiatoday.intoday.in/story/full-list-of-padma-awardees-2016/1/579218.html

McCartney, Patrick. "Downward Facing Dogs, Core Indian Values and Institutionalised Rape of Children." *Sociology International Journal* 2, no. 6 (2018): 748–752.

———. "Politics beyond the Yoga Mat: Yoga Fundamentalism and the 'Vedic Way of Life.' " *Global Ethnographic*, no. 4 (May 2017): 1–18.

———. "Śāntamūrti: The Legitimate Disposition(s) of the 'Temple of Peace' Social Network." *Annual Papers of the Anthropological Institute* 8 (2018): 65–104.

———. "Spiritual Bypass and Entanglement in Yogaland (योगस्तान): How Neoliberalism, Soft Hindutva, and Banal Nationalism Facilitate Yoga Fundamentalism." *Politics and Religion Journal* 13, no. 1 (March 2019): 137–175.

———. "Suggesting Śāntarasa in Shanti Mandir's Satsaṅga: Ritual, Performativity and Ethnography in Yogaland." *Ethnologia Actualis* 17, no. 2 (December 2017): 81–122.

———. "The Unintended Consequences of International Day of Yoga." *Daily O* (blog), June 21, 2018. https://www.dailyo.in/variety/international-yoga-day-soft-power-hindutva-narendra-modi-deen-dayal-upadhyaya-hedgewar/story/1/25021.html

McDaniel, June. *Offering Flowers, Feeding Skulls: Popular Goddess Worship in West Benagal.* New York: Oxford University Press, 2004.

McEvilley, Thomas. "An Archaeology of Yoga." *Res: Anthropology and Aesthetics* 1 (March 1981): 44–77.

McGetchin, Douglas T. *Indology, Indomania, and Orientalism: Ancient India's Rebirth in Modern Germany.* Madison, NJ: Fairleigh Dickinson University Press, 2009.

McGovern, Nathan. "Brahmā: An Early and Ultimately Doomed Attempt at a Brahmanical Synthesis." *Journal of Indian Philosophy* 40, no. 1 (2012): 1–23.

———. *The Snake and the Mongoose: The Emergence of Identity in Early Indian Religion.* New York: Oxford University Press, 2018.

McKean, Lise. *Divine Enterprise: Gurus and the Hindu Nationalist Movement.* Chicago: University of Chicago Press, 1996.

Melton, Glennon Doyle. *Carry On, Warrior: Thoughts on Life Unarmed.* New York: Simon and Schuster, 2013.

"MERU Vlodrop." http://meru-mvu.org/vlodrop

"Mission." Mind & Life Institute. https://www.mindandlife.org/mission

Mittal, Sushil, Gene R. Thursby, and Kathleen M. Erndl, eds. "Śākta." In *The Hindu World*, 140–161. New York: Routledge, 2007.

Montgomery, Dan. "Samaya and the World of Shambhala." *Tricycle: The Buddhist Review*, August 6, 2018. https://tricycle.org/trikedaily/shambhala-samaya

Mujumdar, Dattatraya Chintaman, ed. *Encyclopedia of Indian Physical Culture: A Comprehensive Survey of the Physical Education in India, Profusely Illustrating Various Activities of Physical Culture, Games, Exercises, Etc., as Handed over to Us from Our Fore-Fathers and Practised in India.* Baroda: Good Companions, 1950.

Muller-Ortega, Paul E. "Becoming Bhairava: Meditative Vision in Abhinavagupta's Parātrīśikā-Laghuvṛtti." In *The Roots of Tantra*, edited by Katherine Anne Harper and Robert L. Brown. Albany, NY: SUNY Press, 2002.

———. " 'Tarko Yogāṅgam Uttamam': On Subtle Knowledge and the Refinement of Thought in Abhinavagupta's Liberative Tantric Method." In *Theory and Practice of Yoga: Essays in Honor of Gerald James Larson*, edited by Knut A. Jacobsen, 181–212. Leiden & Boston: Brill, 2005.

———. *The Triadic Heart of Śiva: Kaula Tantricism of Abhinavagupta in the Non-Dual Shaivism of Kashmir*. Albany, NY: SUNY Press, 1989.

Nair, Malini. "The Guru with a Stick." *The Times of India*, August 24, 2014. https://timesofindia.indiatimes.com/home/sunday-times/deep-focus/The-guru-with-a-stick/articleshow/40839884.cms

Nakamura, Hajime. *Indian Buddhism: A Survey with Bibliographical Notes*. Intercultural Research Institute Monograph, no. 9. Hirakata, Japan: KUFS Publication, 1980.

Nakamura, Hajime, and Gaynor Sekimori. *Gotama Buddha: A Biography Based on the Most Reliable Texts*. Tokyo: Kosei Publishing Co., 2000.

Namkhai Norbu, and Adriano Clemente. *Yantra Yoga: the Tibetan Yoga of Movement*. Ithaca, NY: Snow Lion, 2008.

Nanda, Meera. "Ambedkar's Gita." *Economic and Political Weekly* 51, no. 49 (2016): 38–45.

Nayar, Kamala E., Jaswinder Singh Sandhu, and Nānak. *The Socially Involved Renunciate: Guru Nanak's Discourse to the Nāth Yogis*. Albany, NY: SUNY Press, 2007.

Nevrin, Klas. "Krishnamacharya's Viniyoga: On Modern Yoga and Sri Vaisnavism." *Journal of Vaishnava Studies* 14, no. 1 (2005): 65–94.

Newcombe, Suzanne. "Spaces of Yoga: Towards a Non-Essentialist Understanding of Yoga." In *Yoga in Transformation*, edited by Phillip A. Maas and Karin Preisendanz, 549–573. Göttingen: Vienna University Press, 2018.

———. "The Institutionalization of the Yoga Tradition: 'Gurus' B.K.S. Iyengar and Yogini Sunita in Britain." In *Gurus of Modern Yoga*, edited by Mark Singleton and Ellen Goldberg, 147–167. New York & London: Oxford University Press, 2014.

———. "The Revival of Yoga in Contemporary India." In *Oxford Research Encyclopedia of Religion*. Vol. 1. Oxford University Press, May 24, 2017.

Newman, John. "Islam in the Kālacakra Tantra." *Journal of the International Association of Buddhist Studies* 21, no. 2 (1998): 311–371.

———. "Vajrayoga in the Kālacakra Tantra." In *Tantra in Practice*, edited by David Gordon White, 587–594. Princeton, NJ: Princeton University Press, 2000.

Nicholson, Andrew. "Hindu Disproofs of God: Refuting Vedāntic Theism in the *Sāṃkhya-Sūtra*." In *The Oxford Handbook of Indian Philosophy*, edited by Jonardon Ganeri, 598–619. New York: Oxford University Press, 2017.

———. *Unifying Hinduism: Philosophy and Identity in Indian Intellectual History.* New York: Columbia University Press, 2014.

———. *Lord Śiva's Song: the Īśvara Gītā.* Albany, NY: SUNY Press, 2014.

———. "Dialogue and Genre in Indian Philosophy." In *Dialogue in Early South Asian Religions: Hindu, Buddhist, and Jain Traditions*, edited by Brian Black and Laurie L. Patton, 151–169. London & New York: Routledge, 2016.

Nir, Sarah Maslin. "In Queens, Seeking to Clear a Path Between Yoga and Islam." *The New York Times*, April 8, 2012, sec. N.Y. / Region. https://www.nytimes.com/2012/04/09/nyregion/in-queens-seeking-to-clear-a-path-between-yoga-and-islam.html

Norman, Kenneth Roy. "The Pratyeka-Buddha in Buddhism and Jainism." In *Collected Papers* 2, 210–223. Oxford: Pali Text Society, 1991.

Nyberg, Harri. "The Problem of the Aryans and the Soma: The Botanical Evidence." In *The Indo-Aryans of Ancient South Asia: Language, Material Culture, and Ethnicity*, edited by George Erdosy, 382–406, n.d.

O'Brien-Kop, Karen. "Classical Discourses of Liberation: Shared Botanical Metaphors in Sarvāstivāda Buddhism and the Yoga of Patañjali." *Religions of South Asia* 11, no. 2–3 (2017): 123–157.

———. "The 'Other' Yogaśāstra: Reconfiguring the Category of Classical Yoga." Paper presented at the 2018 American Academy of Religion Annual Meeting. Denver, CO, November 17–21. 2018.

O'Flaherty, Wendy Doniger. *The Rig Veda: An Anthology: One Hundred and Eight Hymns.* Harmondsworth: Penguin Books, 2007.

Olivelle, Patrick. "King and Ascetic: State Control of Asceticism in the Ārthaśāstra." In *Festschrift Ludo Rocher*, edited by Richard Lariviere and Richard Salomon, 39–59. Madras: Adyar Library and Research Centre, 1987.

———. *Saṃnyāsa Upaniṣads: Hindu Scriptures on Asceticism and Renunciation.* Oxford: Oxford University Press, 1992.

———. *The Āśrama System: The History and Hermeneutics of a Religious Institution.* New York: Oxford University Press, 1993.

———. *The Early Upanisads: Annotated Text and Translation.* New York: Oxford University Press, 1998.

———. *Upaniṣads.* New York: Oxford University Press, 2008.

Olson, Carl. "Orientalism." In *Studying Hinduism: Key Concepts and Methods*, edited by Sushil Mittal and Gene Thursby, 290–300. New York: Routledge, 2009.

"On the Ground—Sadhguru's Mission." http://isha.sadhguru.org/mission

Openshaw, Jeanne. *Seeking Bāuls of Bengal.* Cambridge: Cambridge University Press, 2004.

"Order of Interbeing History." *Order of Interbeing | Tiep Hien* (blog), July 12, 2011. https://orderofinterbeing.org/about/our-history

Ornish, Dean. *Dr. Dean Ornish's Program for Reversing Heart Disease*. New York: Ballantine Books, 1991.

Osto, Douglas. *Altered States: Buddhism and Psychedelic Spirituality in America*. New York: Columbia University Press, 2018.

Padoux, André. *The Heart of the Yogini: The Yoginihrdaya, a Sanskrit Tantric Treatise*. New York: Oxford University Press, 2013.

———. *The Hindu Tantric World: An Overview*, Chicago: University of Chicago Press, 2017.

———. "What Do We Mean by Tantrism?" In *The Roots of Tantra*, edited by Katherine Anne Harper and Robert L. Brown, 17–24. Albany, NY: SUNY Press, 2002.

Page, Enoch H. "The Gender, Race, and Class Barriers: Enclosing Yoga as White Public Space." In *Yoga, the Body, and Embodied Social Change: An Intersectional Feminist Analysis*, edited by Beth Berila, Melanie Klein, and Chelsea Jackson Roberts, 41–65. Lanham, MD: Lexington Books, 2016.

Panasevich, Jake. "Why Yoga Is More Than a Workout." *US News & World Report* (blog), March 11, 2015. https://health.usnews.com/health-news/blogs/eat-run/2015/03/11/why-yoga-is-more-than-a-workout

"Pandit Rajmani Tigunait, PhD." Himalayan Institute, August 25, 2017. https://www.himalayaninstitute.org/presenter/pandit-rajmani-tigunait

Pant, Bhawanrao Srinivasrao, and Louise Morgan. *The Ten-Point Way to Health: Surya Namaskars*. London: Dent, 1956.

Parel, Anthony. *Gandhi's Philosophy and the Quest for Harmony*. Cambridge: Cambridge University Press, 2008.

Parpola, Asko. *Deciphering the Indus Script*. Cambridge: Cambridge University Press, 2010.

———. *The Roots of Hinduism: The Early Aryans and the Indus Civilization*. New York: Oxford University Press, 2015.

Parsons, William Barclay, ed. *Being Spiritual but Not Religious: Past, Present, Future(s)*. New York: Routledge, 2018.

Patañjali, Hariharananda Aranya, Paresh Nath Mukerji, and Vyasa. *Yoga Philosophy of Patañjali: Containing His Yoga Aphorisms with Vyasa's Commentary in Sanskrit and a Translation with Annotations Including Many Suggestions for the Practice of Yoga*. Albany, NY: SUNY Press, 1983.

"Patricia Walden: Lighting the Way | IYNAUS | Iyengar Yoga: National Association of the United States." https://iynaus.org/yoga-samachar/fall-2011winter-2012/patricia-walden-lighting-way

Patton, Laurie L. *Bringing the Gods to Mind: Mantra and Ritual in Early Indian Sacrifice*. Berkeley: University of California Press, 2006.

Pauwels, Heidi. "Who Are the Enemies of the Bhaktas? Testimony about 'Śāktas' and 'Others' from Kabīr, the Rāmānandīs, Tulsīdās, and Harirām Vyās." *Journal of the American Oriental Society* 130, no. 4 (2010): 509–539.

Pearson, Craig. *The Complete Book of Yogic Flying: The Program of His Holiness Maharishi Mahesh Yogi to Enjoy Bubbling Bliss, Develop Total Brain Functioning and Higher States of Consciousness, and Create National Invincibility and World Peace*. Fairfield, IA: Maharishi University of Management Press, 2008.

Pechelis, Karen. "Introduction: Hindu Female Gurus in Historical and Philosophical Context." In *The Graceful Guru: Hindu Female Gurus in India and the United States*, edited by Karen Pechilis, 3–49. New York: Oxford University Press, 2004.

Pedersen, Kusumita P. "Sri Chinmoy's Work at the United Nations: Spirituality and the Power of Silence." *CrossCurrents* 60, no. 3 (September 2010): 339–351.

Penner, Hans. "The Mystical Illusion." In *Mysticism and Religious Traditions*, edited by Steven T. Katz, 89–116. New York: Oxford University Press, 1983.

Perry, Tony. "Legal Fight against Yoga in Encinitas Schools Is Finished." *Los Angeles Times*, June 12, 2015. http://www.latimes.com/local/lanow/la-me-ln-yoga-legal-fight-20150612-story.html

Phillips, Stephen H. *Yoga, Karma, and Rebirth: A Brief History and Philosophy*. New York: Columbia University Press, 2009.

Pinch, William R. *Warrior Ascetics and Indian Empires*. Cambridge & New York: Cambridge University Press, 2012.

"Plum Village." Plum Village, January 3, 2013. https://plumvillage.org/about/plum-village

Plutarch, Robin Waterfield, and Andrew Erskine. *Hellenistic Lives*. Oxford: Oxford University Press, 2016.

Poceski, Mario. "Contemporary Chinese Buddhist Traditions." In *Oxford Handbook of Contemporary Buddhism*, edited by Michael Kessler Jerryson, 79–99. New York: Oxford University Press, 2017.

Ponzio, Alessio. *Shaping the New Man: Youth Training Regimes in Fascist Italy and Nazi Germany*. Madison: University of Wisconsin Press, 2015.

Potter, Karl H. *Abhidharma Buddhism to 150 A.D.* Princeton, NJ: Princeton University Press, 1991.

Powell, Seth. "Etched in Stone: Sixteenth-Century Visual and Material Evidence of Śaiva Ascetics and Yogis in Complex Non-Seated Āsanas at Vijayanagara." *Journal of Yoga Studies* 1, no. 1 (2018): 45–106.

Powers, John. *A Concise Introduction to Tibetan Buddhism*. Ithaca, NY: Snow Lion, 2008.

Powers, Sarah. *Insight Yoga*. Boston: Shambhala, 2009.

Prebish, Charles S. "Buddhist Councils and Divisions of the Order." In *Buddhism: A Modern Perspective*, edited by Charles S Prebish, 21–35. University Park: Pennsylvania State University Press, 1989.

———. *Religion and Sport: The Meeting of Sacred and Profane*. Westport, CT: Greenwood Press, 1993.

Prebish, Charles S., Kenneth K. Tanaka, and Amy Lavine, eds. "Tibetan Buddhism in America." In *The Faces of Buddhism in America*, 100–115. Berkeley: University of California Press, 1999.

"Preparing for Sadhana." 3HO: Happy, Healthy, Holy. https://www.3ho.org/kundalini-yoga/sadhana/preparing-sadhana

PTI. "Modi Mourns Death of Swami Dayananda Saraswati—Times of India." *The Times of India*, September 24, 2015. http://timesofindia.indiatimes.com/india/Modi-mourns-death-of-Swami-Dayananda-Saraswati/articleshow/49084779.cms

———. "Surya Namaskar Similar to Namaz: Yogi Adityanath." *The Indian Express*. March 29, 2017. http://indianexpress.com/article/india/surya-namaskar-similar-to-namaz-yogi-adityanath-4591630

———. "Swami Atmasthanandaji Maharaj Passes Away, PM Modi Says Personal Loss." *Hindustan Times*, June 19, 2017. http://www.hindustantimes.com/india-news/swami-atmasthanandaji-maharaj-passes-away-pm-modi-says-personal-loss/story-RvTH8E3UpMVMTjsrXbPQVL.html

———. "Yoga Day 2016 Diluted: No 'Suryanamaskar,' Chanting of 'OM' Not Compulsory." *Firstpost*. June 8, 2016. http://www.firstpost.com/india/yoga-day-2016-diluted-no-suryanamaskar-chanting-of-om-not-compulsory-2823704.html

Queen, Christopher S. *Engaged Buddhism: Buddhist Liberation Movements in Asia*. Albany, NY: SUNY Press, 2011.

Qvarnström, Olle. "Hemacandra on Yoga." In *Yoga in Jainism*, edited by Christopher Key Chapple, 139–154. London & New York: Routledge, Taylor & Francis Group, 2016.

———. "Jain Tantra: Divinatory and Meditative Practices in the Twelfth-Century Yogaśāstra of Hemacandra." In *Tantra in Practice*, edited by David Gordon White, 595–604. Princeton, NJ: Princeton University Press, 2000.

Rajneesh, Bhagwan Shree. *Tantra, Spirituality & Sex*. San Francisco & New York: The Rainbow Bridge, 1976.

Ramaswamy, Br. "Swami Dayananda Saraswati." Newsletter, August 2009. http://www.arshavidya.in/Newsletter/Aug09/swamiji-his-life-and-work.pdf

Rao, Mani. *Living Mantra: Mantra, Deity, and Visionary Experience Today*. Cham: Palgrave Macmillan, 2018.

Rao, Velcheru Narayana. "Purāṇa." In *The Hindu World*, edited by Sushil Mittal and Gene R. Thursby, 97–115. New York: Routledge, 2007.

Rastelli, Marion. "Yoga in the Daily Routine of the Pāñcarātrins." In *Yoga in Transformation*, edited by Phillip A. Maas and Karin Preisendanz, 223–257. Göttingen: Vienna University Press, 2018.

Rastogi, Navjivan. "The Yogic Disciplines of the Monistic Śaiva Tantric Traditions of Kashmir: Threefold, Fourfold, and Six-Limbed." In *Ritual and Speculation in Early Tantrism: Studies in Honour of André Padoux*, edited by André Padoux and Teun Goudriaan, 247–280. Albany, NY: SUNY Press, 1992.

Ray, Reginald. "Mahāsiddhas." In *Encyclopedia of Religion*, 5603–5606. Detroit, MI: Macmillan Reference USA, 2005.

Rea, Shiva. *Tending the Heart Fire: Living in Flow with the Pulse of Life*. Boulder, CO: Sounds True, 2014.

Remski, Matthew. "How a #MeToo Facebook Post Toppled a Yoga Icon," January 26, 2020, *Medium Gen*, https://gen.medium.com/how-a-metoo-facebook-post-toppled-a-yoga-icon-c25577185e40.

———. Remski, Matthew *Practice and All Is Coming: Abuse, Cult Dynamics and Healing in Yoga and Beyond*. New Zealand: Embodied Wisdom Publishing, 2019.

———. "Yoga Can Injure You. Here's How to Find a Class That Won't." *The Guardian*, October 27, 2016, sec. Opinion. https://www.theguardian.com/commentisfree/2016/oct/27/yoga-injury-class-regulation-bad-practitioners

Rennie, Bryan S. *Reconstructing Eliade: Making Sense of Religion*. Albany, NY: SUNY Press, 1996.

Rigopoulos, Antonio. *Dattatreya: The Immortal Guru, Yogin, and Avatara: A Study of the Transformative and Inclusive Character of a Multi-Faceted Hindu Deity*. Albany, NY: SUNY Press, 1998.

Rin-chen-rnam-rgyal, Herbert V. Guenther, and Nāḍapāda. *The Life and Teaching of Nāropa*. UNESCO Collection of Representative Works. Oxford: Clarendon Press, 1963.

Rocher, Ludo. *The Puranas*. Wiesbaden: Otto Harrassowitz, 1986.

"Rod Stryker." Himalayan Institute, February 15, 2019. https://www.himalayaninstitute.org/presenter/rod-stryker

Rodrigues, Santan. *The Householder Yogi: Life of Shri Yogendra*. Bombay: Yogendra Publications Fund, 2008.

Roth, Harold David. *Original Tao: Inward Training (nei-yeh) and the Foundations of Taoist Mysticism*. New York & Chichester: Columbia University Press, 1999.

Rueb, Emily S. "Yoga Adjustments Tread a Fine Line of Personal Space." *The New York Times*, February 11, 2011, sec. N.Y. / Region. https://www.nytimes.com/2011/02/13/nyregion/13stretch.html

Ruiz, Fernando Pagés. "The Sticky Business + History of Yoga Mats." *Yoga Journal*, August 28, 2007. https://www.yogajournal.com/yoga-101/sticky-business

Rukmani, T.S. "Śaṅkara's Views on 'Yoga' in the 'Brahmasūtrabhāṣya' in the Light of the Authorship of the 'Yogasūtrabhāṣyavivaraṇa.'" *Journal of Indian Philosophy* 21, no. 4 (1993): 395–404.

———. "The 'Yogasūtrabhāṣyavivaraṇa' Is Not the Work of Śaṅkarācārya the Author of the 'Brahmasūtrabhāṣya.'" *Journal of Indian Philosophy* 26, no. 3 (1998): 263–274.

Samuel, Geoffrey. *The Origins of Yoga and Tantra: Indic Religions to the Thirteenth Century*. Cambridge: Cambridge University Press, 2008.

Sanagaram, Himani Kumar. "Padma Shri Winner Wai Lana Revolutionising Yoga in USA." *NewsGram*, February 4, 2016. https://www.newsgram.com/padma-shri-winner-wai-lana-revolutionising-yoga-in-usa

Sanderson, Alexis. "Śaivism and the Tantric Traditions." In *The World's Religions*, edited by Stewart Sutherland, Leslie Houlden, Peter Clarke, and Friedhelm Hardy, 660–704. London: Routledge, 1988.

———. "Śaivism: Trika Śaivism." In *Encyclopedia of Religion*, edited by Lindsay Jones, 12:8046–47. Detroit, MI: Macmillan Reference USA, 2005.

———. "The Śaiva Age: The Rise and Dominance of Śaivism during the Early Medieval Period." In *Genesis and Development of Tantrism*, edited by Shingo Einoo, 41–349. Japan: Sankibō Busshorin, 2009.

———. "Vajrayāna: Origin and Function." In *Buddhism into the Year 2000: International Conference Proceedings.*, 87–102. Bangkok: Dhammakaya Foundation, 1994.

———. "Yoga in Śaivism (Unpublished Draft)," 1999, 1–42.

"Sant Hazara Singh—Yogi Bhajan's First Teacher." Sikh Dharma International, September 13, 2017. https://www.sikhdharma.org/sant-hazara-singh-yogi-bhajans-first-teacher

Śāntideva, Kate Crosby, and Andrew Skilton. *The Bodhicaryāvatāra*. Oxford & New York: Oxford University Press, 2008.

Santilli, Mara. "Is Your Beat-Bumping Hip-Hop Yoga Class Still Considered 'Real' Yoga?" *Shape Magazine*, October 10, 2017. https://www.shape.com/fitness/trends/fast-paced-yoga-with-music-trend

Sarbacker, Stuart Ray. "Herbs (Auṣadhi) as a Means to Spiritual Accomplishments (Siddhi) in Patañjali's 'Yogasūtra.'" *International Journal of Hindu Studies* 17, no. 1 (2013): 37–56.

———. "Rudolf Otto and the Concept of the Numinous." *Oxford Research Encyclopedia of Religion*, August 31, 2016.
———. "Indo-Tibetan Tantrism as Spirit Marriage." In *Perceiving the Divine through the Human Body: Mystical Sensuality*, edited by Thomas Cattoi and June McDaniel, 29–43. New York: Palgrave Macmillan, 2011.
———. "Meditation as Desired: Smṛti in the Yogasūtra and Cognate Buddhist Sources." Paper presented at the Association for Asian Studies 2011 Annual Conference. Honolulu, Hawaii, March 21–24, 2011.
———. "Power and Meaning in the Yogasūtra of Patañjali." In *Yoga Powers: Extraordinary Capacities Attained Through Meditation and Concentration*, edited by Knut A Jacobsen, 195–222. Leiden: Brill, 2011.
———. "Reclaiming the Spirit through the Body: The Nascent Spirituality of Modern Postural Yoga." *Entangled Religions*, no. 1 (2014): 95–114.
———. *Samādhi: The Numinous and Cessative in Indo-Tibetan Yoga*. Albany, NY: SUNY Press, 2005.
———. "Svādhyāya and Bhakti: Saguṇa Devatā and Nirguṇa Īśvara in Aṣṭāṅgayoga." Paper Presented at the 15th Annual DANAM Conference. Boston, MA, November 17–18, 2017.
———. "Swami Ramdev: Modern Yoga Revolutionary." In *Gurus of Modern Yoga*, edited by Mark Singleton and Ellen Goldberg, 351–371. New York & London: Oxford University Press, 2014.
———. "The Concept of Samadhi: Method and the Study of Meditation in South Asian Religion." University of Wisconsin–Madison, 2001.
———. "The Icon of Yoga: Patañjali as Nāgarāja in Modern Yoga." In *Sacred Matters: Material Religion in South Asian Traditions*, edited by Tracy Pintchman, 15–37. Albany, NY: SUNY Press, 2015.
———. "The Numinous and Cessative in Modern Yoga." In *Yoga in the Modern World: Contemporary Perspectives*, edited by Mark Singleton and Jean Byrne, 161–183. New York: Routledge, 2008.
———. "The Yoga of the Śiva Purāṇa." Paper presented at the IASS 17th World Sanskrit Conference, Vancouver, Canada, July 9–13, 2018.
———. "The Yoga Studio as Locus Numinous." Paper presented at the Yogascapes in Japan Conference, Kyoto, Japan, November 2–3, 2018.
Sarbacker, Stuart Ray, and Kevin Kimple. *The Eight Limbs of Yoga: A Handbook for Living Yoga Philosophy*. New York: North Point Press, 2015.
Schaeffer, Kurtis R. "The Attainment of Immortality: From Nāthas in India to Buddhists in Tibet." *Journal of Indian Philosophy* 30, no. 6 (2002): 515–533.
Schedneck, Brooke. *Thailand's International Meditation Centers: Tourism and the Global Commodification of Religious Practices*. London & New York: Routledge, Taylor & Francis Group, 2017.

"Scheme for Voluntary Certification of Yoga Professionals." http://www.yoga certification.qci.org

Schmidt, Leigh Eric. *Restless Souls: The Making of American Spirituality*. Berkeley: University of California Press, 2012.

Schomer, Karine. *The Sants: Studies in a Devotional Tradition of India*. Delhi: Motilal Banarsidass, 1987.

Schrader, Friedrich Otto. *Introduction to the Pāñcarātra and the Ahirbudhnya Saṃhitā*. Madras: Adyar Library and Research Centre, 1973.

Schrank, Sarah. "American Yoga: The Shaping of Modern Body Culture in the United States." *American Studies* 53, no. 1 (May 22, 2014): 169–181.

———. "Naked Yoga and Sexualization of Asana." In *Yoga, the Body, and Embodied Social Change: An Intersectional Feminist Analysis*, edited by Beth Berila, Melanie Klein, and Chelsea Jackson Roberts, 155–174. Lanham, MD: Lexington Books, 2016.

Schultz, Anna C. *Singing a Hindu Nation: Marathi Devotional Performance and Nationalism*. New York: Oxford University Press, 2013.

Seager, Richard Hughes. *Buddhism in America*. New York: Columbia University Press, 2012.

Sharma, Arvind. *Classical Hindu Thought: An Introduction*. New Delhi & New York: Oxford University Press, 2003.

Shaw, Miranda. *Passionate Enlightenment: Women in Tantric Buddhism*. Princeton, NJ: Princeton University Press, 2011.

Shaw, Sarah. *Buddhist Meditation: An Anthology of Texts from the Pali Canon*. London & New York: Routledge, 2006.

Sherbow, Paul H. "Viśvanātha Cakravartī's View on Yoga." *Journal of Vaishnava Studies* 14, no. 1 (Fall 2005): 209–232.

Shinohara, Koichi. *Spells, Images, and Maṇḍalas: Tracing the Evolution of Esoteric Buddhist Rituals*. New York: Columbia University Press, 2014.

Shipley, Morgan. *Psychedelic Mysticism: Transforming Conciousness, Religious Experiences, and Voluntary Peasants in Postwar America*. Lanham, MD: Lexington Books, 2015.

Shiva, Vandana. "Nature as the Feminine Principle." In *This Sacred Earth Religion, Nature, Environment*, edited by Roger S. Gottlieb, 382–385. New York: Routledge, 2004.

Silk, Jonathan A. "The Yogācāra Bhikṣu." In *Wisdom, Compassion, and the Search for Understanding: The Buddhist Studies Legacy of Gadjin M. Nagao*, edited by Jonathan A. Silk, 265–314. Honolulu: University of Hawai'i Press, 2000.

Singleton, Mark. "Salvation through Relaxation: Proprioceptive Therapy and Its Relationship to Yoga." *Journal of Contemporary Religion* 20, no. 3 (October 2005): 289–304.

———. "The Classical Reveries of Modern Yoga." In *Yoga in the Modern World: Contemporary Perspectives*, edited by Mark Singleton and Jean Byrne, 77–99. London and New York: Routledge, Taylor & Francis Group, 2008.

———. "Transnational Exchange and the Genesis of Modern Postural Yoga." In *Yoga Traveling: Bodily Practice in Transcultural Perspective*, edited by Beatrix Hauser, 37–56. Transcultural Research—Heidelberg Studies on Asia and Europe in a Global Context. Cham & New York: Springer, 2013.

———. "Yoga and Physical Culture: Transnational History and Blurred Discursive Contexts." In *Routledge Handbook of Contemporary India*, edited by Knut A. Jacobsen, 172–184. Abingdon: Routledge, 2016.

———. *Yoga Body: The Origins of Modern Posture Practice*. Oxford & New York: Oxford University Press, 2010.

———. "Yoga, Eugenics, and Spiritual Darwinism in the Early Twentieth Century." *International Journal of Hindu Studies* 11, no. 2 (2007): 125–146.

Singleton, Mark, and Tara Fraser. "T. Krishnamacharya, Father of Modern Yoga." In *Gurus of Modern Yoga*, edited by Mark Singleton and Ellen Goldberg, 83–106, New York: Oxford University Press, 2014.

Singleton, Mark, M. Narasimhan, and M.A. Jayashree. "Yoga Makaranda of T. Krishnamacharya." In *Yoga in Practice*, edited by David Gordon White, 337–352. Princeton, NJ: Princeton University Press, 2012.

Sivananda, Swami. *Essence of Yoga*. Theri-Garhwal, UP: Divine Life Society, 1988.

———. *Yoga Asanas*. Himalalas, India: Divine Life Society, 1979.

———. "Yoga." http://www.dlshq.org/teachings/yoga.htm

———. *Yoga Asanas*. 2nd ed. Himalayan Yoga Series, no. 14. Madras: P.K. Vinayagam, 1935.

Sjoman, N.E. *The Yoga Tradition of the Mysore Palace*. New Delhi: Abhinav Publications, 1999.

Smith, Adam. *Powers of Mind*. New York: Summit Books, 1982.

Smith, Benjamin Richard. "With Heat Even Iron Will Bend: Discipline and Authority in Ashtanga Yoga." In *Yoga in the Modern World: Contemporary Perspectives*, edited by Mark Singleton and Jean Byrne, 140–160. New York: Routledge, 2008.

Smith, Frederick M. *The Self Possessed: Deity and Spirit Possession in South Asian Literature and Civilization*. New York: Columbia University Press, 2006.

Smith, Frederick M., and Joan White. "Becoming an Icon: B.K.S. Iyengar as a Yoga Teacher and a Yoga Guru." In *Gurus of Modern Yoga*, edited by Mark Singleton and Ellen Goldberg, 122–146. New York & London: Oxford University Press, 2014.

Smith, Jonathan Z. "Religion, Religions, Religious." In *Critical Terms for Religious Studies*, edited by Mark C. Taylor, 269–284. Chicago: University of Chicago Press, 1998.

Snellgrove, David L. *Indo-Tibetan Buddhism: Indian Buddhists and Their Tibetan Successors*. Boston: Shambhala, 2002.

Snyder, Stephen, and Tina Rasmussen. *Practicing the Jhanas: Traditional Concentration Meditation as Presented by the Venerable Pa Auk Sayadaw*. Boston: Shambhala, 2009.

"Specialised Yoga Certificate Course." KaivalyaDham Yoga Institute. https://kdham.com/specialised-yoga-certificate-course

Śrī Krishnamacharya the Pūrnācārya. Chennai: Krishnamacharya Yoga Mandiram, 1997.

"Sri OP Tiwari Ji—IYA Governing Council." Indian Yoga Association. http://www.yogaiya.in/profile/sri-op-tiwari-ji

Srinivas, Krishna Ravi. "Intellectual Property Rights and Traditional Knowledge: The Case of Yoga." *Economic and Political Weekly* 42, no. 27/28 (2007): 2866–2871.

Srinivas, Smriti. "Sathya Sai Baba and the Repertoire of Yoga." In *Gurus of Modern Yoga*, edited by Mark Singleton and Ellen Goldberg, 261–282. New York: Oxford University Press, 2014.

Srinivas, Tulasi. "Doubtful Illusions: Magic, Wonder and the Politics of Virtue in the Sathya Sai Movement." *Journal of Asian and African Studies* 52, no. 4 (June 2017): 381–411.

Srinivasan, Doris. "Unhinging Śiva from the Indus Civilization." *Journal of the Royal Asiatic Society of Great Britain and Ireland*, no. 1 (1984): 77–89.

Staal, Frits. *Exploring Mysticism: A Methodological Essay*. Berkeley: University of California Press, 1988.

Stietencron, Heinrich von. "Cosmographic Buildings of India: The Circles of the Yoginīs." In *"Yoginī" in South Asia: Interdisciplinary Approaches*, edited by István Keul, 70–83. London & New York: Routledge & Taylor & Francis Group, 2013.

Strauss, Sarah. *Positioning Yoga: Balancing Acts across Cultures*. Oxford: Berg, 2005.

Strauss, Sarah, and Laura Mandelbaum. "Consuming Yoga, Conserving the Environment: Transcultural Discourses on Sustainable Living." In *Yoga Traveling: Bodily Practice in Transcultural Perspective*, edited by Beatrix Hauser, 175–200. Heidelberg: Springer, 2013.

Streng, Frederick J. "Śūnyam and Śūnyatā." In *Encyclopedia of Religion*, edited by Lindsay Jones, 2nd ed., 13:8855–8860. Detroit, MI: Macmillan Reference USA, 2005.

Strong, John S. *The Buddha: A Short Biography*. Oxford: Oneworld, 2006.

Stuart, Daniel M. "Insight Transformed: Coming to Terms with Mindfulness in South Asian and Global Frames." *Religions of South Asia* 11, no. 2–3 (August 2018): 158–181.

———. "Yogācāra Substrata? Precedent Frames for Yogācāra Thought among Third-Century Yoga Practitioners in Greater Gandhāra." *Journal of Indian Philosophy* 46, no. 2 (April 2018): 193–240.

Sugirtharajah, Sharada. "Colonialism." In *Studying Hinduism: Key Concepts and Methods*, edited by Sushil Mittal and Gene Thursby, 85–97. New York: Routledge, 2009.

Sullivan, Bruce M. *Historical Dictionary of Hinduism*. Lanham, MD & London: The Scarecrow Press, 1997.

Sutherland Goldman, Sally J. "The Voice of Sītā in Vālmīki's Sundarakāṇḍa." In *Questioning Ramayanas: A South Asian Narrative Tradition*, edited by Paula Richman, 223–238. Berkeley: University of California Press, 2001.

Svātmārāma, and Swami Digambara. *Haṭhapradīpikā*. Lonavla, Maharashtra, India: Kaivalyadhama S.M.Y.M Samiti, 1980.

Syman, Stefanie. *The Subtle Body: The Story of Yoga in America*. New York: Farrar, Straus & Giroux, 2010.

Tambiah, Stanley. "The Reflexive and Institutional Achievements of Early Buddhism." In *The Origins and Diversity of Axial Age Civilizations*, edited by S.N. Eisenstadt, 453–471. Albany, NY: SUNY Press, 1986.

Tarthang Tulku. *Tibetan Relaxation: The Illustrated Guide to Kum Nye Massage and Movement —a Yoga from the Tibetan Tradition*. London: Duncan Baird, 2007.

Taves, Ann. "Religious Experience." In *Encyclopedia of Religion*, edited by Lindsay Jones, 2nd ed., 11:7736–7750. Detroit, MI: Macmillan Reference USA, 2005.

"Teachers and Staff." Krishnamacharya Healing and Yoga Foundation. http://www.khyf.net/team

Teltumbde, Anand. *Dalits: Past, Present and Future*, New York: Routledge, 2017.

Thakur, Shreya. "India Rejects Section 377: Sri Sri Ravi Shankar Comes Out In Support." *Republic World*. September 6, 2018. https://www.republicworld com/india-news/general-news/india-rejects-section-377-sri-sri-ravi-shankar-comes-out-in-support

Theodor, Ithamar. *Exploring the Bhagavad Gitā: Philosophy, Structure, and Meaning*. Burlington, VT: Ashgate, 2010.

Tigunait, Rajmani. *At the Eleventh Hour: The Biography of Swami Rama*. Honesdale: Himalayan Institute Press, 2001.

Toland, Sarah. "The Rise of Yoga in the NBA and Other Pro Sports." *SI.Com*. https://www.si.com/edge/2014/06/27/rise-yoga-nba-and-other-pro-sports

Trautmann, Thomas R., ed. *The Aryan Debate*. New Delhi: Oxford University, 2007.

Tulku, Ringu. "Six Yogas of Naropa." *Bulletin of Tibetology*, no. 1–4 (1982): 40–44.

Tweed, Thomas A. "United States." In *Encyclopedia of Buddhism*, edited by Robert E. Buswell, Jr. 2: 864–870. New York: Macmillan Reference, 2003.

Umāsvāti. *That Which Is: Tattvārtha Sūtra*. Translated by Nathmal Tatia. New Haven, CT: Yale University Press, 2011.

Upatissa. *The Path of Freedom: Vimuttimagga*. Translated by N.R.M Ehara, Soma Thera, and Kheminda Thera. Kandy & Sri Lanka: Buddhist Publication Society, 1995.

Urban, Hugh B. "Avatar for Our Age: Sathya Sai Baba and the Cultural Contradictions of Late Capitalism." *Religion* 33, no. 1 (January 2003): 73–93.

———. "Osho, From Sex Guru to Guru of the Rich: The Spiritual Logic of Late Capitalism." In *Gurus in America*, edited by Thomas A. Forsthoefel and Cynthia Ann Humes, 169–192. Albany, NY: SUNY Press, 2005.

———. *Tantra: Sex, Secrecy Politics, and Power in the Study of Religions*. Berkeley: University of California Press, 2003.

———. "The Cult of Ecstasy: Tantrism, the New Age, and the Spiritual Logic of Late Capitalism." *History of Religions* 39, no. 3 (February 2000): 268–304.

———. "The Omnipotent Oom: Tantra and Its Impact on Modern Western Esotericism." *Esoterica: Journal of Esoteric Studies* 3 (2001): 218–259.

Valliere, Paul. "Tradition." In *Encyclopedia of Religion*, edited by Lindsay Jones, 2nd ed., 13:9267–9281. Detroit, MI: Macmillan Reference USA, 2005.

Vanita, Ruth. " 'Free to Be Gay': Same-Sex Relations in India, Globalised Homophobia and Globalised Gay Rights." In *Human Rights in Postcolonial India*, edited by O.P. Dwivedi and V.G. Julie Rajan, 315–331. Basingstoke: Taylor & Francis, 2016.

Varenne, Jean. *Yoga and the Hindu Tradition*. Chicago: University of Chicago Press, 1976.

Vasubandhu, and Louis de La Vallée Poussin. *Abhidharmakośabhāṣyam*. Berkeley, CA: Asian Humanities Press, 1988.

Vasudev, Jaggi. *Inner Engineering: A Yogi's Guide to Joy*, New York: Spiegel & Grau, 2016.

Vasudeva, Somadeva. "The Śaiva Yogas and Their Relation to Other Systems of Yoga." *RINDAS Series of Working Papers: Traditional Indian Thoughts*, no. 26 (2017): 1–17.

———. *The Yoga of the Mālinīvijayottaratantra: Chapters 1–4, 7, 11–17*. Pondichery: Institut français de Pondichéry: Ecole française d'Extrême-Orient, 2004.

Versluis, Arthur. *American Transcendentalism and Asian Religions*. New York: Oxford University Press, 1994.

Vetter, Tilmann. *The Ideas and Meditative Practices of Early Buddhism*. Leiden & New York: E.J. Brill, 1988.

"Vipassana." https://www.dhamma.org/en/schedules/schgiri

"Vipassana Meditation Center—Dhamma Dharā | Vipassana International." https://www.dhara.dhamma.org/about/international

Vitello, Paul. "Hindu Group Stirs Debate in Fight for Soul of Yoga." *The New York Times*, November 27, 2010. https://www.nytimes.com/2010/11/28/nyregion/28yoga.html

Vivekananda, Nikhilananda, and Ramakrishna Vedanta Centre. *Vivekananda: The Yogas and Other Works*. New York & Bourne End: Ramakrishna-Vivekananda Center & Ramakrishna Vedanta Centre, 1984.

Waghorne, Joanne Punzo. "Engineering an Artful Practice: On Jaggi Vasudev's Isha Yoga and Sri Sri Ravi Shankar's Art of Living." In *Gurus of Modern Yoga*, edited by Mark Singleton and Ellen Goldberg, 283–307. New York & London: Oxford University Press, 2014.

Wagoner, Phillip B. " 'Sultan among Hindu Kings': Dress, Titles, and the Islamicization of Hindu Culture at Vijayanagara." *The Journal of Asian Studies* 55, no. 4 (1996): 851–880.

"Wai Lana Biography, Age, Birth Place, Personal Life & 'Oh My Sweet Lord'—Kowaliw.Net."

"Wai Lana Yoga TV Series." Text. Wai Lana, July 17, 2013. https://www.wailana.com/yoga/wai-lana-yoga-tv-series

"Wai Lana's 'Namaste' Music Video Played at United Nations in Celebration of International Yoga Day." *PRWeb*. http://www.prweb.com/releases/2015/Namaste-Wailana/prweb12802457.htm

Wallace, B. Alan. *Contemplative Science: Where Buddhism and Neuroscience Converge*. New York & Chichester: Columbia University Press, 2009.

Wallace, Vesna A. *The Inner Kālacakratantra: A Buddhist Tantric View of the Individual*. Oxford: Oxford University Press, 2001.

Wallach, Luitpold. "Alexander the Great and the Indian Gymnosophists in Hebrew Tradition." *Proceedings of the American Academy for Jewish Research* 11 (1941): 47–83.

Walters, Joanna. " 'Yoga Can Damage Your Body' Article Throws Exponents off-Balance." *The Observer*, January 14, 2012, sec. Life and style. https://www.theguardian.com/lifeandstyle/2012/jan/14/yoga-can-damage-body-row

Wangyal, Tenzin, and Marcy Vaughn. *Awakening the Sacred Body*. Carlsbad, CA: Hay House, Inc., 2011.

Wayman, Alex. *Untying the Knots in Buddhism: Selected Essays*. Delhi: Motilal Banarsidass Publishers, 1997.

Wedemeyer, Christian K. *Making Sense of Tantric Buddhism: History, Semiology, and Transgression in the Indian Traditions*. New York: Columbia University Press, 2013.

Weiss, Richard S. *Recipes for Immortality. Healing, Religion, and Community in South India*. New York: Oxford University Press, 2009.

"Welcome to Bihar Yoga Bharati—Bihar Yoga." http://www.biharyoga.net/uncategorized/welcome

"Welcome to Satyananda Yoga ~ Bihar Yoga—Bihar Yoga." http://www.biharyoga.net

"Welcome to Swami Dayananda Ashram–Arsha Vidya Pitham–Rishikesh." https://www.dayananda.org

Wells, Rusty. *Bhakti Flow Yoga: A Training Guide for Practice and Life*, Boston: Shambhala, 2015.

Wessinger, Catherine. "Hinduism Arrives in America: The Vedanta Movement and the Self-Realization Fellowship." In *America's Alternative Religions*, edited by Timothy Miller, 173–90. Albany, NY: SUNY Press, 1995.

Whicher, Ian. *The Integrity of the Yoga Darsana: A Reconsideration of Classical Yoga*. Albany, NY: SUNY Press, 1998.

White, David Gordon. *Kiss of the Yogini: "Tantric Sex" in Its South Asian Contexts*. Chicago & London: University of Chicago Press, 2003.

———. *Sinister Yogis*. Chicago & London: University of Chicago Press, 2009.

———. "Tantra in Practice: Mapping a Tradition." In *Tantra in Practice*, edited by David Gordon White, 3–38. Princeton, NJ: Princeton University Press, 2000.

———. *The Alchemical Body: Siddha Traditions in Medieval India*. Chicago & London: University of Chicago Press, 2007.

———. *The Yoga Sutra of Patanjali: A Biography*. Princeton, NJ: Princeton University Press, 2014.

Widdess, Richard. "Caryā and Cacā: Change and Continuity in Newar Buddhist Ritual Song." *Asian Music*, 2004, 7–41.

Wilkinson-Priest, Genny. "Does Authorization Matter?" *Elephant Journal*, November 13, 2013. https://www.elephantjournal.com/2013/11/does-authorization-matter-genny-wilkinson-priest

Williams, J. Mark G., and Jon Kabat-Zinn. *Mindfulness: Diverse Perspectives on Its Meaning, Origins and Applications*. New York: Routledge, 2013.

Williams, Paul. *Mahāyāna Buddhism: The Doctrinal Foundations*. London and New York: Routledge, 1998.

Williamson, Lola. *Transcendent in America: Hindu-Inspired Meditation Movements as New Religion*. New York & London: New York University Press, 2010.

Willis, Laurette. *Praisemoves: The Christian Alternative to Yoga*. Eugene, OR: Harvest House, 2006.

Wilson, Liz. *Charming Cadavers: Horrific Figurations of the Feminine in Indian Buddhist Hagiographic Literature*. Chicago: University of Chicago Press, 1996.

———. *Living and the Dead: Social Dimensions of Death in South Asian Religions*. Albany, NY: SUNY Press, 2014.

Wiltshire, Martin G. *Ascetic Figures before and in Early Buddhism: The Emergence of Gautama as the Buddha*. Berlin: Mouton de Gruyter, 1990.

Witzel, Michael. "Indocentrism: Autochthonous Visions of Ancient India." In *The Indo-Aryan Controversy: Evidence and Inference in Indian History*, edited by Edwin F. Bryant and Laurie L. Patton, 341–404. New York: Routledge, 2005.

Woodroffe, John George. *The Serpent Power: Being the Ṣaṭ-Cakra-Nirūpana and Pādukā-Pañcaka: Two Works on Laya-Yoga*. New York: Dover, 2000.

Wright, Robert. *Why Buddhism Is True: The Science and Philosophy of Meditation and Enlightenment*. New York: Simon & Schuster, 2017.

Wujastyk, Dominik. "The Path to Liberation through Yogic Mindfulness in Early Āyurveda." In *Yoga in Practice*, edited by David Gordon White, 31–42. Princeton, NJ: Princeton University Press, 2012.

Yadav, Yatish. "Superstar in Top Padma League." *The New Indian Express*, January 26, 2016. http://www.newindianexpress.com/nation/2016/jan/26/Superstar-in-Top-Padma-League-873638.html

Yamashita, Koichi. *Pātañjala Yoga Philosophy with Reference to Buddhism*. Calcutta: Firma KLM Private Limited, 1994.

"Yoga: The Silk Road to Happiness—Interview with Wai Lana." *Asana—International Yoga Journal* (blog), August 17, 2016. https://www.asanajournal.com/yoga-the-silk-road-to-happiness-interview-with-wailana

"Yoga Alliance Designations." https://www.yogaalliance.org/Credentialing

"Yoga Day: Origin, Theme, Importance, Celebrations, All FAQs Answered." NDTV.com. https://www.ndtv.com/india-news/fourth-international-yoga-day-theme-importance-celebrations-all-you-need-to-know-1870368

"Yoga Federation of India: Rules for National Yoga Sports Championship." http://www.yogafederationofindia.com/rules_nyc.html

Yoga Journal, Yoga Alliance, and Ipsos Public Affairs. "2016 Yoga in America Study." National Study. https://www.yogaalliance.org/Portals/0/2016%20Yoga%20in%20America%20Study%20RESULTS.pdf

"Yoga's Growing Threat of Legal Liability." https://www.counterpunch.org/2014/07/04/yogas-growing-threat-of-legal-liability

"Yogi Gupta | Dharma Yoga Center New York City." https://dharmayogacenter.com/resources/yogi-gupta

Young, Serinity. *Courtesans and Tantric Consorts: Sexualities in Buddhist Narrative, Iconography and Ritual*. New York & London: Routledge, 2004.

Zahler, Leah, Lati Rinpoche, and Denma Lochö Rinbochay. *Meditative States in Tibetan Buddhism*. Boston: Wisdom Publications, 1998.

Zigmund-Cerbu, Anton. "The Ṣaḍaṅgayoga." *History of Religions* 3, no. 1 (1963): 128–134.

Zinser, Lynn. "Title for the Seahawks Is a Triumph for the Profile of Yoga." *The New York Times*, February 4, 2014, sec. Pro Football. https://www.nytimes.com/2014/02/05/sports/football/title-for-the-seahawks-is-a-triumph-for-the-profile-of-yoga.html

Znamenski, Andrei A. *Shamanism: Critical Concepts in Sociology*. London: Routledge Curzon, 2008.

Zysk, Kenneth G. *Asceticism and Healing in Ancient India Medicine in the Buddhist Monastery*. Delhi: Motilal Banarsidass, 2010.

Index

Abhidharmakośa (*bhāṣya*) (Vasubandhu), 103, 135–136
Abhidharma literature, 127, 131, 135–136, 139, 146
abhijñā (higher knowledge), 20, 63, 84–85, 133
Abhinavagupta (philosopher), 29, 149, 157, 167
Abhisamayālaṃkara (Ornament on Clear Understanding), 139
abhiṣeka. *See* initiation (*abhiṣeka*, *dīkṣā*, *upanayana*)
abhyāsa (practice), 99, 113
abrahma (nonchastity), 129. *See also* sexuality and sexual activity (*maithuna*)
absolute reality. *See* ultimate reality (*brahman*)
absorption (*samāpatti*), 84
Ācārāṅgasūtra (Jain text), 11, 70
ācārya (preceptor), 24. *See also* teachers (*guru*, *ācārya*)
accomplished or perfected one (*siddha*, *siddhā*): etymology, 27, 28; liberated soul, in Jainism, 104; Mahāsiddhas and, 170, 178; Nāths and, 169, 170; numinous and cessative goals, 34; in tantric traditions, 56, 156, 178; Vardhamāna as, 71
accomplished posture (*siddhāsana*), 41, 175
accomplishments, powers (*siddhi*, *vibhūti*): *aṣṭasiddhi* (eight accomplishments), 19, 167–168; *haṭhayoga* yields, 12, 20, 21, 171, 172–173, 177; Jain conceptions of, 20, 27, 74, 130, 131; meditation yields, 14, 85, 101–103, 109, 120, 132, 218; in modern yoga, Sivananda on, 216; in sectarian theism, 108, 150, 154, 170, 171. *See also* numinous goals of yoga
accomplishments, powers (*siddhi*, *vibhūti*), Buddhist conceptions of: Buddhahood, attainment of, 75, 78, 86, 137, 140, 143–144; higher knowledge (*abhijñā*), 12, 20, 63, 84–85, 133; Mahāsiddhas, 177–178; Mahāyāna Buddhism, 132, 145; *mantra* in, 145; meditation and, 14; tantric traditions draw from, 168; terminology of, 27, 28; Theravāda Buddhism, 14; Tibetan Buddhism, 180. *See also* Buddhism